KT-365-882

Survey Methods in
Community Medicine

To Eleanor

Survey Methods in Community Medicine

Epidemiological Studies
Programme Evaluation
Clinical Trials

J. H. Abramson
Professor of Social Medicine
The Hebrew University-Hadassah School of Public Health and
Community Medicine
Jerusalem

FOURTH EDITION

CHURCHILL LIVINGSTONE
EDINBURGH LONDON MELBOURNE AND NEW YORK 1990

CHURCHILL LIVINGSTONE
Medical Division of Longman Group UK Limited

Distributed in the United States of America by Churchill
Livingstone Inc., 1560 Broadway, New York, N.Y. 10036, and
by associated companies, branches and representatives
throughout the world.

© Longman Group Limited 1974, 1979, 1984
© Longman Group UK Limited 1990

All rights reserved. No part of this publication may be
reproduced, stored in a retrieval system, or transmitted in any
form or by any means, electronic, mechanical, photocopying,
recording or otherwise, without either the prior written
permission of the publishers (Churchill Livingstone, Robert
Stevenson House, 1–3 Baxter's Place, Leith Walk, Edinburgh
EH1 3AF), or a licence permitting restricted copying in the
United Kingdom issued by the Copyright Licensing Agency
Ltd, 33–34 Alfred Place, London, WCIE 7DP.

First edition 1974
Second edition 1979
Third edition 1984
Fourth edition 1990

ISBN 0-443-04196-2

British Library Cataloguing in Publication Data
Abramson, J. H. (Joseph Herbert), *1924–*
   Survey methods in community medicine : epidemiological
   studies, programme evaluation, clinical trials. – 4th ed.
   1. Public health. Research. Techniques
   I. Title
   614.072

Library of Congress Cataloging in Publication Data
Abramson, J. H. (Joseph Herbert), 1924–
   Survey methods in community medicine : epidemiological
   studies, programme evaluation, clinical trials / J.H.
   Abramson. —4th ed.   p.   cm.
   Companion v. to: Making sense of data / J.H. Abramson,
   1988.
   Includes bibliographical references.
   ISBN 0-443-04196-2
   1. Health surveys. 2. Public health—Research.
   I. Abramson, J. H. (Joseph Herbert), 1924– Making sense of
   data. II. Title.
   [DNLM: 1. Clinical Trials. 2. Community Medicine.
   3. Data Collection—methods. 4. Health Surveys.
   5. Research—methods. W 84.5 A161s]
   RA408.5.A27 1990
   362. 1'0723—dc20
   DNLM/DLC
   for Library of Congress   90–1799
                                                            CIP

Produced by Longman Singapore Publishers (Pte) Ltd.
Printed in Singapore

Preface

The purpose of this book is to provide a simple and systematic guide to the planning and performance of investigations concerned with health and disease and with health care, whether they are studies designed to widen the horizons of scientific knowledge or whether they have more directly practical aims, such as the provision of information needed as a basis for immediate decisions and action. It is not a compendium of detailed techniques of investigation or of statistical methods, but an ABC to the design, conduct and analysis of studies.

For this new edition, the text, notes and references have again been thoroughly revised and updated. Chapters on clinical trials and programme trials have been added, and due attention is now paid to the use of personal computers. The discussion of ethical considerations has been expanded, and a table of random numbers has been added. Case-control and cohort studies are discussed in more detail than previously. The book has grown by over fifty pages.

As in previous editions, the more appropriate title of *Research Methods in Community Medicine*—which would better reflect the book's concern with experimental as well as observational studies—was avoided in order not to repel readers who are interested in conducting investigations aimed at pragmatic purposes, but who conceive of 'research' as an ivory-tower activity far removed from their own mundane activities.

It is hoped that the book will be helpful to doctors and others planning investigations of groups and populations, such as health surveys, prospective studies, comparisons of cases and controls, prophylactic and therapeutic trials, studies of the use of medical services, and other epidemiological and evaluative research. The chapter on community-oriented primary care (added in the third edition) was written to meet the needs of physicians and other health workers who provide primary care for individuals or families in the community and also endeavour to 'treat the community as a patient' by appraising its health needs and establishing and evaluating programmes to meet these needs. The book may also be of use to readers who wish only to enhance their capacity for the judicious appraisal of medical literature.

My book *Making Sense of Data*, a self-instruction manual on the interpretation of data (Oxford University Press, 1988) may be regarded as a companion volume.

Jerusalem, 1990 J.H.A.

Contents

1. First steps

The purpose of most investigations in community medicine, and in the health field generally, is the collection of information that will provide a basis for action, whether immediately or in the long run. The investigator perceives a problem which, in his[1] view, requires solution, decides that a particular study will contribute to this end, and embarks upon the study. If he is blessed with a creative turn of mind and a modicum of luck, and if he plans his study soundly, the findings may well be of wide scientific interest. If he is less inspired, but selects a problem of practical importance, and if he plans his study soundly, the findings will be useful ones, though of less wide interest. If he concerns himself with a problem without theoretical or practical significance, his findings may serve no end but self-gratification; only in this instance may sound planning be unnecessary.

Before planning can start, a problem must be identified. It has been said that 'if necessity is the mother of invention, the awareness of problems is the mother of research'.[2] The investigator's interest in the problem may arise from a concern with practical matters or from intellectual curiosity, from an intuitive 'hunch' or from careful reasoning, from his own experience or from that of others. Inspiration often comes from reading, not only about the topic in which the investigator is interested, but also about cognate topics. An idea for a study on alcoholism may arise from the results of studies on smoking (conceptually related to alcoholism, in that it is also an addiction) or delinquency (both it and alcoholism being, at least in certain cultures, forms of socially deviant behaviour).

While the main purpose is to collect information which will contribute to the solution of a problem, investigations may also have an educational function, and may be carried out for this purpose. A survey can stimulate public interest in a particular topic (the interviewer is asked: 'Why are you asking me these questions?'), and can be a means of stimulating public action. A community self-survey, carried

1

out by participant members of the community, may be set up as a means to community action (but such surveys usually do not collect very accurate or sophisticated information).

This chapter deals with the purpose of the investigation, ethical aspects, and the formulation of the study topic.

CLARIFYING THE PURPOSE

The first step then, before the study is planned, is to clarify its purpose — the 'why' of the study. (We are not speaking here of the researcher's psychological motivations—a quest for prestige, promotion, the gratifications of problem-solving, etc. of which he may or may not be aware, and is sometimes better off unaware.) Is it 'pure' or 'basic' research with no immediate practical applications in health care, or is it 'applied' research? Is the purpose to obtain information that will be a basis for a decision on the utilization of resources, or is it to identify persons who are at special risk of contracting a specific disease in order that preventive action may be taken; or to add to existing knowledge by throwing light on (say) a specific aspect of aetiology; or to stimulate the public's interest in a topic of relevance to its health? If an evaluative study of health care is contemplated, is the motive a concern with the welfare of the people who are served by a specific practice, health centre or hospital, or is the main purpose to see whether a specific treatment or kind of health programme is good enough to be applied in other places also?

The reason for embarking on the study should be clear to the investigator. In most cases it will in fact be clear to him from the outset; but sometimes the formulation of the problem to be solved will be less easy. In either instance, if an application is made for facilities or funds for the study he may have to describe this purpose in some detail, so as to justify the performance of the study. He will need to review previous work on the subject, describe the present state of knowledge, and explain the significance of the proposed investigation. This is the 'case for action'.

Preconceived ideas introduce a possibility of biased findings, and the researcher should be honest with himself in clarifying his purposes. If he proposes to study a health service because he thinks the service is atrocious, and he wants to collect data that will help him to condemn it, he should subsequently take special care to ensure objectivity in the collection and interpretation of information. In such a case he would be well advised to 'bend over backwards' and consciously set out to seek information to the credit of the service. Regrettably, not all evaluative studies are honest.[3]

ETHICAL CONSIDERATIONS

Before embarking on a study the investigator should satisfy himself that it is ethical to do it, and that it can be done in an ethical way. Ethical questions arise in both experimental and non-experimental studies.

There is an obvious ethical problem if an experiment to test the benefits or hazards of a treatment is contemplated. However beneficial the trial may turn out to be for humanity at large, some subjects may be harmed either by the experimental treatment or by its being withheld. There is also an ethical problem in *not* performing a clinical trial, since this may lead to the use of an ineffective or hazardous treatment. 'Where the value of a treatment, new or old, is doubtful, there may be a higher moral obligation to test it critically than to continue to prescribe it year-in-year-out with the support merely of custom or wishful thinking'.[4] But, it has been pointed out, 'the thesis that controlled clinical investigations constitute an ethical imperative addressed to individual physicians and patients can only be maintained if, and to the extent that, it is possible to conduct controlled trials in an ethically justifiable way'.[5] The heinous medical experiments conducted on helpless victims in this century should never be forgotten.[6]

For an experimental study to be ethical, the subjects should be aware that they are to participate in an experiment, should know how their treatment will be decided and what the possible consequences are, should be told that they may withdraw from the trial at any time, and should freely give their *informed consent*. In clinical settings these requirements are not always easily accepted, and are sometimes circumvented by medical investigators who feel that they have a right to decide their patient's treatment. Studies have shown that patients (especially poorly educated ones) who sign consent forms are often ignorant of the most basic facts. Special problems concerning consent arise in trials where a total community is exposed to an experimental procedure or programme (see p 301), and when experiments (such as trials of new vaccines) are performed in developing countries.[7]

Ethical objections to clinical trials are reduced if there is genuine doubt[8] about the value of the treatment tested, and if controls are given a good established treatment. 'The essential feature of a controlled trial is that it must be ethically possible to give each patient *any* of the treatments involved'.[9]

Decisions on the ethicality of trials are not simple.[10] Bradford Hill has said that there is only one Golden Rule, namely 'that one can make no generalization . . . the problem must be faced afresh with every proposed trial'.

In non-experimental studies[11] ethical problems are usually less acute, unless the study involves hazardous test procedures or intrusions on privacy. But here too there is a need for informed consent[12] if participants are required to answer questions, undergo tests that carry a risk (however small), or permit access to confidential records. The investigators should give an honest explanation of the purpose of the survey when enlisting subjects, and respondents should be told what their participation entails and be assured that they are free to refuse to answer questions or continue their participation. Pains should be taken to keep information confidential. Any promises made to participants, say about anonymity or the provision of test results, should of course be kept.

Of particular importance is the question of what action should be taken if a survey reveals that participants would benefit from medical care or other intervention. A horrible illustration is the Tuskagee study in Alabama. This was a study which began in 1932, with the aim of throwing light on the effects of untreated syphilis. Some 400 untreated black syphilitics (mostly poor and uneducated) were identified and then followed up; their course was compared with that of apparently syphilis-free age-matched controls. Treatment of syphilis was withheld. By 1938–1939 it was found that a number of the men had received sporadic treatment with arsenic or mercury, and a very few had had more intensive treatment. In the interests of science 'fourteen young untreated syphilitics were added to the study to compensate for this'. Treatment was withheld even when penicillin was found to be effective and it became easily available in the late 40s and early 50s. Participants received free benefits, such as free treatment (except for syphilis), free hot lunches, and free burial (after a free autopsy). By 1954 it was apparent that the life expectancy of the untreated men aged 25–50 was reduced by 17%. By 1963, 14 more men per 100 had died in the syphilitic than in the control group. In 1972 there was a public outcry, and compensation payments were later made.

In many countries informed consent is mandatory for studies of human subjects unless there are valid contraindications, such as qualms about alarming fatally ill patients with doubts about the efficacy of treatment. Many institutions have ethical committees that review and sanction proposed studies. Some investigators feel that this control is too permissive, but there are many who think it is too restrictive ('stops worthwhile research');[13] a fanciful account of the rise and fall of epidemiology between 1950 and 2000 AD—printed in 1981[14]— attributes the fall to ethical committees and regulations designed to protect the confidentiality of records.

At a different ethical level, consideration should be given to the justification for any proposed study in the light of the availability of resources and the other ways in which these might be used. Does the possible benefit warrant the required expenditure of time, manpower and money? Is it ethical to perform the study at the expense of other activities, especially those that might directly promote the community's health?

An honest endeavour to clarify the purpose of the study may lead to second thoughts—is the study really worth doing? A great deal of useless research is conducted. This wastes time and resources, and exposes the scientific method to ridicule.[15]

How well the study is planned and performed is also important: 'Scientifically unsound studies are unethical. It may be accepted as a maxim that a poorly or improperly designed study involving human subjects—one that could not possibly yield scientific facts (that is, reproducible observations) relevant to the question under study—is by definition unethical. Moreover, when a study is in itself scientifically invalid, all other ethical considerations become irrelevant. There is no point in obtaining "informed consent" to perform a useless study'.[16]

FORMULATING THE TOPIC

When the purpose and moral justification of the study are clear, the investigator can formulate the topic he proposes to study, in general terms. In many cases this is easily done and almost tautological. For example, if the reason for setting up the study is that infant mortality is unduly high in a given population and there is insufficient information on its causes for the planning of an action programme, the topic of the study can be broadly stated as 'the causes of infant mortality in a defined population in a given time period'. If the reason for the investigation is that health education on smoking has been having little effect, and that it is considered that certain new methods may be more effective, the investigation will be a comparative study of defined educational techniques for the reduction of smoking.

In other instances the formulation of the topic may be less easy, since the researcher may have difficulty in deciding precisely what study is needed to solve the research problem, taking account of practical limitations. As an illustration, a problem arose in a tuberculosis programme; the extent of public participation in X-ray screening activities fell short of what was desired, and there were indications that the tuberculosis rate was higher among people who did not come for screening. It was decided to seek information that would help to improve the situation, but considerable thought was required before a study topic could be formulated. The alternative topics were the reasons for non-participation and those for participation. For a variety of reasons it was decided that the latter approach would be more useful. [17]

As another example, a researcher interested in the possibility that eating fish reduces the risk of coronary heart disease has several alternative approaches. He may for instance decide to study the previous dietary habits of people with and without coronary heart disease; or he may follow up groups of people whose diets differ, to determine the occurrence of the disease during a defined period; or he may examine statistics on the disease rates and average fish consumption of different countries. His decision will be based both on the ease with which the required information can be obtained and on the probability of obtaining convincing evidence, one way or the other.

At this early stage, the formulation of the topic of study may be regarded as a provisional one. When planning and the pretesting of methods get under way, it frequently happens that unpredicted difficulties come to light, requiring a change in the topic or even leading to a decision that there is no practical way of solving the research problem.

NOTES AND REFERENCES

1. The investigator may, of course, be of either sex. Throughout, please read 'he' as 'he or she', and 'his' as 'his or her'. E.g. (the first two sentences of Chapter 4): 'Having decided *what* to study, and knowing *why* he or she wants to study it, the investigator can now formulate his or her study objectives. That is, he or she can state what knowledge he or she wants the study to yield—*what questions* is he or she setting out to answer?'
2. Geitgey D A, Metz E A 1969 Nursing Research 18: 339.
3. A dishonest evaluation of health care may be *eyewash* (an appraisal limited to aspects that look good), *whitewash* (covering up failure by avoiding objectivity, e.g. by soliciting testimonials), *submarine* (aimed at torpedoing a programme,

regardless of its worth), a *postponement ploy* (noting the need to seek facts, in the hope that the crisis will be over by the time the facts are available), etc. Providers of care who evaluate services that they themselves provide should take pains to confute the criticism that this is like 'letting the fox guard the chicken house'. Spiegel A D, Hyman H H 1978 Basic health planning methods. Aspen Systems, Germantown, Maryland, pp 324, 355.

4. Green F H K, cited by Hill (1977) (see note 9).
5. Roy D J 1986 Controlled clinical trials: an ethical imperative. Journal of Chronic Diseases 39: 159.
6. Seidelman (1988) cites the horrors committed by Mengele and other Nazi physicians as warnings against 'ethical compromise where human life and dignity become secondary to personal, professional, scientific, and political goals'. Seidelman W E 1988 Mengele Medicus: medicine's Nazi heritage Milbank Quarterly 66: 221.
7. Proposed International Guidelines for Biomedical Research Involving Human Subjects have been published by the World Health Organization and the Council for International Organizations of Medical Sciences (Geneva: CIOMS, 1982). The guidelines state that in community-based research—e.g. health services research and trials undertaken on a community basis—'individual consent on a person-to-person basis may not be feasible, and the ultimate decision to undertake the research will rest with the responsible public health authority. Nevertheless, all possible means should be used to inform the community concerned of the aims of the research, the advantages expected from it, and any possible hazards or inconveniences. If feasible, dissenting individuals should have the option of withholding their participation. Whatever the circumstances, the ethical considerations and safeguards applied to research on individuals must be translated, in every possible respect, into the community context'.

   Regarding *research in developing countries*, the international guidelines state: 'Rural communities in developing countries may not be conversant with the concepts and techniques of experimental medicine... Where individual members of a community do not have the necessary awareness of the implications of participation in an experiment to give adequately informed consent directly to the investigators, it is desirable that the decision whether or not to participate should be elicited through the intermediary of a trusted community leader. The intermediary should make it clear that participation is entirely voluntary, and that any participant is free to abstain or withdraw at any time from the experiment'.
8. A clinical experimenter must be genuinely uncertain about the relative value of treatments offered, since he is ethically bound to offer every patient what he believes to be the best available treatment. This requirement may make a trial or its continuance impossible. For some investigators it may be enough to know that there is genuine uncertainty 'in the clinical community', whatever their own views. Freedman B 1987 Equipoise and the ethics of clinical research. New England Journal of Medicine 317: 141.
9. Hill A B 1977 A short textbook of medical statistics. Hodder and Stoughton, London, p 223.
10. The basic principle is neatly summarized in the following exchange: 'Mr Ederer: "If you could give only one bit of advice to a clinician planning a clinical trial, what would you tell him?" Dr Davis: "A one-word answer might be 'don't'. If you are determined to do it, my advice would be from the beginning put yourself in the patient's position and develop the protocol so you would be happy to be one of the subjects. If you cannot do that, you'd better not start."' Davis M D 1975 American Journal of Ophthalmology 79: 779.

    See the Helsinki declaration and the British Medical Research Council's statement on investigations of human subjects; Hill A B 1977 A short textbook on medical statistics. Hodder and Stoughton, London, pp 248–253. For a more detailed discussion of ethical problems, see Freund F A (ed) 1972 Experimentation with human subjects. George Allen & Unwin, London. Lebacqz K 1983 discusses the conflicts that may arise between the three basic guiding principles of respect for persons, beneficence and justice in Clinical Trials: Issues and Approaches (Shapiro S H, Louis T A eds) Marcel Dekker, New York, pp 81–98. Mackillop W J & Johnston P A 1986 call for empirical studies—how, for example, are experimental subjects actually procured? (Ethical problems in clinical research: the need for empirical studies of the clinical trials process. Journal of Chronic Diseases 39: 177).

11. *Ethical aspects of epidemiological research* are discussed by Susser M, Stein Z, Kline J 1978 Ethics in epidemiology. Annals of the American Academy of Political and Social Science 437: 128; Stolley P D, Schlesselman J J 1982 Planning and conducting a study. In: Schlesselman J J (ed) Case-control studies: design, conduct, analysis. Oxford University Press, New York, pp 69–104; Waters W E 1985 Ethics and epidemiological research. International Journal of Epidemiology 14: 48.

12. A specimen 'informed consent' form for use in an interview survey is provided by Stolley & Schlesselman (1982; see note 11).

13. Waters 1985 (see note 11).

14. Rothman K J 1981 The rise and fall of epidemiology, 1950–2000 A.D. New England Journal of Medicine 304: 600.

15. 'Time, talent, and money are sometimes squandered on the measurement of the trivial, the irrelevant, and the obvious. . . . A friend of mine who has a gift for felicitous expression has distinguished between "ideas" research on the one hand and "occupational therapy for the university staff" on the other, and once referred to a research project as "squeezing the last drop of blood out of a foregone conclusion"' (Lord Platt 1967 Medical science: master or servant. British Medical Journal 2: 439). See an amusing compilation by Hartston (1988) of actual research results (Do rats prefer tennis balls to other rats? Can pigeons tell Bach from Hindemith? Does holy water affect the growth of radishes?) that serves 'to drop a gentle hint that there might be too much research going on, and much of that is taken far too seriously'. Hartston W 1988 The drunken goldfish: a celebration of irrelevant research. Unwin Hyman. Useless research is satirized in the Journal of Irreproducible Results (P O Box 234, Chicago Heights, Illinois 60411); see Scherr G H (ed) 1983 The best of the Journal of Irreproducible Results: improbable investigations and unfounded findings. Workman Publishing, New York.

16. Rutstein D D in Freund (1972) (see note 10), pp 383–401.

17. Rosenstock I M, Hochbaum G M 1961 Some principles of research design in public health. American Journal of Public Health 51: 266.

2. Types of investigation

Before discussing the detailed planning of a study we will consider the various types of investigation and their nomenclature. The primary distinction is between surveys and experiments.

EXPERIMENTS

Since a survey is most easily defined negatively, as a 'non-experimental investigation', we will start by defining an experiment.

An *experiment* is an investigation in which the researcher, wishing to study the effects of exposure to or deprivation of a defined factor, himself decides which subjects (persons, animals, towns, etc.) will be exposed to, or deprived of, the factor. Experiments are 'studies of deliberate intervention' by the investigators.[1] If the investigator compares subjects exposed to the factor with subjects not exposed to it, he is conducting a *controlled experiment*; the more care he takes to ensure that the two groups are as similar as possible in other respects, the better controlled is his experiment. In a controlled experiment on the effect of vitamin supplements, for example, he will himself decide who will and who will not receive such supplements; in a survey, by contrast, he would compare persons who happened to be taking vitamin supplements with persons not taking such supplements.

A study is a true experiment only if decisions about exposure to the factor under consideration (e.g. to whom will vitamin supplements be offered?) are made by the experimenter. A researcher who wants to conduct an experiment does not always have full control over the situation, and may be unable to make such decisions. He may be able, however, to construct a study that resembles an experiment although in this respect it falls short of being a true one. For example, it may be possible to make observations before and after some intervention not under the investigator's control (medical treatment, exposure to a health education programme, etc.) and to make parallel observations in an unexposed group. The study may then be called a *quasi-experiment*[2] (although some experts prefer to regard such studies as non-experimental). This term is also sometimes used if the allocation to experimental and control groups (even if under the experimenter's control) is not random (see *Randomization*, p 285).

Although they are sometimes given the unflattering appellation of 'pseudo-experiments', quasi-experiments are often well worth doing when a true experiment is not feasible (see pp 301 and 304); but their findings must be interpreted with caution—it is difficult to be sure that the outcome is in fact attributable to the intervention.

The term *natural experiment* is often applied to circumstances where, as a result of 'naturally' occurring changes or differences, it is easy to observe the effects of a specific factor. A famine may permit a study of the effects of starvation. Snow's classic comparison of cholera rates in homes with different water sources, some more contaminated than others, in London in the middle of the last century may be termed a 'natural experiment'.[3] 'Natural experiments' are surveys or, at most (if they examine the effects of man-made changes), quasi-experiments. They have also been termed 'experiments of opportunity'.

Manipulations of animals or human beings are not synonymous with experiments. An investigator who studies bacteriuria in pregnancy by needling the bladders of pregnant women through their abdominal walls in order to collect urine for examination is conducting a survey, not an experiment. An experiment is always a study of change.

SURVEYS

A *survey* is an investigation in which information is systematically collected, but in which the experimental method is not used. There is no active intervention by the investigators. To stress this feature, the term 'observational study'[4] is sometimes used. In this book the term 'survey' is used in a broad sense to cover non-experimental studies of any kind; the term is sometimes used more narrowly.[5] Surveys are not necessarily brief operations; they may involve long-term surveillance (see p 22) or repeated interviews or examinations.

Surveys may be descriptive or analytic. A *descriptive* survey sets out to describe a situation, e.g. the distribution of a disease in a population in relation to sex, age and other characteristics. An *analytic* (or *explanatory*) survey tries to explain the situation, i.e. to study the

Types of investigation

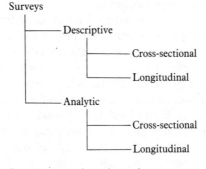

Surveys
- Descriptive
  - Cross-sectional
  - Longitudinal
- Analytic
  - Cross-sectional
  - Longitudinal

Experiments and quasi-experiments

---

determinative processes (Why does the disease occur in these persons? Why do certain persons fail to make use of health services? Can the decreased incidence of the disease be attributed to the introduction of preventive measures?). This is done by formulating and testing hypotheses. These may have various sources.[6] They may be based, inter alia, on the findings of previous descriptive surveys. The distinction between a descriptive and analytic survey is not always clear, and a single survey can combine both purposes. A broad descriptive survey may be so planned, for example, that it also provides information for the testing of a specific hypothesis. An analytic survey may be used to explain a local situation in a specific population in which the researcher is interested, or to obtain results of more general applicability, e.g. new knowledge about the aetiology of a disease.

Surveys, whether descriptive or analytic (or mixed), can be usefully categorized as cross-sectional or longitudinal, depending on the time period covered by the observations. A *cross-sectional* ('instantaneous', 'simultaneous', 'prevalence') survey provides information about the situation that exists at a single time, whereas a *longitudinal* ('time-span') survey provides data about events or changes during a period of time. A study in which children are measured in order to determine the distribution of their weights and heights, or to compare children of different ages, is cross-sectional; the children are examined once, at about the same time (not necessarily on the same day). A study in which the same children are examined repeatedly in order to appraise their growth is longitudinal. If the influence on child growth of parents' smoking habits is investigated in any of these studies, the study is an analytic one. The term 'cross-sectional' is also used in other senses, e.g. for studies of total populations or representative samples ('cross-sections') of them.[7]

A longitudinal study in which a group of individuals (however selected) is followed up for some time may be called a *cohort* ('follow-up', 'panel') study; but the term 'cohort study' is often used more restrictively, to refer to a type of analytic study (see p 15); 'cohort study' should not be confused with 'cohort analysis'.[8] A study of the occurrence of new cases of a disease is an *incidence* study, and a follow-up study of persons born in a defined period is a *birth-cohort* study.

Surveys may use previously recorded data, or observations made after the start of the study. These kinds of data are best termed *retrolective* and *prolective* respectively (from the Latin root of the word 'collect')[9] rather than 'retrospective' and 'prospective', to avoid confusion with other meanings of the latter terms (see below).

EPIDEMIOLOGICAL STUDIES

Epidemiology is the science concerned with the occurrence, distribution and determinants of states of health and disease in human groups and populations. Epidemiological studies may deal with the distribution of diseases or health-relevant characteristics in groups (descriptive surveys) and with the factors influencing this distribution (analytic surveys, experiments and quasi-experiments).

Epidemiological studies have three main uses. First, they serve a diagnostic purpose. Just as the doctor caring for an individual requires a diagnosis of the state of health of his patient, so the doctor or other health worker caring for a community (or other defined group of people) requires a *community diagnosis*[10] or *group diagnosis*. Epidemiological studies provide the required information about the determinants of health in this specific community or group. Secondly, epidemiological studies can throw light on aetiology, the natural history of disease and growth and development. Such knowledge is of general interest, and has far wider applicability than in a specific local situation. And thirdly, epidemiological studies contribute to the evaluation of health care both in specific local situations (How well is this tuberculosis case-finding programme working?) and in general (Does this vaccine prevent disease?).

All three of these uses have a clear relevance to community medicine. Epidemiological studies have an obvious role in answering what Kark has called the cardinal questions that face practitioners of community medicine.[11]

What is the state of health of the community?

What are the factors responsible for this state of health?

What is being done about it by the health care system and by the community itself?

What more can be done, what is proposed, and what is the expected outcome?

What measures are needed to continue health surveillance of the community and to evaluate the effects of what is being done?

The role of epidemiological studies in community-oriented primary care, whose practitioners endeavour to integrate their care of individuals with the care of the community as a whole, will be described in Chapter 32.

Surveys of population health, it has been said, 'can be both the alpha and omega of health care by being the vehicle for both the discovery of need and the evaluation of the outcome of care and treatment'.[12]

Epidemiological and evaluative studies lend an organized structure to the practice of community medicine, and can be referred to as SHAPE activities (surveillance of health and programme evaluation).

Descriptive epidemiological surveys may be cross-sectional (How many blind people are there in the population?) or longitudinal.[13] Longitudinal surveys investigate *change*, e.g. studies of child growth and development or the 'natural history' of disease (What is the course of events after infection with AIDS virus?)

Analytic surveys may be group-based or individual-based. A *group-based* analytic survey is a comparison of groups or populations. It is a study of a group of groups, not a group of individuals. As an example, a group of countries could be compared with respect to their death rates from cirrhosis of the liver, on the one hand, and the average consumption of alcohol and various nutrients on the other.[14] Such studies are sometimes termed *ecological* or 'correlation' studies. We could also compare data for the same population at different times, e.g. by analysing the changing mortality rate from a disease in a single country in relation to changes in average fat intake and per capita tobacco consumption;[15] such studies are sometimes called *trend* studies. They are based on a comparison of successive descriptive cross-sectional studies. Inferences drawn from group-based studies are often misleading and are usually regarded as hints rather than definite conclusions. If we find that populations with a high consumption of beer tend to have a high death rate from cancer of the

Types of epidemiological study

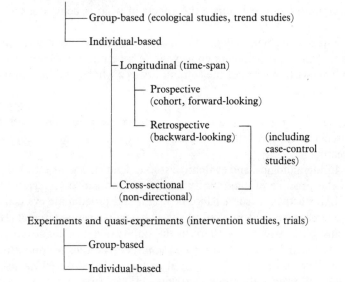

Descriptive surveys

—— Longitudinal (studies of change)

—— Cross-sectional

Analytic surveys

—— Group-based (ecological studies, trend studies)

—— Individual-based

—— Longitudinal (time-span)

—— Prospective
(cohort, forward-looking)

—— Retrospective
(backward-looking)   (including
case-control
studies)

—— Cross-sectional
(non-directional)

Experiments and quasi-experiments (intervention studies, trials)

—— Group-based

——Individual-based

rectum,[16] this does not necessarily mean that *individuals* who drink more beer are prone to develop this tumour; this should be tested in an individual-based survey, or maybe in a rather pleasant experiment. If a comparative study of 18 developed countries in Europe and North America has demonstrated a strong positive correlation between infant mortality and the number of doctors per 10 000 population,[17] this does not necessarily mean that infants should be kept away from doctors.

Group-based studies should, however, by no means be scorned. Doll & Peto have pointed out that although the striking correlations observed between colon cancer and meat consumption and between breast cancer and fat consumption, when countries are compared, may not mean that eating meat or fat is a major aetiological factor, they certainly show that the large international differences in the rates of these neoplasms are not chiefly genetic in origin, and suggest that these cancers are largely avoidable.[18] Trend studies often produce results of considerable interest, like the doubling of the rate of fractures of the proximal femur in Oxford between 1956 and 1983.[19]

Individual-based analytic surveys are of course (like all epidemiological studies) surveys of groups; but they utilize information
about each individual in the group. In their simplest form, such
surveys are performed to test a hypothesis that a specific causal
factor is a determinant of a specific disease (or other outcome), by
measuring each individual's exposure to the postulated causal factor
and the presence of the disease in each individual.

Most individual-based analytic surveys can be categorized as
prospective, retrospective or cross-sectional. This is a simple and
useful classification. These studies can, however, be classified in
other ways, and there is no generally agreed nomenclature. The
terms 'prospective', 'retrospective' and 'cross-sectional' are sometimes used with meanings other than those explained below.[20] To
avoid confusion, other connotations of these terms will be mentioned,
and less ambiguous alternative names for these three kinds of study
will be suggested.

A *prospective* study is a follow-up study in which people who are
(respectively) exposed and not exposed to the postulated causal
factor(s), or who have different degrees of exposure, are compared
with respect to the subsequent development of the disease (or other
outcome under study). The subjects may be chosen for follow-up
because of their exposure or non-exposure to the causal factor, or
they may be selected in some other way (say, because they live in
a specific neighbourhood) and then characterized with respect to
their exposure status. Inclusion in the study is not determined by the
presence of the disease. This kind of survey resembles an experiment,
except that exposure or non-exposure is not controlled by the investigator. The characteristic feature is that (like experiments)
these surveys are 'forward-looking' in their *directionality*, i.e. when
analysing the findings and reasoning about causal relationships, the
investigator starts with the cause and goes forward to the outcome
(Fig. 2.1). The term *cohort study* is often used as a synonym for
'prospective study'; the term *forward-looking study* may also be used.
These names avoid confusion with the common use of the word
'prospective' to refer to the use of observations made after the start
of the study (prolective data; see p 12).

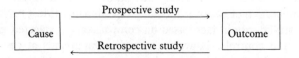

Fig. 2.1 Difference between prospective and retrospective studies.

In this scheme a *retrospective* study is also defined in terms of its directionality, with reference to the way the findings are analysed and inferences are drawn. It is a *'backward-looking'* study that starts with the outcome and goes back to the postulated cause: people with the disease are compared with those free of the disease, to determine whether they differ in their past exposure to the causative factor. A hypothesis that sudden frights during pregnancy are a cause of congenital anomalies could be examined retrospectively by comparing the histories of mothers of malformed and normal babies, or prospectively by comparing the occurrence of malformations among the offspring of mothers who did and did not have shocks during pregnancy. Samples of diseased and disease-free persons may be chosen for comparison, or the subjects of a retrospective study may be selected in some other way; they may, for example, be a random sample of a population, whose members are then investigated to determine whether the disease is present, so that people with and without the disease can be compared. Note that a retrospective study does not necessarily use previously recorded (retrolective) data.

Some epidemiologists base the definition of a retrospective study on the way that study subjects are selected, rather than on directionality, i.e. as a study where selection is based on the occurrence of putative outcomes, e.g. a comparison of groups of cases and controls.[20] It has been suggested that to avoid confusion, studies should be classified both according to their directionality and according to the criteria used in selecting subjects (by exposure, by outcome, or in some other way).[20]

Opponents of classifications based on directionality (who aver that these are 'founded on nonsense')[21] say that they reason from cause to effect even when they compare cases and controls — 'the case-control design can be considered a more efficient form of the follow-up study, in which the cases are those that would be included in a follow-up study and the controls provide a fast and inexpensive means of inferring the person-time experience according to exposure in the population that gave rise to the cases';[22] 'the key distinction is that a case-control study involves gathering data on only a (disease-selective) subset of the source population'.[23]

The term *case-control study* is often used instead of 'retrospective study' to avoid the confusion engendered by the word 'retrospective' or the implication of backward-looking directionality. Most backward-looking studies are in fact based on comparisons of selected groups of cases and controls. However, not all comparisons of cases and controls are backward-looking. In some the time relationship between the variables is uncertain (as in a comparison of metabolic indicators in obese and non-obese subjects), so that the approach is non-directional rather than backward-looking; others use a forward-looking approach, as in a comparison of the birth weights of children born to samples of women who do and do not bleed during pregnancy; and others have nothing to do with the testing of an aetiological hypothesis (as in evaluative studies of screening or diagnostic tests). In this book 'case-control study' will refer to studies in which cases (of the outcome condition) are compared with controls in order to investigate a causal hypothesis; they may be backward-looking or non-directional, or may combine both these approaches (for different causal factors). Other terms used for what we have called retrospective studies include 'case-base' (or 'case-referent'), 'case-comparison', 'case history' and 'trohoc'[24] studies. The term *case-base* study gives emphasis to the comparison of cases with the population from which they are drawn.[25]

Prospective and retrospective studies are 'time-span' (longitudinal) studies, since directionality is possible only if the measurements of cause and outcome refer (or are believed to refer) to different points in time. In this classification a *cross-sectional* study is defined as one where the measurements of cause and outcome refer to the same or approximately the same point in time, and there is no inbuilt directionality. A common reason for the lack of directionality is that both the postulated causal factor and the postulated outcome have been present for some time before the study, and it is not certain which came first (the 'cart-or-horse' problem). A study of the relationship between obesity and physical inactivity (measured at the same time) is an example. Also, in some instances it may not be conceptually clear that one of the variables can be considered a cause of the other.

By this definition, cross-sectional studies may be case-control comparisons or based on samples of other kinds. It may be preferable to call them *non-directional*, to avoid confusion with other uses of the term 'cross-sectional', which is sometimes applied to studies in which information about cause and outcome is *collected* at the same time, or to studies of total populations or representative samples of them.

In some studies data that refer to a single point in time are treated as if they referred to different times. Reported disease in the subject's relatives, for example, may be taken as evidence of his prior exposure to genetic or other familial factors; or in a study of the association between lead poisoning and behavioural problems in school, the lead content of milk teeth may be used as an indicator of lead poisoning in early childhood.[26] A backward-looking or forward-looking approach may then be used. In these instances, nomenclatural confusion may be avoided by calling them *quasi-retrospective* or *quasi-prospective* studies.[1]

The *timing* of the study (*when* it is conducted, in relation to the time of exposure to the suspected cause and the time of occurrence of the outcome) is of obvious importance, since the accuracy of information on prior events may be affected by the availability or quality of past records or by bias in recalling or reporting these events. But timing does not play a role in the classification we have used. A prospective (or cohort) study is not necessarily a study of outcomes that occur after the start of the investigation; it may deal with outcomes that occurred before the study was started. An example is a comparison of the mortality experience of obese and non-obese persons, based upon their weight when they originally took out life insurance policies, and their survival since then until the time of the study. A study of this sort may (among other terms)[27] be called a *historical prospective study*. As in ordinary ('concurrent') prospective studies, the information about exposure to the causal factor is usually, however, recorded before the appearance of the outcome. In a retrospective study, exposure to the suspected cause is generally measured only after the appearance of the outcome; but sometimes information about exposure is available from previous records. Information about the exposure and the outcome may be collected at the same time. A cross-sectional study may be based on retrolective or prolective data.

Prospective, retrospective and non-directional approaches may be combined in the same study, and numerous hybrid designs can be identified. One of these is the *nested case-control* or *ambidirectional* study, in which new cases of a disease are identified in a follow-up study of a population and are then compared with controls drawn from the same population. In some studies, distinctions based on directionality are artificial or blurred: in studies of population samples, for example, the results can often be analysed using either a forward- or backward-looking approach.[28]

Each kind of study has its advantages and disadvantages.[29] Backward-looking and non-directional studies are generally simpler to perform; they usually require less time and fewer subjects, and avoid the difficult task of following up the subjects. But the fact that information about exposure to the 'cause' is generally obtained when the disease is already present may produce various kinds of bias. There may, for example, be 'rumination bias' (cases may ruminate about causes for their illnesses, and this may influence their report of prior exposures) or 'exposure suspicion bias' (the investigator's knowledge that the illness is present may stimulate an especially intensive search for evidence of exposure).[30] Prospective studies are in many ways preferable. They generally leave less doubt about the time relationships between exposure and the disease, and can more easily provide information about the degree of risk associated with exposure, the natural history of the disease, and other effects of the exposure. They may, however, be impracticable if the disease is rare or if it develops long after exposure to the cause. For example, the hypothesis that severe diarrhoea is conducive to the development of cataract many years later is more easily tested retrospectively[31] than prospectively.

Epidemiological experiments that are designed to test cause–effect hypotheses may be termed *intervention studies*. They can be performed only if it is feasible and ethically justified to manipulate the postulated cause. 'The bearing of children, exposure to hazards, or personality type, are not normally subject to experiment'.[32] Like surveys, intervention studies may be group-based or individual-based. If the effect of fluoride on dental caries is investigated by fluoridating the water supplies of some towns and comparing the subsequent occurrence of dental caries in these towns with that in control towns, this is a group-based experiment; data are not available on the fluoride consumption of each individual. On the other hand, when the hypothesis that the administration of oxygen to premature infants caused retrolental fibroplasia (a blinding disease) was tested by administering oxygen continuously to some babies and not to others,[33] this was an individual-based experiment.

Experiments and quasi-experiments conducted to appraise the value of treatments, preventive procedures and health care programmes are generally termed *trials*.

EVALUATIVE STUDIES

Evaluative studies[34] are those that appraise the *value* of health care— they set out to measure how 'good' care is. (The criteria used will be discussed in Chapter 5.)

Evaluative studies are of two main types. These may be termed *reviews* and *trials*, and are distinguished by their different purposes.

A *programme review* is motivated by concern with the welfare of the specific patients, community or population to whom care is given, and it evaluates the care given to them. It may evaluate a particular programme that operates in a defined setting, with well defined aims such as case-finding, immunization, the control of hypertension, fluoridation of water supplies, etc. (A programme may be defined as 'any enterprise organized to eliminate or reduce one or more problems').[35] It may also evaluate a specific health service (a national or regional service, a health centre, a group practice, a hospital, etc.), a part or aspect of a service, or even the work of an individual practitioner, and may be called a 'service review'.

Types of evaluative study

1. Programme reviews
2. Trials
   a. Of care given to groups and populations:
      Programme trials
   b. Of care given to individuals:
      Clinical trials
      Trials of screening and diagnostic tests

An essential feature of a programme review is that the findings should be helpful to whoever makes decisions about the specific programme or service. It follows that the evaluation can be conducted within the framework of the assumptions accepted by the decision maker or makers, e.g. the assumption that the performance of certain procedures will have beneficial effects. These assumptions, on which the programme is based, are not necessarily questioned or tested. The evaluation results can be useful without necessarily being found convincing by those who doubt the validity of the assumptions on which the programme is founded. Programme and service reviews are akin to a physician's periodic reviews of the treatment given to a specific patient, which enable him to decide whether to continue, modify or stop therapy. These assessments are an indispensable part of the clinical process, although the clinician can seldom obtain convincing evidence of the extent to which changes in the patient's condition can be attributed to the treatment.

A *trial*, by contrast, sets out to obtain generalizable knowledge, that can be applied in other settings, about the value of a *type* of health care. To meet its purpose a trial must yield conclusions that are well enough substantiated to be generally convincing. It is not enough merely to demonstrate a beneficial effect, but there must be evidence that the effect can be attributed to the care given. To this end, pains must be taken to eliminate or allow for the possible influence of other factors.

It is important to distinguish between programme reviews and programme trials, since the questions they ask and the methods they use are different. In a review, basic assumptions are not in question, and definitive tests of cause–effect hypotheses are not required; it is wasteful and may be self-defeating to use excessively rigorous study techniques. A trial, on the other hand, may be inconclusive if methods are insufficiently rigorous. There are other differences as well, which also have implications for the planning of the study. To be useful, a review must usually be rapid and (if possible) ongoing. Changes in circumstances, personnel and policy result in frequent changes in the procedures used in a service, and there may be little practical benefit in evaluating a programme as it used to be some years previously. If appraisal is rapid, it can give early warning of inadequacies and provide an up-to-date factual basis for decisions. Speed is less important in a trial. Further, a review is carried out in a service-oriented setting—this is the review's *raison d'être*. Evaluation may not be seen as an important element, and little time and resources may be available for special information-collecting procedures. A trial, on the other hand, is more likely to be conducted as a specific investigative procedure. Not infrequently the programme is set up specially, as a test or demonstration.

Programme reviews are generally descriptive surveys. Programme trials may be experiments or quasi-experiments.

An evaluation of a programme may be of a hybrid type, e.g. when a programme trial is conducted in the context of a service review. This may happen if there is a call for the appraisal of an innovative feature of the service, or if certain of the assumptions on which the service is based are questioned, or if there is a wish to generalize from the experience of the service. In such instances there will be a need for the demanding methods of study that are appropriate to a trial, as well as for the less rigorous ones needed for a review of other aspects of the service. Difficulties often arise when a programme trial is conducted in the setting of an established service, since evaluation and service may make competing demands.

A *clinical trial* appraises the worth of a form of care—preventive, curative, educational, etc.—given to individuals, rather than to a group or population; it may be an experiment or a quasi-experiment. Trials may also be conducted to evaluate screening and diagnostic tests (see pp 160–163).

While clinical and programme trials require separate consideration (see Chs 30 and 31), there is a degree of overlap between them, as some programme trials are based on a comparison of individuals who are exposed and not exposed to the programme under study.

Individual-based programme trials of this sort do not differ in their design from other clinical trials.

Some trials have double objectives: when testing a new form of treatment, the aim may be both to appraise its value for individuals and to evaluate the programme whereby it is provided to the public.

The use of case-control studies for the evaluation of preventive and therapeutic procedures is discussed on page 292.

The term *'inbuilt evaluation'* may be used if the evaluation is planned in advance and the requisite information is collected in a systematic way as an integral part of the provision of a service.

Medical audit is a technique used mainly in service reviews, whereby the quality of a service is evaluated by appraising the quality of the care given to individuals. It will be discussed in more detail in Chapter 20.

SURVEILLANCE

Surveillance denotes the maintenance of an ongoing watch over the status of a group or community. It yields information about new and changing needs, and provides a basis for appraising the effects of health care (see p 317). A watch may be kept on health status—in terms of mortality, morbidity, nutritional status, child growth and development, or other indices—and on environmental hazards, health practices, and other factors that may affect health.

Demographic surveillance[36] refers to ongoing measurement of the size of the population, its age and sex composition, and other demographic characteristics. Apart from other purposes, this is a prerequisite for the measurement of a community's health, since it provides information about the *denominator population.*

There is considerable confusion about the use of the terms 'surveillance' and 'monitoring', and they are often used interchangeably. *Monitoring* is probably best used to refer to the maintenance of an ongoing watch over the activities of a health service, e.g. the provision of answers to questions such as 'what are we doing at the present moment?'; 'what does it cost in resources to do what for whom?'[37]

Surveillance and monitoring may be based on ongoing data collection (often as a byproduct of the provision of a service) or a trend study, i.e. comparison of repeated cross-sectional surveys. The term 'inbuilt surveillance' may be applied if a health service has set up routine procedures for this purpose, such as the ascertainment and recording of births, deaths and movements, the notification of infectious diseases, and the use of records designed for the easy retrieval of diagnostic information, with periodic analysis of these data.

OTHER TERMS

The term *exploratory study* is often applied to a descriptive survey designed to increase the investigator's familiarity with the problem he wishes to study. The aim may be to formulate a problem for more precise investigation, to develop hypotheses, to clarify concepts, or to make the investigator more familiar with the phenomenon he wishes to investigate or with the setting in which he will study it. Such a study is sometimes called a *pilot study*; however, this term is better confined to another connotation, namely a dress rehearsal of an investigation performed in order to identify defects in the study design. A descriptive survey in which a very large number of characteristics are studied, i.e. in which the net is thrown wide, performed in the hope that the results will provide hypotheses for subsequent testing, is sometimes unflatteringly referred to as a *fishing expedition*.

A *methodological study* is one performed with the purpose of collecting information on the feasibility or accuracy of a research method (see Ch 15 and 16). In community medicine the aim of such a study is usually the evaluation of an investigative procedure for use in community diagnosis.

A *morbidity survey* is a study, usually descriptive, of the occurrence and distribution of a disease, or diseases, in a population. It may be a *prevalence study*, concerned with all cases of the disease present in the population at a given point in time or during the period of the survey, or an *incidence study*, concerned only with new cases (patients, or episodes of illness) occurring or diagnosed during a given period. A *two-stage morbidity study* is one in which screening tests (see p 38) are used to identify persons who may have the disease, and the presence of the disease is then determined by more exact tests.

The term *household survey* usually refers to a descriptive survey of illnesses and disability, performed by interviewing persons in their own homes, often by questioning a single informant about other members of his household.

KAP studies are studies of knowledge, attitudes and practices.

Health practice research (health services research, operational research) is concerned with organizational problems—with the planning, management, logistics and delivery of health care services. It deals with manpower, organization, the utilization of facilities, the quality of health care, cost, the relationship between need and demand, and other topics. It makes use of systems analysis, computer simulation, and other sophisticated techniques of operations research.[38]

NOTES AND REFERENCES

1. Bailar et al (1984) define longitudinal studies as prospective or retrospective, depending on whether the selection of study subjects is based on the occurrence of putative causes or outcomes. They subclassify prospective and retrospective investigations as follows: studies of deliberate intervention by the investigators, observational studies (including studies of deliberate interventions not under the control of the investigators), and pseudolongitudinal (pseudoretrospective and pseudoprospective) ones. (Bailar J C III, Lewis T A, Lavori P W 1984 A classification for biomedical research reports. New England Journal of Medicine 311: 1482). The latter studies are called 'quasi-retrospective' and 'quasi-prospective' in this book.
2. *Quasi-experiments* are discussed by Campbell D T, Stanley J C 1966. Experimental and quasi-experimental designs for research. Rand McNally, Chicago. Campbell D T 1969 Factors relevant to the validity of experiments in social settings. In: Schulberg H C, Sheldon A, Baker F (eds) Program evaluation in the health fields. Behavioral Publications, New York. Cook T D, Campbell D T 1979 Quasi-experimentation: design and analysis issues for field settings; Rand McNally, Chicago, Illinois. Kleinbaum D G, Kupper L L, Morgenstern H 1982 Epidemiologic research: principles and quantitative methods. Lifetime Learning Publications, Belmont, California, p 44.
3. Snow J 1855 On the mode of communication of cholera. Churchill, London. Facsimile edition 1965: Hafner, New York.
4. The term 'observational study' does not imply that methods other than observation (questionnaires, documentary sources) are not used. Another term for non-experimental studies is 'naturalistic': Polgar S, Thomas S A 1988 Introduction to research in the health sciences. Churchill Livingstone, Melbourne, p 71.
5. The term 'survey' is sometimes used in a narrow sense to refer to specific types of non-experimental study, such as questionnaire-based ones (Blum M L, Foos P W 1986 Data gathering: experimental methods plus. Harper and Row, New York, p 255), descriptive studies of population characteristics (Polgar & Thomas 1988; see note 4), field surveys, household surveys (see p 23), cross-sectional studies (see p 11); Kleinbaum et al 1982; see note 2), or studies of public opinion.
6. How hypotheses about a possible cause are generated 'is little understood. They are products of their times, what is in the air, of what is known and being thought important, and of the prepared mind and individual imagination . . . *Where* epidemiological hypotheses come from is also interesting: they emerge—from everywhere . . . and from nowhere in particular'. Morris J N 1975 Uses of epidemiology, 3rd edn. Churchill Livingstone, Edinburgh, pp 233–249.
7. Fleiss J L 1981 Statistical methods for rates and proportions, 2nd edn. Wiley, New York, p 20.
8. Cohort analysis refers to the investigation of data concerning people born in various specific time periods (e.g. 1910–1919) with a view to learning about the morbidity, mortality, etc. of each birth cohort or its various subgroups, and to comparing people born in different periods. This may reveal a cohort effect—i.e. there may be differences in morbidity, mortality, etc. when people of the same age in different birth cohorts are compared, as a result of differences in the experience of different cohorts. In a cross-sectional survey 50-year-olds may be shorter and have a lower mean IQ than 30-year-olds, not because they are older, but because they belong to different cohorts with different prior experiences.

9. Feinstein A R 1981 Clinical biostatistics: LVII. A glossary of neologisms in quantitative clinical science. Clinical Pharmacology and Therapeutics 30: 564.
10. The principles and methods of *community diagnosis* are described by Morris (1975; see note 6; Chapter 2); Tapp J W 1974 Community diagnosis. In Kane R L (ed) The challenges of community medicine, Springer, New York, pp 13–26. For discussions and examples of community diagnosis in the context of community-oriented primary care, see Kark S L 1981 The practice of community-oriented primary health care. Appleton-Century-Crofts, New York; and the references cited in note 1, p 324. The use of epidemiological information as a basis for the planning and evaluation of health services is discussed in some detail by Dever G E 1980 Community health analysis. Aspen, Germantown, Maryland.
11. Kark 1981; see note 10.
12. Acheson R M, Hall D J 1976 In: Acheson R M, Hall D, Aird L (eds) Seminars in community medicine, vol. 2: health information, planning, and monitoring. Oxford University Press, London, pp 145–164.
13. For a detailed discussion of studies in which the same variable is examined repeatedly, see Cook N R, Ware J H 1983 Design and analysis methods for longitudinal research. Annual Reviews of Public Health 4: 1.
14. Qiao Z-K, Halliday M L, Coates R A, Rankij J G 1988 Relationship between liver cirrhosis death rate and nutritional factors in 38 countries. International Journal of Epidemiology 17: 414. The authors found that a higher average intake of protein, vitamins A and B2 and calcium (none of which was related to average alcohol consumption) was associated with a lower mortality from liver cirrhosis. They concluded that these relationships were not necessarily causal, but indicated a need for further studies.
15. After analysing trends in New Zealand, for example, Jackson & Beaglehole (1987) concluded that changes in fat and tobacco consumption provided a biologically plausible explanation for at least part of the decline in coronary mortality between 1968 and 1980. Jackson R, Beaglehole R 1987 Trends in dietary fat and cigarette smoking and the decline in coronary heart disease in New Zealand. International Journal of Epidemiology 16: 377.
16. Breslow N E, Enstrom J E 1974 Geographic correlations between cancer mortality rates and alcohol-tobacco consumption in the United States. Journal of the National Cancer Institute 53: 631.
17. Cochrane A L, St Leger A S, Moore F 1978 Health service 'input' and mortality 'output' in developed countries. Journal of Epidemiology and Community Health 32: 200.
18. Doll R, Peto R 1981 The causes of cancer. Oxford University Press, Oxford, pp 1204–1205.
19. Boyce W J, Vessey M P 1985 Rising incidence of fracture of the proximal femur. Lancet i: 150.
20. Kramer & Boivin 1987 review the confusion in the classification and nomenclature of epidemiological study designs. To 'unconfound' the situation they suggest a three-way classification by (1) the *directionality* in which exposure and outcome are investigated (cohort, case-control, or cross-sectional); (2) *sample selection* criteria (by exposure, outcome, or other criteria), and (3) *timing* of the study proper with respect to the calendar times of exposure and outcome, the categories being *historical* (exposure and outcome occurred before the study), *concurrent* (both exposure and outcome occur during the study) and *mixed* (exposure before the study, outcome during the study). Kramer J S, Boivin J F 1987 Toward an 'unconfounded' classification of epidemiologic research design. Journal of Chronic Diseases 40: 683.
   Debates on alternative classifications appear in the Journal of Clinical Epidemiology 1988 41: 705 and 1989 42: 819. For defences of the utility of

directionality as an axis of classification, see the following papers in that journal: Kramer M S, Boivin J-F 1988 The importance of directionality in epidemiologic research design: 41: 717; Kramer M S, Boivin J-F 1989 Directionality, timing and sample selection in epidemiologic research design: 42: 827; Abramson J H 1989 Classification of epidemiologic research: 42: 819; and Feinstein A R 1989 Directionality and scientific inference: 42: 829.

21. Miettinen O S 1988 Steps to deconfound the fundamentals of epidemiologic study design. Journal of Clinical Epidemiology 41: 709.

22. Rothman K J 1986 Modern epidemiology. Little, Brown, Boston, p 64. The 'person-time' concept is explained in note 3, p 99.

23. Greenland S, Morgenstern H 1988 Classification schemes for epidemiologic research designs. Journal of Clinical Epidemiology 41: 715.

24. *Trohoc*, a term proposed as an unambiguous replacement for 'retrospective' (Feinstein 1981; see note 9), is 'cohort' spelt backwards, and makes many epidemiologists shudder.

25. The 'case-base' or 'case-referent' approach is strongly championed by some epidemiologists: Miettinen O S 1985 Theoretical epidemiology: principles of occurrence research in medicine. Wiley, New York, chapter 4; Miettinen 1988 (see note 21); Axelson O 1985 The 'case-control' study: valid selection of subjects. Journal of Chronic Diseases 38: 553.

Miettinen explains this approach as follows: 'Given a study population's experience over time, or a *study base*, it is necessary to ascertain the relevant facts about the occurrence of the illness in this experience. One approach to this is to employ a simple *census*, that is, to ascertain all of the relevant facts on all members of the study population... An alternative to this approach is one of combining census and sampling. First one uses a census of the base population ... to identify all cases. Then a second census is conducted on the cases to ascertain other facts (concerning the determinants, modifiers and confounders) on them. Finally, a sample of the base is used to obtain information of the latter type about it. This alternative to the census approach may be considered the *census-sample* or *case-base* approach. It may also be termed the *case-referent* approach, since the study base, which the sample represents, is the direct referent of the empirical pattern of occurrence in the study. On the other hand, the term "case-control" approach is a misnomer, as the base sample is no more a control series than a census of the base (referent) is'. Miettinen O S 1985 The 'case-control' study: valid selection of subjects. Journal of Chronic Diseases 38: 543.

Other epidemiologists are less convinced, and suggest that the main issue is the appropriate selection of controls: Schlesselman J J 1985 Valid selection of subjects in case-control studies. Journal of Chronic Diseases 38: 549; Feinstein A R 1985 The case-control study: valid selection of subjects. Journal of Chronic Diseases 38: 551.

26. Needleman H L, Gunnoe C, Levison A et al 1979 Deficits in psychologic and classroom performance of children with elevated dentine lead levels. New England Journal of Medicine 300: 689.

27. A historical prospective study may be called a *non-concurrent prospective study*, a *retrospective cohort study*, a *prospective study in retrospect*, or a *retrospective design with forward directionality* (all this in the interest of greater clarity).

28. Kramer & Boivin 1987 (see note 20)

29. The uses of retrospective and prospective studies are discussed in all textbooks of epidemiology. Chapters describing the uses and limitations of cross-sectional studies (Abramson J H, p 89), cohort studies (Feinleib M, Detels R, p 101) and case-control studies (Greenberg R S, Ibrahim M A, p 123) will be found in the Oxford Textbook of Public Health 1985 vol 3: Investigative methods in public health (Holland W W, Detels R, Knox G, eds). Oxford University Press, Oxford. For an especially thorough treatment of the pros and cons of a large number of study designs, including hybrid designs, see Kleinbaum et al (1982)

(see note 2), Chapter 5. Case-control studies are discussed in detail in a symposium edited by Ibrahim M A 1979 Symposium on the case-control study. Journal of Chronic Diseases 32: 1 and by Schlesselman J J 1982 Case-control studies: design, conduct, analysis. Oxford University Press, New York and Breslow N 1982 Design and analysis of case-control studies. Annual Reviews of Public Health 3: 29.

30. Sackett D L 1979 Bias in analytic research. Journal of Chronic Diseases 32: 51.
31. An association between severe diarrhoea and cataract has been shown by case-control studies in India and England. Minassian D C, Mehra V, Jones B R 1984 Dehydrational crises from severe diarrhoea or heatstroke and risk of cataract. Lancet i: 751; van Heyningen R, Harding J J 1988 A case-control study of cataract in Oxfordshire: Some risk factors. British Journal of Ophthalmology 72: 804.
32. Susser M, Stein Z, Kline J 1978 Ethics in epidemiology. Annals of the American Academy of Political and Social Science 437: 128.
33. Kinsey V E, Hemphill F M 1955 American Journal of Ophthalmology 40: 166.
34. For a short introduction to evaluative studies, see Rundall T G 1986 Evaluation of health service programs. In: Last J M (ed) Maxcy–Rosenau public health and preventive medicine, 12th edn. Appleton-Century-Crofts, Norwalk, Connecticut, pp 1831–1847 or Spiegel A D, Hyman H H 1978 Basic health planning methods. Aspen Systems, Germantown, Maryland, Chapter 7.
35. Kane R L, Henson R, Deniston O L (1974) In: Kane R L (see note 10).
36. Accurate information on the size and composition of the population served is seldom easy to obtain. It is usually not possible to obtain suitable data from official censuses, and a community health service may have to develop its own data-gathering mechanism. If the population served is too large for accurate surveillance, a 'defined area' may be demarcated for this purpose (see p 311). If the service is provided to specific people (not to all comers or to all residents in a neighbourhood), a register of eligible persons will provide the requisite information.

   For information on microcomputer programs (EasWesPo, DemProj, MCPDA, MortPak and others) for demographic analyses, including the estimation of fertility rates, population projections and life tables from simple demographic survey data, write to Project Director, Software and Support for Population Data Processing, Department of Technical Cooperation for Development, Room DC2-1570, United Nations, New York 10017.
37. The meanings of the terms 'surveillance' and 'monitoring' are discussed by Acheson & Hall (1976; see note 12), p 126. 'Monitoring' often denotes not only watching, but using the observations as a basis for continual modification of goals, plans or activities; Knox E G (ed) 1979 Epidemiology in health care planning. Oxford University Press, Oxford, pp 18–19, 127–129. Its use in programme evaluation is briefly reviewed by Rundall (1986) In: Last J (see note 34), pp 1837–1839.
38. For a brief introduction to health services research, see Lewis C E Health services research: asking the painful questions. In: Kane (1974; see note 10), pp 69–86. Morris (1975; see note 6) defines operational research as 'the systematic study, by observation and experiment, of the working of health services as well as of health'. Operational and system studies are described by Cretin S 1985 Operational and system studies. In: Holland W W, Detels R, Knox G (eds) Oxford Textbook of Public Health, vol 3: Investigative methods in public health. Oxford: Oxford University Press, pp 222–236. The principles of decision analysis are reviewed by McNeil B J, Pauker S G 1984 Decision analysis for public health: principles and illustrations. Annual Reviews of Public Health 5: 135.

3. Stages of an investigation

The stages of an investigation may be listed in a logical sequence, in which each phase is dependent on the preceding phase.

1. Preliminary steps
   a. Clarifying the purpose
   b. Formulating the topic
2. Planning
3. Preparing for data collection
4. Collecting the data
5. Processing the data
6. Interpreting the results
7. Writing a report

After the investigator has clarified the purpose of the study and formulated its topic in general terms (see Ch. 1), he can prepare a detailed plan (Chs. 4–22). He can then prepare to collect data by testing the methods and making whatever practical arrangements are needed (Ch. 23). The data are then collected (Ch. 24) and processed (Ch. 25.). The researcher can then sit down to make sense of his findings and decide on their theoretical and practical implications (Chs 26–28). Finally he prepares a report to communicate the findings to others (Ch. 29).

In practice, this scheme is seldom followed rigidly, even by the most obsessional of researchers. There are two main reasons for this. First, it may be convenient for certain stages to overlap. For example, some of the preparations for the collection of data may be made before the study plan is complete, or it may be possible to collect and even analyse some types of information before other aspects have been fully planned. Secondly, and more important, the various phases may be influenced not only by the preceding phases, but also by subsequent ones. As one example, unforeseen snags may appear when the methods are tested, or even after data collection has commenced, sending the investigator 'back to the drawing board'. As another example, in the above scheme the interpretation of findings follows their processing, which seems logical; but a basic element of the scientific method is that inferences are drawn from facts, and these inferences are then tested by obtaining further facts; this means that usually, except in the simplest of investigations, the researcher inter- prets the data that have been processed, decides what further analyses are needed, interprets the new facts, and so on; processing and inter- pretation have a two-way influence on each other, and usually proceed hand in hand.

REVIEWING THE LITERATURE

'Reviewing the literature' does not appear in the above scheme, not because it is unimportant, but because it is so important throughout the study that it cannot be seen as a separate stage. The published experiences and thoughts of others may not only indicate the presence and nature of the research problem, but may be of great help in all aspects of planning and in the interpretation of the findings. At the outset of his study the investigator should be or should become acquainted with the important relevant literature, and he should continue with directed reading throughout; he should know how to make effective use of library facilities,[1] and should file his references in an organized way, manually[2] or using a personal computer (PC or microcomputer).[3] (This is only one of the many ways in which a PC can streamline the conduct of a study.)[4] It is of limited use to wait until a report has to be written, and then read and cite (or merely cite) a long list of publications to impress the reader with one's erudition—a procedure that may defeat its own ends, since it is often quite apparent that the papers and books listed in the extensive bibliography have had no impact on the investigation.

Papers should be read with a healthy scepticism.[5] If the title and abstract suggest that the paper may be of interest, you should ap- praise the methods used in the study [which requires the kind of familiarity with research methods and their pitfalls that this book attempts to impart (advert)], assess the accuracy of the findings, judge whether the inferences are valid, and decide whether the study has relevance to your own needs and interests. Do not expect any study to be completely convincing, or reject a study because it is *not* completely convincing—avoid '*I am an epidemiologist' bias* (repudia- tion of any study containing any flaw in its design, analysis or interpretation) and other forms of what Owen (1982) has called 'reader bias'.[6]

THE PLANNING PHASE

1. Formulation of study objectives
2. Planning of methods
   a. Study population
      Selection and definition
      Sampling
      Size
   b. Variables
      Selection
      Definition
      Scales of measurement
   c. Methods of collecting data
   d. Methods of recording and processing

Needless to say, the value of any investigation depends on sound planning, which may necessitate a considerable amount of effort. The closer the attention to detail, the better the prospects of a fruitful study. The planning phase may take more of the investigator's time, or even of the total duration of the investigation, than any other phase of the study.

A dilemma frequently faced by investigators seeking research funds is that the success of the application may depend on the quality of the study plan, so that a considerable investment of time is required for planning, without any assurance that the study will actually be performed.

The first step in planning is to formulate the objectives of the investigation. The investigator already knows *why* he is undertaking the study, and has formulated the topic in general terms (see Ch. 1). He must now decide what his detailed study objectives are, i.e. precisely what knowledge he wishes the study to yield. (Note that the term 'objective' is sometimes used to indicate what we have called the 'purpose' of the study on page 2; we are specifically excluding this connotation.) His decision on what he wishes to learn from the study determines the further planning of the investigation, and the methods of the study can be judged by their appropriateness to these study objectives. The formulation of objectives will be discussed in Chapters 4 and 5.

The second step is to plan the methods. Consideration must be given to:

1. *The study population* (see Chs 6–8): Whom is it proposed to study? Will a sample or samples be used? How will sampling be done? What will be the sample size?
2. *The variables to be studied* (Chs 9–13). What characteristics will be measured? How will the variables be defined? What scales of measurement will be used?
3. *Methods of data collection* (Chs 14–20): Will data be collected by direct observation, from documentary sources, or by interviews or self-administered questionnaires? What are the detailed procedures and questions to be used?
4. *Methods of recording and processing* (Chs 21–22): How will the data be recorded? What data-processing techniques will be used? What is the analysis plan?

Chapters 3–22 have relevance to the planning of both non-experimental and experimental studies. Specific aspects of the planning of trials will be discussed in Chapters 30 and 31.

The various elements of planning are interdependent, and should be regarded as different aspects on which attention must be focused, rather than as discrete entities. A decision on the characteristics to be measured, for example, may depend not only on the study objectives, but on the nature of the study population and on the practicability of various methods of data collection; or a detailed consideration of the methods required to satisfy the study objectives may lead to a re-formulation of the objectives.

Some investigators see their main planning task as the design of a 'form'—a schedule on which findings will be recorded, or a questionnaire—and make this their first (and sometimes only) planning activity. This approach cannot be recommended.

It is usually helpful to commit the study plan to writing, whether briefly or in detail, since human memory is fallible. The study objectives and an outline of the methods will in any case require to be described in the report of the study. If an application is made for research funds the objectives and methods may have to be stated in a detailed study protocol.

It may not be frivolous to suggest that, as the plan of the study begins to take form and a clearer picture emerges of the effort and cost involved, the investigator should ask himself whether the investigation is still seen as worthwhile—is its performance warranted by the importance of the problem which was its starting-point? It is better to scrap a study at the outset than to decide afterwards that it was not worth doing.

MUST A STUDY BE PERFECT?

In the pages which follow, a great deal of attention will be paid to various aspects of sound planning—the careful choice of definitions, the use of standardized and accurate methods of collecting information, etc. The better the techniques of investigation, the greater are the prospects of producing useful findings, and the more certain the researcher can be that his findings will be reproducible. However, there are very few perfect studies. Almost invariably, practical difficulties, oversights and accidents produce methodological imperfections. What is important is that the investigator should be aware of these imperfections, examine their impact, and take them into account in interpreting his findings; if this is done, the study will still be a sound and possibly a useful one. While striving for perfection, the investigator should from the outset realize that his reach will almost certainly be shorter than his grasp, and be prepared to make compromises with reality. In fact, an undue insistence on impeccable techniques at all costs may well ruin a study. There is much truth in the statement that 'in science as in love a concentration on technique is quite likely to lead to impotence'.[7]

NOTES AND REFERENCES

1. Pertinent publications may be sought in cumulative indexes, such as Index Medicus (its Bibliography of Medical Reviews is especially helpful), or journals of abstracts (e.g. Excerpta Medica), or by a computerized (e.g. MEDLINE) search. If a key source is known, use the Science Citation Index to identify recent papers that cite it; with luck, some of these will have extensive relevant bibliographies. A convenient way of keeping up-to-date is by scanning the weekly issues of Current Contents, which reproduce the contents pages of hundreds of journals. For a simple guide to the use of Index Medicus and MEDLINE, see Sackett D L, Haynes R B, Tugwell P 1985 Clinical epidemiology: a basic science for clinical medicine. See Little, Brown Boston, pp 271–283. Haynes R B, McKibbon K A, Fitzgerald D, Guyatt G H, Walker C J, Sackett DL 1986 How to keep up with the medical literature. Annals of Internal Medicine 105: 149, 309, 574, 636, 810 & 978.

   Hewitt & Chalmers 1985 explain how to use MEDLINE in the following articles: Hewitt P, Chalmers TC 1985 Using MEDLINE to peruse the literature. Controlled Clinical Trials 6: 75. Perusing the literature: methods of accessing MEDLINE and related databases. Clinical Trials 6: 168. Using MEDLINE for perusing the literature: software and search interface of interest to the medical professional. Controlled Clinical Trials 6: 198. Use of a personal computer to make access to MEDLINE is described by Haynes et al 1986; see above p 810 and Hewitt & Chalmers 1985; see above p 198.

2. A card index of references is a great help (one reference per card). Full bibliographical details should be included (names of all authors, first and last page numbers, etc.) so that the article will not have to be hunted again when a bibliography is prepared for the report. If photocopies, reprints or tear-out copies of articles are collected they should be filed and indexed in an orderly way. The planning of a filing system is described in detail by Haynes et al (1986; see note 1), p 978.

3. As a rule, only public-domain and user-supported software for IBM PC and compatible computers will be mentioned by name in this book (commercial programs can afford their own advertising). These programs may be freely copied, and are available free or at low cost from computer clubs, bulletin board systems, software libraries, and other sources (consult a computer magazine). In some cases the full version is available only after payment of a registration fee. Remarks on named programs may well be out-of-date by the time you read them.

   To make a file of references, use any database program that has good sorting and searching capabilities (usually based on author's name, words in the title, or key words) and a large field for your notes. *PC-File Plus* and *PC-File db* are examples. Instant Recall (a speedy pop-up program) indexes every single word in free-format entries, and text is easily transferred to or from ASCII files; the database of the free-distribution version cannot exceed 80 Kbytes (a fuller version is sold commercially under another name). *Papers (Scientific Paper Database)* can store long notes as well as bibliographic details; it has good search facilities; text can be imported from ASCII files. *MedLit* is designed as a medical literature data-base; entries can be typed in, or imported from MEDLINE; but there is no place for notes, and the free version can take only 150 references. *RefList* maintains a master list of references (without notes) for a single purpose, viz. helping writers to prepare bibliographies and text citations; it can modify the format of references. Commercial programs are listed by Haynes et al (1986; see note 1), p 978; also, see Hewitt & Chalmers (1985; see note 1), p 198.

4. The uses of microcomputers in research are reviewed by Madron T W, Tate C N, Brookshire R G 1985 (Using microcomputers in research. Sage Publications, Newbury Park, California (and by Schrodt P A 1987) Microcomputer methods for social scientists, 2nd edn. Sage Publications, Newbury Park, California). Schrodt provides down-to-earth advice for PC tyros. (Examples: 'Computers and liquids . . . do not mix . . . Even tears have been known to short-circuit a keyboard . . . There is one and only one source of reliable information about ·software: word of mouth . . . The secret to getting the full potential out of a program has been enshrined in the acronym RYFM, which, for public consumption, may be translated as 'Read your factfilled manual'.)

   There is increasing experience with the use of microcomputers in surveys in developing countries; this may require special computer–literacy courses and the use of equipment that contends with electric power problems (voltage regulators, battery-powered computers). The main problem is the lack of a local hardware and software support system. See Frerichs R R, Miller R A 1985 Introduction of a microcomputer for health research in a developing country — the Bangladesh experience. Public Health Reports 100: 638; Gould J B, Frerichs R R 1986 Training faculty in Bangladesh to use a microcomputer for public health: followup report. Public Health Reports 101: 616; Frerichs R R, Tar K T 1989 Computer-assisted rapid surveys in developing countries. Public Health Reports 104: 14.

   However helpful a computer may be, it cannot work magic. A description of one computer program claims that it 'is designed to allow anyone, no matter how knowledgeable or ignorant of statistical and survey methods, to conduct a useful and correctly designed survey. It has everything you need' (PC Magazine 1989, 8: 254). If only that were true!

5. For guides to the critical reading of clinical journals see Sackett et al (1985; see note 1), pp 285–321 or a series of papers in Canadian Medical Association Journal

1981 124: 555, 703, 869, 985, 1156; 1984 130: 377. If you like using checklists, they are provided by Polgar S, Thomas S A 1988 Introduction to research in the health sciences. Churchill Livingstone, Melbourne, p 279 and (for case-control studies) by Lichtenstein M J, Mulrow C D, Elwood P C 1987. Guidelines for reading case-control studies. Journal of Chronic Diseases 40: 893. Checklists should be used with circumspection, to avoid confusing 'the *possibility* that a bias might exist with the actual occurrence of the bias in the study at hand': Vandenbroucke J P 1987 A checklist for observational research. Journal of Chronic Diseases 40: 1067.

6. Other forms of 'reader bias' listed by Owen . . . (1982) include *rivalry bias* (pooh-poohing a study published by a rival), *personal habit bias* (over-rating or under-rating a study to justify the reader's habits, e.g. a jogger favouring a study showing the health benefits of running), *prestigious journal bias* (over-rating results published in a prestigious journal), *esteemed professor bias* ['more readily accepting the conclusion of the reader's professor, who spoke only the truth (and looked like Moses)'], *pro-technology bias* (over-rating or under-rating a study owing to the reader's enchantment with medical technology) and *anti-technology bias*; Owen R 1982 Reader bias. Journal of the American Medical Association 247: 2533.

7. Berger P L 1969 Invitation to sociology: a humanistic perspective. Penguin Books, Harmondsworth, p 24.

4. Formulating the objectives

Having decided *what* to study, and knowing *why* he wants to study it, the investigator can now formulate his study objectives. That is, he can state what knowledge he wants the study to yield—*what questions* is he setting out to answer? Serendipity apart—and accidental discoveries are less uncommon than some researchers may care to admit[1]—he will not learn anything he has not set out to learn.

The explicit formulation of study objectives is an essential step in the planning of a study. It may be an exaggeration to say that 'a question well-stated is a question half-answered',[2] but a question that is poorly stated or unstated is unlikely to be answered at all. The specification of objectives determines the whole subsequent planning of the study. 'If you don't know where you're going, it is difficult to select a suitable means for getting there.'[3] In fact, 'if you're not sure where you're going, you're liable to end up someplace else'.[3]

The objectives of a descriptive survey of a specific group or population—a survey carried out with a diagnostic purpose—are usually easy to formulate. The investigator needs only to state the characteristics he wants to measure. These may be diseases, deaths, or other 'disagreeable Ds' (disabilities, discomforts, dissatisfactions, deviations from statistical or social norms); they may be positive aspects of health (e.g. physical fitness, life expectancy); or they may be somatic or psychological characteristics (body weight, biological markers,[4] behaviour patterns, etc.) that are not necessarily negative or positive, but are seen as elements of health status or expressions of health. There are numerous health indicators and health indices, serving different ends and appropriate in different circumstances.[5] The investigator may also want to study other characteristics of the group (demographic, biological, behavioural, social or cultural), or environmental features. He may also be interested in the health services provided to the population, or in their use.

These objectives are easily stated, e.g. 'to determine the infant mortality rate in population Y during period Z', 'to measure the incidence rate of rabies', 'the prevalence rate of scabies', 'the case fatality rate of tabes', 'to determine the distribution of serum cholesterol values', etc.

Objectives may be stated in general terms, e.g. 'to measure the prevalence of disability (in population Y at time Z)', or may be phrased more specifically, e.g. in terms of mobility, capacity to work, ability to perform activities of daily living, or other selected functions. The more specifically the objectives are stated, the more helpful they will be in the further planning of the study. A formulation that is too general, e.g. 'to study the health status of . . .' will not be helpful at all. If general objectives are stated, more specific ones should be listed as well. Careful thinking about specific objectives may help to ensure that the study meets its purposes.

Even in a simple descriptive survey there is usually interest in obtaining separate information for different groups—for specific age groups, for the two sexes, for ethnic groups or parts of a city, etc. The objective might be stated as 'to measure X in population Y by age, sex (etc.)'. In a survey of the 'community diagnosis' type, findings may provide pointers to the different health needs of different parts of the population. If alcoholics are concentrated in one neighbourhood, that neighbourhood may need a special programme.

Not uncommonly, a survey centres not on the characteristic (say, disease D) in which interest actually lies, but on something that is known to be associated with this characteristic. The main circumstances in which the study may focus on an associated characteristic or characteristics (C) are as follows:

1. If it is easy to obtain information about C and difficult to obtain information about D, C may be used as a *proxy measure* of D. As an example, an investigator may be interested in the occurrence of prostatic hypertrophy in a community; if rectal examinations to establish the diagnosis are not feasible, he may investigate the prevalence of a specific symptom pattern (frequency, nocturia, hesitancy, weak stream, terminal dribbling) believed to be associated with the disease.[6] It may be possible to estimate the prevalence rate of D from the prevalence rate of C.[7] If C is a poor proxy measure many individuals will be misclassified, and problems of interpretation may arise (see p 159).

2. The presence of C may be of use as a *screening test*—that is, to discriminate between people who are likely and those who are unlikely to have D. Once people who have C (say a high casual

blood pressure measurement) have been identified, they can be invited to be examined more fully in order to determine whether D (hypertensive disease) is present. To warrant such use of the association, C must be easier to study than D; C and D must be present at the same time; and certain other conditions (see pp 161–162) must be met. The study objective might be stated as 'to identify people with positive screening tests for D'.

3. If C precedes D in time, it may be of use as a *risk marker*—that is, to distinguish between people who are likely and those who are unlikely to develop D in the future. The presence of C identifies vulnerable individuals or groups (*at risk* or *high risk* groups) who are especially likely to develop the disorder, and who hence have a special need for preventive care. C *points to* the increased risk, it does not necessarily *cause* it. It may be a cause, or it may be a precursor or early manifestation of the disorder, or it may itself be an effect or correlate of the factor that increases the risk. In a study of elderly men, for example, the risk markers for dying within the next 5 years were found to include impaired memory and inability to work.[8] These are unlikely to *cause* mortality—any special care given to these high-risk men would be directed at other factors. On the other hand, a risk marker may itself be a cause of the increased risk—the same study showed that a high diastolic blood pressure was another indicator of mortality risk, and presumably a reason for the high risk. A study might aim to 'determine the prevalence of a (specified) risk marker' or 'to identify people who are at special risk of a (specified) disorder'. *Health hazard appraisal*[9] is a particular instance of the use of risk markers.

4. C may also be of interest because it is a *cause* of D—that is, its presence or degree influences the risk of developing D. If C is amenable to change, and if a change in C will reduce the risk of D, there may be a case for intervention directed at C. In such instances C is possibly best termed a *modifiable risk factor* (the adjective 'modifiable' refers both to the factor and to the risk). The unqualified term '*risk factor*' is generally used, but unfortunately this has more than one meaning; it is also often used to denote *any* cause of a disorder (modifiable or not), and sometimes to denote a risk marker. A causal factor may or may not be of use as a risk marker, and it may or may not be modifiable. The general objective of a study of modifiable risk factors might be formulated as 'to determine the prevalence of' or 'to identify people who have' specified factors.

STUDYING ASSOCIATIONS BETWEEN VARIABLES

Information about associations between variables—that is, about whether and how different characteristics 'hang together'[10]—may be sought both for practical purposes and because of interest in processes affecting health and disease. Analytic surveys, both those that aim to explain the health status of a specific population and those that seek new knowledge about aetiology and natural history, have the examination of associations between variables as their main function, as do many methodological studies—e.g. those that test the value of screening and diagnostic tests and risk markers—and all experiments.

Possible formulations of the study objective, when an association is to be investigated, include 'To examine the association between infant mortality rates and region', 'To determine whether there is a difference between the rates in regions A and B', and 'To test the hypothesis that the rates in regions A and B differ'. *Hypotheses* are suppositions that are tested by collecting facts that lead to their acceptance or rejection. They are not assumptions that are to be taken for granted, neither are they beliefs that the investigator sets out to prove. They are 'refutable predictions' (T H Huxley wrote of 'the great tragedy of Science—the slaying of a beautiful hypothesis by an ugly fact').

A hypothesis may be stated as a positive declaration (sometimes called the *research hypothesis*), e.g. 'The infant mortality rates in regions A and B are different' or 'The rate is higher in region A than in region B', or as a negative declaration (null hypothesis), e.g. 'There is no difference between the rates' or 'The rate is not higher in region A than in region B'. Statistical testing of an association requires the formulation of a null hypothesis, which is tested against a specific alternative;[11] this alternative ('that there is a difference between the two regions', or 'that the rate is higher in region A') is the 'research hypothesis'. If statistical testing is intended it is advisable to make the hypotheses as specific as possible at this stage, and not to leave them implicit (as in 'to study the association between mortality and region').

In a retrospective survey designed to examine a possible causal relationship between smoking and a disease, typical specific hypotheses might be that the proportion of smokers is higher among cases than among controls, that the proportion of heavy smokers is higher among cases than among controls, that the average age at starting smoking is earlier among cases than among controls, etc. In a prospective study set up for the same purpose the hypotheses would relate to the incidence of the disease among persons with different smoking habits. The value of epidemiological hypotheses is enhanced if they deal not only with the combined occurrence of the postulated cause and effect (i.e. when one is present, does the other tend to be present?), but also with the quantitative *dose–response* relationship between cause and effect (e.g. when there is more intensive exposure to the cause, is the disease more frequent or more severe?) or with the *time–response* relationship (the relationship to the time interval since exposure).

As will be seen later (in Ch. 27), if we want to know *why* there is an association between two variables, we will usually need analyses that take account of the way the association is influenced by other characteristics. The selection of these other variables will be discussed on pages 94–96. If the investigator wishes he may make mention of them when formulating the study objectives, e.g. by saying that the association will be tested 'holding sex and ethnic group constant' or 'controlling for' these variables, or that the hypothesis will be tested separately in each sex and ethnic group, or by listing the 'modifying' and 'confounding' variables that he will take into account (these terms will become clearer later). Remember there is still lots of time for these decisions; the planning of the study is still in its early stages, and study objectives can be rethought and reformulated as often as we wish. Remember too that these complications are of course unnecessary in a simple descriptive survey.

Study objectives

1. Do they meet the purpose of the study?
2. Are they clear?
3. Are they expressed in measurable terms?

It is usually helpful to formulate the study objectives explicitly in writing. For convenience they are often first given in fairly general terms, e.g. 'to measure smoking habits' or 'to examine the association between smoking and a (specified) disease', and each of these general objectives is followed by an explicit statement of the relevant specific objectives, including the testing of specific hypotheses. The stated objectives should satisfy three requirements. First, they must meet the purpose of the study. This is usually easily achieved in a descriptive survey, but in planning an analytic survey or experiment there may be considerable difficulty in the formulation of a hypothesis; this is where the creative researcher comes into his own. Secondly, the objectives should be phrased clearly—unambiguously and very specifically—leaving no doubt as to precisely what has to be measured. Thirdly, they should be phrased in measurable terms. That is, the objectives should be realistic (answerable questions, testable hypotheses) and formulated in operational terms, which can be applied in practice. 'Any fool can ask a question; the trick is to ask one that can be answered.'[12]

A few imaginary and actual examples follow.

1. A survey of diabetes was conducted in an English community. Its first objective was '1. To establish exactly the number of diabetics'. This is a clear statement; but the formulation is incomplete, since the investigators also measured the prevalence *rate* of diabetes and established the age and sex distribution of cases. The second objective was '2. To discover the undiagnosed cases of diabetes'. This is not a complete statement, as the investigators also wanted to answer questions about the hitherto unknown cases. It should go on: 'and to compare their age and sex distribution with that of known cases'. The next objective was '3. To investigate the possible hereditary factors'. This is far too non-specific to be helpful as a blueprint in planning the study. Did the investigators intend to examine familial clustering among the people they examined? Did they want to see if prevalence was higher among the offspring of consanguineous marriages? Did they want to look for an association with the occurrence of genetic markers, such as human leucocyte antigens? Or (as was actually the case) did they want to compare the frequency of positive family histories of diabetes among known diabetics, newly discovered diabetics, and non-diabetics, controlling for age and sex? One last example from this study: '6. To repeat the whole survey at a future date'. This is hardly a study objective.

2. A report on a national study of cerebral palsy in adolescence and adulthood[13] states: 'The primary objectives of the study were: 1. To learn about the extent and nature [of the problem] and the specific needs of cerebral palsied youngsters and adults through a sociomedical study. 2. To collect epidemiological data on the cerebral palsied'. These formulations may be useful as starting points in planning a study, or as summary statements in a report, but would not be very useful as blueprints. Much further detail is needed for this purpose. (The study itself is a good one, and it is

clear that the investigators actually did have specific and well thought out objectives.) Another stated objective, 'To evoke the interest of local communities and public agencies in the problems and needs of the cerebral palsied', is a laudable *purpose* for a study, but not what we have called a study objective. It might be stated as an objective of an action programme.

3. The objective of a study was stated to be 'to study the effects of vaccination against measles'. This formulation is completely non-specific, and could have given the investigator little help in the planning of his study. Was he interested in the development of serological changes, or in differences in antibody titre between groups of vaccinated and non-vaccinated children, or in differences in the subsequent incidence of measles? In fact, and to this reader's surprise, the study turned out to be a descriptive survey of the incidence of fever, pain at the injection site, and other manifestations immediately after vaccination.

4. A hypothesis including the word 'cause', such as one that the habitual drinking of coffee is a cause of cancer of the bladder, must be made more specific before it can be tested. Is it proposed to determine whether the incidence rate of the disease in different countries or at different times is correlated with the average consumption of coffee per head (group-based analytic surveys), or to determine whether patients drink more coffee than controls (a cross-sectional or retrospective survey), or to determine whether the incidence of new cases is higher among persons who drink much coffee than among those who take less coffee, and lowest among those who drink no coffee at all (a prospective survey or a rather unlikely experiment)? 'Controlling for age, sex, smoking habits (etc.)' would probably be specified in the hypothesis.

5. The hypothesis that 'there is an association between a specified disease and diet' is not sufficiently specific. The investigator may aim to compare the dietary histories of cases and controls, or compare incidence rates in vegetarians and others, or seek correlations between national disease rates and food consumption data. Neither is it stated in operational terms. In what aspect of diet is the investigator interested: in the average daily intake of calories, proteins, fats and other specific nutrients, or in the average amounts consumed of milk, meat, and other specific foodstuffs, or in the number of days a week that meat, fish, etc. are usually eaten, or in the average number of meals taken per day? It may be felt that such decisions can be postponed until later in the planning phase. There is no great harm in this, but it is arguable that since

these decisions may be very close to the nub of the research problem, they should be made at an early stage of planning. They are of a different order of importance from decisions on various methods of measurement, such as the choice of a technique for measuring the daily caloric intake (questioning, self-maintained dietary records, weighing of dishes and leftovers, etc.). Similar considerations arise when other vague terms are used, such as 'nutritional status', 'disability', 'emotional health', or 'stress'.

NOTES AND REFERENCES

1. 'One sometimes finds what one is not looking for' (Sir Alexander Fleming, the serendipitous discoverer of penicillin). Other discoveries based on unplanned 'chance' observations (immunization with attenuated pathogens, anaphylaxis, the connection between the pancreas and diabetes, etc.) are listed by Beveridge W I B 1957 in The Art of Scientific Investigation 3rd edn. Vintage Books, New York. This useful book, which stresses that 'the most important instrument in research must always be the mind of man', concentrates on the 'mental skills' of scientific investigation, such as the ability to recognize the importance of a chance or unexpected observation, to interpret the clue and develop a hypothesis, and to follow up the initial finding in a systematic way.
2. Isaac S, Michael W B 1977 Handbook in research and evaluation for education and the behavioural sciences. EdITS, San Diego, p 2.
3. Mager R F 1975 Preparing instructional objectives. Fearon, Belmont, California.
4. *Biological markers* are biochemical, molecular, genetic, immunological or other indicators (often quantitative) of past exposure, biological changes, disease processes, or predisposition to disease. Examples: lead content of blood, creatinine clearance, human leucocyte antigens, alpha-fetoprotein, antibody titres. Their uses in epidemiological research are discussed by Schulte P A 1987 Methodologic issues in the use of biologic markers in epidemiologic research. American Journal of Epidemiology 126: 1006.
5. *Health indicators*: a 'shopper's guide'—a 'list of things to think about' when choosing a measure of health status—is provided by Ware J E Jr, Brook R J, Davies A R et al 1981 Choosing measures of health status for individuals in general populations. American Journal of Public Health 71: 620. See Ware J E Jr 1984 Methodological considerations in the selection of health status assessment procedures. In: Wenger N K, Mattson M E, Furberg C D, Elinson J (eds) Assessment of quality of life in clinical trials of cardiovascular therapies. LeJacq Publishing (Waymarket-Doyma, New York), p 87. Murnaghan J H 1981 Health indicators and information systems for the year 2000. Annual Reviews of Public Health 2: 299 pays special attention to health indicators in developing countries. Purposes of health indicators are discussed by the above authors and by Jette A M 1980 Journal of Chronic Diseases 33: 567; Jette distinguishes between indicators of the status of a population and indicators of the status of individuals (some indicators serve both purposes).
   For descriptions of specific health indicators and their uses, see Holland W W, Ipsen J, Kostrzewski J (eds) 1979 Measurement of levels of health. WHO, Copenhagen; Jette (1980; see above) and the periodical Clearinghouse on Health Statistics.
   'Health index' may be a synonym for 'health indicator', or may refer to a numerical index based on two or more indicators, such as the Health Problem Index ('Q value') devised by the Division of Indian Health in the USA. This is

based mainly on the mortality rate, the average age at death, and the numbers of outpatient visits and hospital days per head; see Haynes M A 1972 in Reinke W A (ed) Health planning: qualitative aspects and quantitative techniques. Johns Hopkins University, Baltimore, Md, p 158.

6. Kark S L, Gofin J, Abramson J H et al 1979 Prevalence of selected health characteristics of men: a community health survey in Jerusalem. Israel Journal of Medical Sciences 15: 732.

7. For methods of estimating the confidence limits of the prevalence of a disease in a population from the prevalence of a proxy attribute in the population or a sample, see Peritz E 1971 Estimating the ratio of two marginal probabilities in a contingency table. Biometrics 27: 223 (correction note: 27: 1104) and Rogan W J, Gladen B 1978 Estimating prevalence from the results of a screening test. American Journal of Epidemiology 107: 71.

8. Abramson J H, Gofin R, Peritz E 1982 Risk markers for mortality among elderly men: a community study in Jerusalem. Journal of Chronic Diseases 35: 565.

9. *Health hazard appraisal* (or *health risk appraisal*), which is becoming increasingly popular, is the use of a battery of information on health-related behaviour and personal characteristics in order to estimate an individual's chances of acquiring specific diseases, of dying, etc. It has been mainly used to enable individuals to identify hazards and to motivate them to lessen them. The technique offers promise as a tool for use in community medicine, both for identifying high-risk individuals and as a way of gauging a group or population's risk of preventable diseases and other outcomes. Many programmes over-reach existing scientific knowledge in order to accomplish the former aim. An important criticism is that the message generated for the client is based on the sometimes questionable assumption that changes made by the individual will necessarily change the risk—i.e. that risk markers are modifiable risk factors. Health hazard appraisal may be offered as an incentive to make participation in a health survey attractive. Schoenbach V J, Wagner E H, Karon J M 1983 The use of epidemiologic data for personal risk assessment in health hazard/health risk appraisal programs. Journal of Chronic Diseases 36: 625; Gordis L (ed) 1988 Epidemiology and health risk assessment. Oxford University Press, New York; Fielding J E 1987 The health of health risk appraisal. Health Services Research 22: 441.

10. See note 1, p 263.

11. See note 10, p 264.

12. Lemkau P V, Pasamanick B 1957 Problems in evaluation of mental health programs. American Journal of Orthopsychiatry 27: 55.

13. Margulec I (ed) 1966 Cerebral palsy in adolescence and adulthood: a rehabilitation study. Jerusalem Academic Press, Tel Aviv, p 8.

5. The objectives of evaluative studies

When we evaluate a treatment or other form of health care we are making a value judgement. To reduce the subjective element in this judgement we should base the appraisal on facts, using explicit criteria. An evaluative study sets out to collect these facts.

The basic questions that are commonly asked in evaluative studies are listed on p 48. These questions specify the dimensions of care that are commonly appraised, whether as separate issues or as components of global appraisals. They provide a framework for decisions on specific study objectives. In these questions 'care' refers to whatever action is being evaluated — care directed at individuals or populations, screening and other diagnostic activities, or nonpersonal health programmes.

We will discuss each of these basic questions separately, and consider its role as a basis for the formulation of clear-cut study objectives. (Study objectives of clinical and programme trials will be discussed further in Chs 30 and 31).

The need for objective data should be reflected in the wording of the specific study objectives. These should not use terms requiring value judgements. In an appraisal of the desirability of routine medical examinations of schoolchildren, for example, the specific objectives might be to determine the prevalence of previously undiagnosed chronic disorders or the proportion of identified disorders that were already known or under treatment. Words like 'good', 'bad', 'should' and 'ought' have no place in the specific study objectives of evaluative studies.

REQUISITENESS

The first question is the *requisiteness* ('relevance', 'appropriateness'[1]) of care. To what extent is care *needed*? It can hardly be of value if there is no need for it. This question may be asked in reviews of well established programmes and services, which may have outlived their need. It is not asked in trials—the need for care is a precondition for a trial rather than a question the trial sets out to answer.

The basic questions of evaluative studies

1. Requisiteness
   To what extent is care needed?
2. Quality
   a. How satisfactory is the *outcome*?
      Attainment of desirable effects (*effectiveness*)?
      Absence of undesirable effects (*harmlessness*)?
   b. How satisfactory is the *performance of activities* by the providers of care?
   c. How satisfactory are *compliance* and the *utilization of services* by the recipients of care?
   d. How satisfactory are *facilities* and *settings*?
3. Efficiency
   How efficiently are resources used?
4. Satisfaction
   How satisfied are the people concerned?
5. Differential value
   How do the above features differ in different categories or groups or in different circumstances?

The appraisal by health professionals of the need for care generally requires, inter alia, facts about the nature, extent and severity of the problem or problems that the programme aims to solve, and of other problems that compete for the available resources, as well as facts about the availability of resources. Account may also be taken of *perceived need* (as stated by patients or public) and *expressed demand* (e.g. requests for care, as reflected by the use of services, waiting-lists for treatment, etc.). When formulating study objectives, thought should be given to the specific facts required to permit appraisal of the need for care.

QUALITY

The quality of health care may be judged from information about effects (*outcome evaluation*), about the performance of activities (*process evaluation*), or about facilities and settings (*structure evaluation*). In each instance, the question asked is 'How satisfactory'? and the evaluative study aims to yield the objective facts required to answer this question.

A full appraisal of *outcome* (Question 2a) depends on the balance between desirable and undesirable effects. *Effectiveness*[2] refers to the degree of achievement of desirable effects. These may be expressed at the individual level (recovery from disease, restoration of function, etc.) or at the group or community level (changes in mortality and morbidity rates, changes in a community's knowledge or practices, environmental changes, etc.).

Effectiveness is sometimes distinguished from *efficacy*. While definitions vary, 'efficacy' may be used to refer to the benefits observed when a procedure is applied as it 'should' be, and with full compliance by all concerned. The term is usually reserved for benefits at the individual level, as measured by a clinical trial. 'Effectiveness' then refers to the benefits observed at the population level, or among people to whom the procedure or service is offered. 'Efficacy' answers the question, '*can* the procedure or service work?' whereas 'effectiveness' answers the question, '*does* it work?'[3] A programme for the control of hypertension in a community would use drugs known to be efficacious; the community programme might or might not be effective.

Clear-cut explicit criteria of effectiveness (or efficacy) are readily available if the activities under evaluation have well defined predetermined goals, i.e. situations or conditions whose attainment was set up as an aim. (We will refer to these as 'goals' rather than 'objectives', so as not to confuse them with study objectives; some authors distinguish between the 'goals' and 'objectives' of health care programmes.[4]) The extent of accomplishment of these aims is an objective measure of effectiveness. With this method of evaluation in mind, effectiveness is sometimes defined as 'the extent to which pre-established objectives are attained as a result of activity'.[2]

This 'goal attainment' approach (which will be further discussed on p 300) can be used only if predetermined goals are known or can be inferred, and if it is possible to measure their attainment. For the latter purpose, they must be expressed in clear and specific terms. It is not easy to appraise the effectiveness of an antenatal programme it its goal is expressed in such general terms as 'to promote the health of the mother and baby'. If the goals are 'to reduce the stillbirth rate', 'to reduce the number of babies born with Down's syndrome', etc., evaluation is easier. It is especially easy if precise quantitative targets[4] are stated—e.g. 'to reduce the stillbirth rate to 15 per 1000 births'.

If the goal attainment model cannot be used, the investigator will need to formulate his own criteria, or to use standards[5] or criteria formulated by expert consultants (see Ch. 19). The need for such (additional) criteria should be considered even when the goal attainment model is used, so as to avoid the danger of 'tunnel vision'—if the investigator concentrates only on the preset goals, he may not see beneficial outcomes that were not specified as goals, and may be blind to adverse effects.

When possible, *end results*—i.e. effects on health status—should be used as criteria of effectiveness, even if the production of these effects is not a direct aim of the procedure or programme under evaluation. A highly 'successful' case-finding programme may merit a negative evaluation if the detection of new cases resulted in no improvement in health status. The ultimate criterion of effectiveness is the extent to which the underlying problem is alleviated or prevented. This is sometimes referred to as the *adequacy* of the intervention. A programme that deals with only a small part of a large problem may be regarded as inadequate, however effectively it does what it *does* do.

Adverse effects[6] may be missed unless they are sought. These include not only side-effects of medication ('The children crippled by thalidomide are on their slow procession through the special schools for the handicapped, following those made deaf by streptomycin who succeeded the infants blinded by oxygen'[7],) but over-dependence, anxiety, and other less obvious effects. An editorial entitled 'The menace of mass screening' in a public health journal points to the morbidity caused among children with innocent heart murmurs who falsely perceive themselves as having heart disease, and the disability caused to children as a result of being identified as carriers of the sickle-cell trait.[8] Being labelled as hypertensive may produce symptoms of depression.[9]

An appraisal of the *performance of activities* (Question 2b) requires information on the services provided—what kinds, and how much? If there is a programme plan that lays down what activities *should* be performed, these requirements provide ready-made yardsticks. If the stated intention was to make contact with every known blind person at least once a year, or to examine the developmental status of all year-old children, or to X-ray the chests of all patients with pneumonia after their treatment, to what extent were these things done? In some programmes, *coverage*[10] may be a useful criterion—what proportion of the people who can or should receive a service (the target population) actually receive it? A third approach, especially in studies of the quality of medical care, is to make a detailed formulation of the activities that it is believed *should* be carried out, usually in relation to a specific diagnosis or other medical problem, and to compare actual performance with this set of standards[5] (see 'Medical audit' in Ch 20).

A further basis for evaluation is provided by information on the activities of patients or public (Question 2c)—the *utilization of services* (what services, and how much?), the degree of *compliance* with advice or instructions (taking of medicines, keeping of appointments, persistence with treatment, etc.) and the degree of *community participation* in the programme. Clear-cut criteria are not usually available. The appraisal of activities (by providers and recipients of care) may be extended to studies of knowledge and attitudes that may influence overt behaviour, and of relationships and communication between providers and recipients.

Finally, information on *facilities and settings* (Question 2d) also provides a basis for the appraisal of quality. Are equipment, accommodation, suitably qualified personnel, laboratory facilities etc. available? Recommended norms[5] are sometimes used as criteria, e.g. for numbers of hospital beds. How accessible are services to those who need them? (What are the organizational and fiscal arrangements? Transport facilities? Are there language barriers? etc.) Is the service accountable, and to whom? Are there organizational arrangements to permit continuity of care, teamwork and co-ordinated functioning, co-ordination and co-operation with other agencies (including arrangements for patient referrals and information transfer), and community participation?

Numerous schemes of evaluation have been proposed,[11] and it may not greatly matter which is used. But beware of schemes that focus only on an appraisal of the structural and organizational context within which health care is provided, while neglecting the actual care given and its effects. Appraisals of such attributes as the availability, accessibility, comprehensiveness and co-ordination of services, continuity of care, and accountability—if based on hard facts rather than impressions—may indicate whether the setting is conducive to a satisfactory quality of care. But (unless inadequacies are striking) firm conclusions about the quality of care generally require evaluation of the process and outcome of care as well.

EFFICIENCY

Efficiency[12] (*or economic efficiency*) is a measure of the cost in resources that is incurred in achieving results. It is determined by the balance between what is put in (in time, manpower, equipment, etc. or their monetary equivalent—the collection of this information is a major task of a study of efficiency) and what is got out. It may be expressed as the average cost per unit of care (cost per test, per day in hospital, per patient treated, etc.) in comparison with the cost of other programmes or with recommended standards.[5] More usefully, the input can be compared with measures of effectiveness (*cost-effectiveness analysis*). The output is sometimes translated into monetary terms (*cost–benefit analysis*). These methods permit comparisons of the costs of alternative ways of achieving similar ends, and of the benefits that may be obtained at the same cost by different means. As an example, a comparison of three ways of reducing heart disease by controlling cholesterol levels in children—A: population-wide intervention centred on health education; B: universal screening, and C: selective screening for children with a family history of coronary heart disease—indicated that A would cost 2.6 times as much per year as B, and 17.5 times as much as C. But A would save 6.8 times as many years of life as B, and 32.6 times as many as C. A was thus the most cost-effective—its cost per year of life saved would be 32% of that of B, and 45% of that of C.[12]

If efficiency is to be appraised, the task of the study is to collect the required facts on inputs and outputs.

SATISFACTION

If patients or public are satisfied with their health care, this does not necessarily mean that their care is of high quality. Satisfaction does, however, enhance the prospects of compliance and the proper utilization of services, and it is also an important additional end-result in its own right. The measurement of satisfaction requires a survey of attitudes or of overt acts from which attitudes can be inferred, such as changes of physician, or the lodging of complaints.

Attention may also be paid to the satisfaction of health professionals. Although the gratification of health workers can hardly be regarded as a central purpose of health care, 'it is reasonable to assume that the best technical care cannot be maintained if the persons who provide it are unhappy with the work they do and the conditions under which it is done'.[13]

DIFFERENTIAL VALUE

Care may differ in value in different categories of patients or population groups, or in different circumstances. This possible non-uniformity appears as a separate item in our list (Question 5) because of its importance and the frequency with which it is forgotten. This question could actually be asked as an extension of each of the other questions: To what extent is care needed by various groups of the population? How do effectiveness and safety vary in different categories of patients or population groups? Are services equally accessible to all parts of the population?—equality of service may be one of the touchstones in evaluating a programme.[14] Why is the rate of hysterectomies (670 000 were performed in the USA in 1985) consistently twice as high among young women in the southern USA as it is in the northeastern states?[15] Who is getting better care? Are the people who use the service the ones who need it?—women with a low risk of cancer of the cervix may participate in a screening programme, while high-risk groups may stay away.[16] Who is more compliant, who is less compliant? And so on. If such questions are to be asked, they must be formulated as study objectives.

OBJECTIVES OF PROGRAMME REVIEWS

In trials (see Ch 30 and 31) the central issue is usually the outcome of the programme or treatment under evaluation. In programe reviews, which evaluate an ongoing programme and do not seek generalizable knowledge that can be applied elsewhere (see p 20), interest generally centres on the process rather than the outcome of care, and on requisiteness (especially in long-established programmes), the availability of equipment and other facilities, the public's satisfaction, and differences between population groups or categories in their need for care, use of services, and coverage.

The assumption that the planned activities of the programme are beneficial is generally not in question; the issue, rather, is whether they are conducted as planned, and their performance is used as a criterion of the quality of care. Data on activities can usually be obtained far more readily and rapidly than data on outcome, often as a byproduct of routine work, i.e. from inbuilt monitoring procedures. If there is no record of what activities were planned—as is often the case in a clinical service—arbitrary standards may be applied, e.g. by using medical audit techniques (see p 196).

This emphasis on measures of 'process' and 'structure' does not mean that measures of outcome have no place in a programme review. On the contrary, information on outcomes may be valuable even without rigorous evidence that they are actually consequences of the programme. It is usually believed that changes (or their absence) are, at least to some extent, reflections of the effectiveness of the programme. They are hence often used as a basis for decisions on the need for continuation or modification of the programme. At the very least, they may indicate whether there is a need for more detailed evaluative study.

Short-term outcomes are usually the easiest to measure. Measurement of long-term outcomes may require information about members of the target population with whom there is no routine contact, or with whom contact has ceased. It may also involve a long-term follow-up, with its attendant difficulty and delay. However, if surveillance procedures are available to provide data on relevant end-results, such as mortality rates, case fatality rates, or changes in the health status of patients or the population, this information is often especially helpful. If the programme has predetermined outcome goals, information on their accomplishment is of course particularly meaningful.

In a programme review the appraisal of efficiency, like that of quality, has special features. Although detailed studies of inputs may be undertaken, emphasis is often put on simple observations that can be used as a basis for decisions aimed at enhancing efficiency. Such observations relate especially to evidence of wasteful operation—the avoidable use of expensive or ineffective drugs, over-staffing, delays, the underexploitation of expensive equipment, superfluous activities, unnecessary hospitalization, unduly long institutional care, etc. Use is not necessarily made of explicit standards in appraising these observations. If cost-effectiveness studies are undertaken, cost is usually balanced against estimates or subjective appraisals of effectiveness, or against the performance of assumedly beneficial activities (used as a proxy measure of effectiveness).

The formulation of study objectives usually presents no difficulties in a simple programme review. If cause–effect hypotheses are to be tested (are the outcomes attributable to the programme?) the methods of a programme trial (Ch. 31) must be used.

NOTES AND REFERENCES

1. 'Program directors are concerned with appropriateness when they ask, "Are our program objectives worthwhile and do they have a higher priority than other possible objectives of this or other programs?" ', Deniston O L, Rosenstock I M, Getting V A 1968 Evaluation of program effectiveness. Public Health Reports 83: 323; reprinted in Schulberg H C, Sheldon A, Baker F (eds) 1969 Program Evaluation in the Health Fields. Behavioural Publications, New York, pp 219–239. See Acheson R M 1978 The definition and identification of need for health care. Journal of Epidemiology and Community Health 32: 10.

2. A distinction may be made between *effectiveness evaluation*—does the programme meet its stated (immediate) objectives?—and *impact evaluation*—are there long-lasting effects on the ultimate problems the programme is intended to remedy? Veney J E, Kaluzny A D 1984 Evaluation and decision making for health service programs. Prentice-Hall, Englewood Cliffs, N J; Rundall T G 1986 Evaluation of health services programs. In: Last J M (ed) Maxcy—Rosenau public health and preventive medicine, 12th edn. Appleton-Century-Crofts, Norwalk, Connecticut, pp 1831–1847.
3. Sackett D L 1980 Evaluation of health services. In: Last J M (ed.) Maxcy–Rosenau public health and preventive medicine, 11th edn. Appleton-Century-Crofts, New York, p 1800.
4. A distinction is sometimes made between *goals* and *objectives*: 'goals are expressions of desired conditions of health status and health systems expressed as quantifiable, timeless aspirations', whereas 'objectives should express particular levels of expected achievement ... by a specific year'; Bureau of Health Planning and Resources Development 1970 Guidelines concerning the development of health systems plans and annual implementation plans. U S Department of Health, Education & Welfare. Using these definitions, a goal might be to keep the mortality rate from road accidents to less than 15 per 100 000 per year, whereas an objective might be to reduce it to a given level by a given time; Dever G E A 1980 Community health analysis. Aspen, Germantown, Maryland, pp 169–176.
5. *Norms* and *standards* prescribed by an authority as 'what is desirable' may be used as criteria for evaluating facilities, performance, outcome, and cost. A distinction is sometimes made between norms and standards; definitions of 'norms', 'standards' and 'criteria' are discussed by Donabedian A 1981 Criteria, norms and standards of quality: what do they mean? American Journal of Public Health 71: 409. Standards may be normative or empirical (see p 196). They may specify a 'minimum' (minimum acceptable), an 'ideal' level, the 'desired achievable' level, or a 'maximum'.
6. Methods of studying adverse reactions to therapy are briefly reviewed by Sartwell P E 1974 Iatrogenic disease: an epidemiologic perspective. International Journal of Health Services 4: 89. The 'current iatrogenic pandemic' is described and copiously documented by Illich I 1977 Limits to medicine: medical nemesis: the expropriation of health. Penguin Books, Harmondsworth.
7. Morris J N 1975 Uses of epidemiology, 3rd edn. Edinburgh, Churchill Livingstone, p 92.
8. Bergman A B 1977 American Journal of Public Health 67: 601.
9. A community survey in California identified people who were normotensive and not receiving medical care for hypertension, but had previously been told they were hypertensive. These 'mislabelled' people had more symptoms of depression and reported being in poorer health than other normotensives. Possible confounding by age, sex, education, marital status and ethnicity was controlled by matching, and the presence of other disorders was controlled in the analysis. The mislabelled hypertensives had as many symptoms of depression as correctly labelled hypertensives. Bloom J R, Monterossa S 1981 Hypertension labeling and sense of well-being. American Journal of Public Health 71: 1228.
   A study of a US national sample yielded similar findings: normotensives whose doctors had told them they had high blood pressure had lower 'general wellbeing' scores than other normotensives, as did 'correctly labelled' hypertensives, whether under treatment or not. Monk M 1980 Psychologic status and hypertension. American Journal of Epidemiology 112: 200.
10. The evaluation of health service *coverage* is discussed by Tanahashi T 1978 Bulletin of the World Health Organization 56: 295. Hart J T 1982 (British Medical Journal 284: 1686) stresses the importance of 'measuring what we do not do—the gap between what is done and what could and should be done', and the potential for such studies in general practices with stable populations.

11. A number of *evaluation schemes* are summarized by Spiegel A D, Hyman H H 1978 Basic health planning methods. Aspen Systems, Germantown, Maryland.
12. The principles of *economic evaluation* of health programmes are discussed by Drummond M F, Stoddart G L 1985 (Principles of economic evaluation of health programmes. World Health Statistics Quarterly 38: 355), and their application in developing countries by Mills A 1985 (Economic evaluation of health programmes: application of the principles in developing countries. World Health Statistics Quarterly 38: 368).

    For a review of *cost–benefit* and *cost-effectiveness* studies, see Drummond M F 1985 (Survey of cost-effectiveness and cost–benefit analyses in industrialized countries. World Health Statistics Quarterly 38: 383) who points out that the less tangible costs of illness (i.e. other than impaired productivity) are seldom taken into account, and that estimates of the effects of preventive programmes are often speculative because of the paucity of epidemiological evidence. (Many of these studies are reminiscent of the method of weighing a pig attributed to John Burns: Find a plank that is absolutely straight, balance it at dead centre so that it is absolutely level, place the pig on one end, and pile stones on the other end until the plank is exactly level again. Then carefully guess the weight of the stones. This is the weight of the pig.)

    The cited study of options for controlling children's cholesterol levels made extensive use of *sensitivity analysis*, by seeing how results would be affected by different estimates of the risk associated with cholesterol level, the stability of cholesterol level, the degree of compliance, the change of cholesterol with diet, and the costs of screening and dietary intervention; these variations did not affect the ranking of the three programmes; Berwick D M, Cretin S, Keeler E 1985 Cholesterol, children, and heart disease: an analysis of alternatives. Pediatrics 68: 721.
13. Donabedian A 1966 Evaluating the quality of medical care. Milbank Memorial Fund Quarterly 44 (3, part 2): 166.
14. Cochrane A L 1972 Effectiveness and efficiency. Nuffield Provincial Hospitals Trust, London. Also, see Mooney G 1987 What does equity in health mean? World Health Statistics Quarterly 40: 296.
15. Pokras R, Hufnagel V G 1987 Hysterectomies in the United States, 1965–84. Vital and Health Statistics series 13 no. 92. Hysterectomy is the most frequently performed surgical operation in the USA (670 000 in 1985).
16. Kleinman J C, Kopstein A 1981 Who is being screened for cervical cancer? American Journal of Public Health 71: 73.

6. The study population

At an early stage in the planning of any investigation decisions must be made concerning the study population, i.e. the group of individual units (whether they are persons, families, medical records, certificates, nursery schools, specimens of milk, or dustbins) to be investigated. In the discussion that follows emphasis will be placed on human study populations.

The required decisions are:

1. *What is the study population?* — Or, if there is more than one (e.g. groups of cases or controls, or groups of people who differ in their exposure to a suspected health hazard), what are the study populations? The population or populations should be clearly and explicitly defined in terms of place, time, and any other relevant criteria.[1] Procedures to be used for finding and selecting cases, controls or other study subjects should be specified. (Methods of selecting controls will be discussed in Chs 7 and 30.)
2. *Will sampling be used?* If so, how will the selection from the study population be done? How big should the sample or samples be? How many controls are needed (see Ch. 8)?

If a sample is chosen, the group or population from which it is selected may be called the 'study population', the 'sampled population' or the 'parent population'. If the study population (all or some of whose members are to be investigated) is believed to be typical of a broader population to which it is possible to generalize the findings, the latter population may be termed the *reference* population.[2] As an example, the study population may comprise the elderly people in a given neighbourhood, all or a sample of whom may be studied; the investigators may decide they can apply the findings to elderly people in the whole city or nation.

SELECTING THE STUDY POPULATION

Often the investigator will have implicitly chosen his study population when he defined the topic of his investigation, through his interest in a specific community, a specific health programme, or the testing of a treatment for a specific category of patient. In other instances he may require purposefully to select a study population. Appropriateness and practicability should be taken into account.

The appropriateness of the study population refers mainly to its suitability for the attainment of the objectives of the study. If the hypothesis is that cancer is related to the consumption of carrots, is the population one where it can be expected that there will be sufficient variation in carrot intake to permit the hypothesis to be tested? On the other hand, there may be too much variation in a population, and the objectives may be such that they can be best met by restricting the study to a selected category, such as one sex or a single age group or families of a standard size and composition, in order to avoid the effects of characteristics that may confound the association which is to be studied. Maybe the study would best be performed in a very special kind of population—among vegetarians or monks—or in an occupational group subjected to seasonal emotional stress; the choice of a suitable study population is one of the factors making for originality in research. Paradoxically, some aetiological processes may best be investigated in a population where the disease under study is rare; it would be difficult to study the possibility that asymptomatic urinary tract infection may be an occasional cause of anaemia in a population with a high prevalence of anaemia due to hookworm disease or dietary iron deficiency.

A specific study population may also be chosen because it is believed to be typical of a broader reference population to which the investigator wishes to generalize the findings.

Practical questions also arise. Is the proposed study population one about which it will be possible to obtain the required information? Is it an 'accessible' population to which the investigator already has an *entrée*? Is it likely to co-operate in the study, or will it be a resistant one, possibly as a result of having been over-researched in the past? If patients with a specific disease are to be studied, will it be possible to identify enough cases to yield useful conclusions? If a long-term follow-up study is planned, is the population so mobile that it may be difficult to maintain contact with the subjects? A preliminary exploratory survey may sometimes be required in order to answer such questions.

SPECIFIC FEATURES OF THE STUDY POPULATION

The specific features of the study population may affect the validity of subsequent generalizations from the findings. For example:

1. *Volunteer populations.* Persons who volunteer to enter a study or submit to a procedure may differ in many respects from those who do not so volunteer, and therefore the findings in a volunteer population do not necessarily apply to the population at large. In some circumstances people who are anxious about their health may be those most likely to volunteer; in others, they may be the most reluctant. It is wrong to evaluate an immunization procedure by immunizing volunteers and then comparing them with persons who have not been immunized.

2. *Hospital or clinic populations.* Persons receiving medical care are obviously not representative of the general population or, necessarily, of all ill persons. People with rheumatoid arthritis who are treated in hospital may differ from those receiving ambulant care, and both groups may differ from patients with this disease who do not receive medical care for it. Expectant mothers who receive care from physicians may have different characteristics from those who do not—they may have higher incomes and include fewer teenagers,[3] or differ in other ways. Furthermore, the chance of entering a clinic population may vary for different diseases (or other characteristics) and for various combinations of characteristics, and this may produce spurious associations. For example, if people who have two specific diseases at the same time have an especially high chance of hospitalization, a study of hospital patients may reveal an association between the two diseases even if there is no such association in the population as a whole. If the two diseases carry different chances of hospitalization, a third characteristic (another disease, or a suspected aetiological factor) might turn out to be more frequently associated with one of the two diseases than with the other. Cigarette smoking, bunions, or some other factor might be found more frequently among hospital patients with bronchitis than among those with coronary heart disease, in the absence of any such association in the population as a whole. This problem of the interplay of admission rates, which is referred to as *Berkson's bias*[4] (admission rate bias) may arise in any population (not only hospital or clinic populations) in which individuals with different characteristics have different chances of inclusion. The use of hospital or clinic patients in case-control studies is discussed on page 70.

3. *Populations with good medical records.* It is often tempting to carry out studies in specific practices or clinics in which practitioners maintain good clinical records or are prepared to keep especially detailed records for the purposes of the study. This may be an essential condition for some studies, e.g. surveys of the work of general practitioners. But the doctors who are selected in this way may be singular in other respects also, and their practices may be atypical.

4. *People living at home.* A study population comprising people living at home necessarily excludes those who are in hospitals, old folks' homes, and other institutions; there may thus be a selective exclusion of persons with diseases and other conditions of interest to the investigator. Young adults who are unfit for army service may be over-represented, in a country where such service is compulsory.

5. *Patients notified as having a disease.* Even if notification is compulsory, it is unlikely that all cases are notified, and the notified cases may not be representative. Socially unacceptable diseases, such as venereal disease, may be more fully notified by public agencies than by private physicians. A study in the USA showed under-reporting (particularly by private physicians) of hepatitis B patients who were homosexual.[5]

6. *Autopsy populations.* Persons submitted to autopsy are obviously not necessarily representative of all decedents. Also, Berkson's bias may occur. It played a role in a well known epidemiological blunder, the discovery in 1929 of an apparent 'antagonism' between tuberculosis and cancer, which led to the institution of a 'programme for treating cancer patients with tuberculin'.

7. *Groups characterized by their behaviour or occupation* (smokers, joggers, migrants, bus drivers, etc). It is often worth considering the selective factors that may have led to membership in these groups or exclusion from them, especially if health status may have played a role. This has been called 'membership bias'.[7] Persistent cigarette smokers may be healthier than ex-smokers, not because smoking is salubrious, but because people stop smoking because of illness. The mental health status of immigrants may be a reflection of the characteristics that led to migration, rather than of the stresses or rewards of migration. Since ill health interferes with work, workers are ipso facto healthier, on average, than non-workers (this is termed the *healthy worker effect*). Since having children may keep women away from work, working women may be relatively infertile (the *infertile worker effect*).[8] Membership bias

may crop up in unexpected places: a follow-up study in Finland showed that poor health at the age of 14 was predictive of a heavier coffee consumption at the age of 18, suggesting a 'sick drinker effect'.[9] If there are many cases where ill health has led to, for example, the adoption of a sedentary occupation, or retirement from work, or weaning from the breast, relationships that are subsequently detected between health and sedentary work, retirement or breast feeding may be misinterpreted.

8. *Populations in which the same individuals appear more than once.* If the same individuals appear more than once in a study population, the findings in these individuals may have an undue effect on the results.[10] This may arise in a study of the correlates of gastroenteritis, based on an investigation of all cases of this disease treated in hospital, including repeated hospitalizations of the same patients. A list of women who received antenatal care may include repeated pregnancies of the same women, and patients who consult their doctor frequently will be over-represented in a study based on records of medical visits. If the study is concerned with people rather than with episodes it may be decided to limit each person to a single appearance, e.g. by using the first episode or a randomly chosen one.

'HIDDEN' STUDY POPULATIONS

When an investigator sets out to compare populations, e.g. different villages or a group of cases and a group of controls, it is obvious that he is dealing with more than one study population. It is less obvious that the investigator is also dealing with two study populations in any epidemiological survey that makes use of rates.[11] These populations are firstly, the persons with a defined disease or other characteristic, who constitute the numerator for the calculation of the rate; and secondly, the total population at risk, who constitute the denominator. If the former group is completely contained within the latter and the same information is required about both groups, and this information can be collected in the same way for all persons in the population at risk, then no special problem arises. This is not the case, however, if different methods of obtaining information are required for the numerator and denominator populations, or if additional information is required about one of these populations. In these instances, although a single study population may have been specified, there are in effect two populations, to which separate consideration must be given in planning the study.

For example, in a study of the correlates of infant mortality, a single study population may be chosen (defined in terms, say, of geographical area and time). But information is actually required both about the babies who died (the numerator of the infant mortality rate) and about those who were born alive (the denominator). For a conventional infant mortality rate, which is based on births and deaths in the same year, these are two overlapping populations: some of the infants who died in 1990 were born in 1989. In practice it is often necessary to use different procedures to obtain information about the two populations, e.g. by the use of death and birth certificates respectively. Some data may be wanted for the numerator population only (e.g. age at death, cause of death), and the study plan should take this into account. If specific infant mortality rates are to be calculated, i.e. taking sex, birth rank and other characteristics into account, thought should be given to the practicability of obtaining parallel data about both populations. The biggest problem in such studies is often the unavailability of data about the denominator population.

A further instance of a 'hidden' study population may be given. It is often impossible to interview or examine all members of the study population or sample. Especially in a study requiring the co-operation of the persons to be investigated there may be many 'non-respondents'. When there is incomplete coverage of the study population or sample there is a possibility of bias. In a study of cardiovascular disease in California, for example, non-respondents were especially likely to be smokers, and were much less likely to have a family history of heart disease.[12] In Sweden, over half the non-participants in a health survey study said their reason was that they were ill, or in regular contact with a doctor; social insurance records revealed that non-participants in another Swedish study had over five times as many sickness benefit days, on average, as did participants.[13] It may thus be difficult to apply the findings to the study population, let alone to make generalizations to a wider population.

In order to test for bias, the demographic and other relevant characteristics of the individuals included and omitted (the respondents and non-respondents) should, if possible, be compared. From a practical point of view this means that during the planning phase the investigator should think of the non-respondents as a separate study population, since specific efforts may be required to obtain the requisite information about all or a representative sample of them. Similarly, members of the study population who are unwilling to participate in a trial may be seen as a 'hidden' study population.

SELECTING CASES FOR A CASE-CONTROL STUDY

There are at least three important considerations when deciding how to choose cases for a case-control study.

First, for a number of reasons it is best to use new ('incident') cases of the disease, rather than existing ('prevalent') cases varying in duration. The time lapse since exposure to the suspected causal factors is shorter, and it may be easier to obtain information about these factors. The time relationship between onset of the disease and exposure to these factors may be clearer than in long-established cases. Also, the use of new cases avoids *prevalence—incidence bias*:[7] if prevalent cases are used, patients who recover rapidly are likely to be under-represented, and those who die soon after onset (e.g. sudden deaths from coronary heart disease) will not be represented at all; so that if a difference in exposure to some factor is detected between cases and controls, it may be difficult to infer that the factor is a cause of the disease rather than a determinant of its subsequent course.

Secondly, it is generally hoped that associations that are found with the disease will apply not only to the specific study population investigated, but to a wider reference population, e.g. to all cases of the disease, or all severe cases. It is therefore important to consider whether the cases will be suitable representatives of the reference population the investigator has in mind. Cases drawn from clinical sources, rather than from a case-finding survey in a population, may not be representative of all cases, since there may be under-representation of those with no symptoms or with mild or atypical ones (over 25% of myocardial infarctions, for example, are not diagnosed clinically)[14] and of members of population groups with a low availability or use of medical services. Cases drawn from a hospital or consultative clinic may not be typical of all cases under clinical care; and cases drawn from a teaching hospital may not be representative of all hospital cases (*referral filter bias*[7]).

A third consideration is that the results of a case-control study using clinic or hospital cases may be affected by Berksonian bias (see p 59) if the postulated causal factor has an independent effect on the risk of entering the clinic or hospital population. There is no Berkson's bias if the case and control groups are both chosen from the community. If clinic or hospital cases are used, special precautions are needed when choosing controls in order to minimize this bias (see p 70).

Practical constraints (the availability of cases, the accessibility of disease registers and other records, etc.) usually enforce compromises.

But if the investigator is aware of the study's shortcomings he can take account of them when analysing the data and interpreting the findings.

The need for clear diagnostic criteria will be discussed in Chapter 11, and methods of sampling in Chapter 8.

It is often decided to specify *eligibility criteria*, determined mainly by the investigator's concept of the reference population—he may want to focus the study on elderly people or fertile women. He may also decide to restrict the study to a certain category of subject in order to avoid effects that might be confused with the effects of the factor under study; for example, the study may be restricted to non-smokers, so as to avoid effects connected with smoking. Confusion of effects ('confounding') may be significant if something that strongly influences the incidence of the disease, i.e. that helps to determine whether the subject will be a case or a control, is also strongly associated with the causal factor under study. Restriction of eligibility is one way—although not the only or necessarily the best one—of dealing with this problem (see page 258). Care must obviously be taken not to exclude cases because of characteristics or behaviour that may be consequences of the factor under study.

Subjects are sometimes excluded on the grounds that they could not have been exposed to the causal factor under study; for example, post-menopausal women and those who were sterilized many years previously might be excluded from a case-control study of the short-term effects of oral contraceptives. Such decisions will reduce the cost of the study (unless it is difficult to identify ineligible subjects). Other advantages have been questioned.[15]

All eligibility criteria will of course limit the generalizability of the findings—the findings of a case-control study of non-smokers may not be applicable to smokers. Needless to say, eligibility criteria applied to the cases must also (where relevant) be applied to the controls. Eligibility criteria should preferably be decided in advance, even if they can be applied only after the collection of data.

NOTES AND REFERENCES

1. A written record should be kept of the criteria for inclusion in the study population. These should be stated explicitly; e.g. if residents of a stated neighbourhood are to be studied, what is a 'resident'? (6 months' stay is often used as a criterion). If unforeseen problems of definition arise subsequently (e.g. students who live at home at weekends only) the new decisions should also be recorded, so that they can be applied uniformly.
2. The term 'target population', is best avoided in this context, since it is sometimes used for the sampled population and sometimes for the reference population. In

the context of health care, it refers of course to the population at which a programme is directed.

3. Peoples-Sheps M D, Kalsbeek W D, Siegel E 1988 Why we know so little about prenatal care worldwide: an assessment of required methodology. Health Services Research 23: 361.

4. Real-life examples of *Berkson's bias*, from surveys in Ontario, include the detection of a strong association between diseases of the respiratory and locomotor systems in hospital data but not in the general population, and the finding that fatigue was positively associated with allergic and metabolic disease in the general population, but negatively in hospital data: Roberts R S, Spitzer W O, Delmore T, Sackett D L 1978 An empiric demonstration of Berkson's bias. Journal of Chronic Diseases 31: 119. In a clinic, the rate of neurological disorders in boys was found to be double that in girls; this unusual finding was attributed to the fact that the ratio of boys to girls was 4:1 in this clinic; Brown G W 1976 Berkson fallacy revisited: spurious conclusions from patient surveys. American Journal of Diseases of Children 130: 56. Algebraic explanations of Berkson's fallacy are given by Fleiss J L 1981 Statistical Methods for Rates and Proportions, 2nd end. John Wiley, New York, pp 8–13.

5. Alter M J, Mares A, Hadler S C et al 1987 The effect of underreporting on the apparent incidence and epidemiology of acute viral hepatitis. American Journal of Epidemiology 125: 133

6. Lilienfeld A M, Lilienfeld D E 1980 Foundations of epidemiology, 2nd edn. Oxford University Press, New York, pp 203–204; Mainland D 1963 Elementary Medical Statistics, 2nd edn. W B Saunders, Philadelphia, pp 121–122.

7. For lists and descriptions of possible biases, see Sackett D L 1979 Bias in analytic research. Journal of Chronic Diseases 32: 51; Schlesselman J J, Stolley P D 1982 Sources of bias. In: Schlesselman J J (ed) Case-control studies: design, conduct, analysis. Oxford University Press, New York, pp 124–143.

8. Joffe M 1985 Biases in research in reproduction and women's work. International Journal of Epidemiology 14: 118

9. Hemminki E, Rahkonen O, Rimpela M 1988 American Journal of Epidemiology 127: 1088.

10. Bias due to the over-representation of frequent attenders in a study that is based on records of medical visits can be controlled by a weighting procedure. This is described by Shepard D S, Neutra R 1977 American Journal of Public Health 67: 743, who show how estimates of the numbers and characteristics of hypertensive patients attending a medical clinic can be derived from a study of visits.

11. See Note 2 p 99, on rates.

12. Criqui M H, Barrett-Connor E, Austin M 1978 Differences between respondents and non-respondents in a population-based cardiovascular disease study. American Journal of Epidemiology 108: 367

13. Janzon L, Hanson B S, Isacsson S-O et al 1986 Factors influencing participation in health surveys: results from prospective population study 'Men born in 1914' in Malmo, Sweden. Journal of Epidemiology and Community Health 40: 174; Bergstrand R, Vedin A, Wilhelmsson C et al 1983 Bias due to non-participation and heterogeneous sub-groups in population surveys. Journal of Chronic Diseases 36: 725.

14. Over 25% of myocardial infarctions found at routine examinations in the Framingham study had not been recognized as such by the patient or attending doctor. Half were 'silent', and half caused atypical symptoms. The chances of subsequent heart failure, stroke, and death were the same for unrecognized and recognized infarctions. Kannel W B, Abbott R D 1984 Incidence and prognosis of unrecognized myocardial infarction: an update of the Framingham Study. New England Journal of Medicine 311: 1144.

15. For a debate on the 'exposure-potential rule', see Poole C 1986 Exposure opportunity in case-control studies. American Journal of Epidemiology 123: 352; Schlesselman J J, Stadel B V 1987 Exposure opportunity in epidemiologic studies. American Journal of Epidemiology 125: 174; Poole C 1987 Critical appraisal of the exposure-potential restriction rule. American Journal of Epidemiology 125: 179.

7. Control groups

CONTROL GROUPS IN SURVEYS

Controls are never needed in studies in which hypotheses are not tested, and are sometimes superfluous in studies that do test hypotheses. In Bradford Hill's words, 'If we survey the deaths of infants in the first month of life and find that so many are caused by dropping the baby on its head on the kitchen floor I am not myself convinced that we need controls to convince us that it is a bad habit. If, on the other hand, so many of the deaths are found to be of infants whose mothers had influenza during pregnancy then I should shriek for controls before I was satisfied that the two events were related'.[1]

The selection of controls in analytic epidemiological surveys (see pp 68–74) depends on the nature of the survey. In a cohort (prospective) study of the association between a postulated cause and a disease (or other outcome), the incidence of the disease among people exposed to the causal factor is compared with the incidence in a control group (or 'comparison' or 'contrast' group) of unexposed people, or in a total population. In a case-control study the cases are compared with controls who do not have the disease.

If it was decided to restrict the study to a specific population category (e.g. a specific age–sex group) or to apply eligibility criteria (see p 64), these decisions should (where relevant) be applied to the controls also.

A sampling procedure may be needed (see Ch. 8), and it may be decided to *match* the controls with the members of the study group (i.e. with the subjects exposed to the causal factor, in a cohort study; or with the cases, in a case-control study).

However the controls are selected, all the possibly relevant characteristics of the study and control groups should later be compared, to determine whether there are differences that may explain the findings of the study.

SELECTING CONTROLS FOR A COHORT STUDY

The ideal control group for a cohort study is one that would have the same disease rate as the group exposed to the suspected causal factor, if this factor were unassociated with the disease. The closest approximation to this ideal is achieved in a cohort study of a total population (or a representative sample of a total population), where inclusion in the study is not influenced by exposure to the factor. Such a study has built-in controls (an *internal comparison group*). A well known example is the cohort study of British physicians that provided one of the first clear demonstrations of the effect of smoking on lung cancer mortality.[2] In cohort studies of total populations the use of two groups, 'exposed' and 'non-exposed', can often be replaced by a categorization of subjects according to their amount of exposure (number of cigarettes per day, duration of smoking, etc.), so that the dose–response relationship (see p 261) can be examined.

If an *external comparison group* of unexposed people is used, the controls should if possible be selected from the same general population as the exposed group; if the exposed people are members of a special population (e.g. workers in a factory) the controls should be drawn from the same special population. Failing this, the comparison population should be one that is as similar as possible to the population of which the exposed persons are members, with respect to factors (other than the exposure) that may influence the risk of incurring the disease.

Since it may not be possible to find a completely satisfactory control group, it is frequently decided to use two or more groups drawn from different sources, and to see whether the various comparisons yield similar conclusions. In a study of workers exposed to a specific occupational hazard, for example, one comparison might be with disease incidence in the general population—a comparison that is probably biased by the 'healthy worker effect' (see p 60). Another might be with workers in some other industry. Sometimes both internal and external comparison groups are used—the exposed workers might also be compared with non-exposed workers in their own industry.

The choice of control groups is sometimes constrained by the need to ensure that the same methods of investigation, especially for case detection, are applied as in the exposed group or groups. It is advisable to gather information—for both exposed and non-exposed subjects—about all factors that may affect the risk of the disease, so that their influence can be taken into account when the findings are analysed and interpreted.

The need to define 'non-exposure' may sometimes lead the investigator to give closer thought to the meaning of 'exposure', and to formulate the research hypothesis more precisely. What control group is required in a cohort study of the effect of smoking? This depends on the definition of smoking. Are 'non-smokers' people who have never smoked at all, or those who have never smoked regularly, or those who do not smoke at present, or those who have not smoked for a given number of years, or those who have not smoked (say) at least 20 cigarettes a day for a continuous period of at least 10 years?

SELECTING CONTROLS FOR A CASE-CONTROL STUDY

A case-control study compares the exposure of cases and controls to a suspected causal factor. The purpose of the controls is to provide an estimate of what the exposure of the cases to this factor would be, if there were no association between the factor and the disease. Ideally, cases and controls should therefore come from the same source population. The controls should be representative of disease-free people in this population (rather than of *all* disease-free people).

If the study includes all the cases in a defined population, or a representative sample of them, the choice of controls thus presents no special problems—a sample of people without the disease can be chosen from the same population (see Ch. 8). The population might be the residents of a defined neighbourhood or region, the registered patients of a general practice, the children in a school, workers in a factory, etc. In a nested case-control study, where new cases are identified in a follow-up study of a cohort, the controls are drawn from the same cohort.

Complete or reasonably complete identification of cases may be achieved by a survey in which members of a defined population are investigated, and in some other circumstances. The disease may, for example, be one that always, or almost always, leads to hospitalization, e.g. (in many countries) ectopic pregnancy. A community health service that provides ongoing care for a defined population is particularly likely to possess accumulated information about diseases occurring in this population, especially severe or long-term ones.

The choice of suitable controls is more problematic if the cases are not representative of all cases in a population. Clinically identified cases may be unrepresentative, since people who seek medical care for the disease may differ from those who do not. Hospital cases, in particular, may be a biased sample of all patients with the disease, and cases drawn from one hospital may differ from those in other hospitals. In these instances it is difficult to define the selected sub-population from which the cases are drawn, and from which the controls should also be drawn (the controls should be representative of people who would have been selected as cases if they had developed the disease). Berksonian bias is an additional problem in studies of hospital or clinic cases; it may occur if the chance of entering the hospital or clinic is influenced by the postulated causal factor (see p 59).

Use is often made of *hospital or clinic controls* who have other diseases. These controls are usually drawn from the same clinical source as the cases, to ensure that they represent the same catchment population and are subject to the same selective factors as the cases. It should be remembered, however, that the probability of reaching a specific institution may vary for different diseases, depending on the reputation of various specialists, the availability of other services, etc. This problem is avoided if cases and controls have the same clinical picture, e.g. in a study of women referred for breast biopsies of suspicious nodules, in which confirmed cases of breast cancer are compared with those not found to have cancer or precancerous conditions.[3]

The use of hospital controls is a convenient solution, but has a drawback: the controls (being ill) are obviously a selected group, not necessarily representative of people without the disease under study. If the analysis reveals (or fails to reveal) interesting differences between the cases and controls, this may have more to do with the epidemiology of the diseases of the control patients than with the disease under study. This problem is minimized if patients with diseases known or suspected to be associated with the postulated causal factor are not used as controls—patients with lung cancer would not be good controls in a study of smoking and cervical cancer. Patients admitted because of traffic accidents or for elective surgery are often used as controls, in the hope that they represent the healthy population.

An alternative possibility is the use of controls taken from the population from which the cases are drawn (*population controls*, community controls, neighbourhood controls). This method has obvious advantages, but only if the source population is well defined and the cases are representative of all the cases in this population. It has disadvantages too; these include its cost and inconvenience, the probability of a higher non-response rate than there would be for hospital controls, difficulties in ensuring that the controls will be investigated in the same way as the cases, and the possibility that the controls will differ from hospital patients in their motivation to recall and report past events.

Use may also be made of controls identified through their relationship with the cases, e.g. friends, neighbours, spouses, siblings, fellow-workers or classmates. Such controls will tend to resemble the cases in their circumstances, lifestyles or (for blood relatives) genetic characteristics. This similarity may be an advantage, since the reduction of irrelevant differences between cases and controls may make it easier to test the study hypothesis. But it may also blur the very difference sought by the study—if friends tend to share smoking habits, it becomes more difficult to detect differences between the smoking habits of cases and controls. Blood donors, hospital visitors[4] and other special groups can also be used as controls.

When deciding on a control group, attention must of course be paid to the feasibility of obtaining information comparable to that collected about the study group. An issue sometimes raised in studies where information about dead cases is obtained from relatives is whether dead controls (who died of other causes) should be sought, so as to ensure comparability.[5]

If hospital cases are used in a case-control study, the best hope for avoiding Berkson's bias is to use hospital controls who have a comparison condition that has the same probability of hospitalization as the disease under study; the direction of the bias depends on whether the probability of hospitalization is higher for the disease under study or for the comparison condition. It is usually found that drawing controls from all hospital patients who are free of the disease under study underestimates the association between the disease and the causal factor, and use of population controls overestimates it.[6]

It is seldom easy to find a source of controls that is both convenient and free of possible bias. Each instance must be considered on its merits, and a careful choice made of the lesser of the alternative evils. It is often best to use two or more control groups (of different kinds), and to see whether different comparisons yield the same conclusion.

In some case-control studies there is no need to seek controls. These are 'control-initiated' studies, undertaken when an investigator has a data set that can be used as the control data, and then seeks suitable cases for comparison.[7]

MATCHING

If there are differences between the characteristics of study and control groups, they may sometimes obscure or distort the associations being studied. If the groups are large, such differences can be handled by appropriate computations during the analysis of the findings (see p 258). To avoid or reduce these differences, however, it may be decided to 'match' the control group with the study group, thus ensuring similarity with respect to possible confounding factors that may distort the findings.

Matching reduces the confounding effect, and (under certain conditions)[8] adds to the precision with which the association under study is estimated. Its use also simplifies the statistical analysis. But matching should not be undertaken when it is unnecessary, since it also has disadvantages:

1. It complicates the selection of controls, and may be costly. The study may suffer delay if large numbers of potential controls have to be screened, or if a pool of potential controls is not immediately available (e.g. if the controls are patients suffering from a specific condition, and it is necessary to wait for the appearance of a suitable candidate).
2. It may lead to the exclusion of subjects if enough suitable controls cannot be found. If there are numerous matching variables, many subjects may be 'wasted' in this way, and the study group may become less representative of the reference population.
3. A confounding variable that has been controlled by matching can no longer be studied as an independent variable. If cases and controls are matched for age it becomes impossible to study the relationship of the disease to age: a comparison of the ages of the cases and controls will provide information only on the effectiveness of the matching procedure. Also, it becomes difficult to reach useful conclusions on associations with variables that are closely linked with age. Note, however, that the effect of age as a *modifier* (see p 55) of other relationships can still be examined; i.e. it is possible to see whether an association—between, say, drinking and coronary heart disease—is consistent in different age groups.
4. The groups may inadvertently be made so similar that the difference that the investigation was designed to seek may be masked ('matched out'); this is sometimes called *overmatching*.
5. Unnecessary matching (i.e. in the absence of a strong confounding effect) may impair the precision with which the

association can be measured.[8] This is also sometimes called 'overmatching'.

Matching is useful if three conditions are met (the first two are prerequisites for a strong confounding effect):

1. There is likely to be a marked disparity between the groups if the characteristic is not 'held constant' by matching.
2. The characteristic is believed to be strongly associated with whatever is being compared in the groups (e.g. disease incidence in a prospective study, or exposure to a causal factor in a case-control study).
3. The groups are small, so that the handling of confounding effects during the analysis may be unfeasible or inefficient.

Matching can be done in two ways:

1. Each control may be selected so as to be similar to a specific member of the study group (*individual matching*). This may be done by formulating matching criteria and then seeking suitable controls for each subject. A large pool of potential controls may be needed if there are more than two or three matching variables and a very close match is demanded on each variable. Individual matching may also be achieved by selecting a spouse, sibling, friend, neighbour[9] or fellow-worker, a child born on the same day in the same hospital, a patient in the same hospital ward, etc.
2. The controls may be so selected that, as a group, they are in some respects (e.g. age and sex) similar to the study group (*group matching*). For *frequency matching* the potential controls are divided into strata (say age–sex groups) and an appropriate number of individuals is then selected from each stratum. *Mean matching* ('balancing') tries to produce groups with similar mean values.

The control and study groups need not be equal in size; if individual matching is used, two or more controls can be selected for each subject. There may be good reasons for having unequal groups.[10]

Whatever method is used, clear-cut rules[11] should be laid down, in order to ensure objectivity when deciding whether a match is sufficiently close and when choosing between two or more individuals who meet the matching criteria.

CONTROLS IN EXPERIMENTS

'I was a 90 lb weakling, and look at me now!' is not convincing evidence of the effectiveness of a course of treatment, as the change may well have been due to processes of adolescence or other factors quite unrelated to the treatment. To be reasonably convincing, 'before–after' studies of this sort (without external controls) must be replicated, or extended in time so as to see what happens when the treatment is withdrawn.

In most experiments separate control groups are used. The findings in the experimental group are compared with those in a control group not exposed to the experimental procedure. Infant mortality dropped after the introduction of a programme; but what happened in other (similar) regions? This approach is often the best available method of evaluating a programme or procedure. In the absence of an external control group we run the risk that we may think that a change is a specific effect of the intervention that we are testing, when actually it is not.[12] The main circumstances that may confuse the issue are:

1. *Changes that are due to other causes.* People may recover from illnesses for reasons quite unconnected with the care they receive. Changes happen because people age, they mature, they adapt to disability, they become integrated into new social settings, and external events and changes exert their influence on them. Food prices may alter, foodstuffs low in calories or saturated fats may become readily available, there may be a publicity campaign about cigarette smoking, a new medical service may be started, a war may break out or come to an end, etc.

2. *Non-specific effects caused by the intervention or the experiment.* The administration of (say) a drug may produce a *placebo effect* that is due not to any pharmacological action but to the mere fact that a medicine was taken. If the subjects know that they are participating in an experiment, this awareness may in itself produce changes (the *guinea pig effect*). This is part of the possible influence of the experimental situation as a whole—the examinations and other procedures, the feedback of investigation findings, the special relations with investigators, etc.—that is sometimes called the *Hawthorne effect.* This name comes from a study of industrial efficiency at the Hawthorne Plant in Chicago in the 1920s,[13] which showed that work output increased when experimental changes were made to working conditions, even when these were worsened. Production rose both when illumination was improved and when it was reduced to the brightness of a moonlight night. In a

study of smoking by schoolchildren, the Hawthorne effect was considered as a reason for the relatively low rates observed in schools that had been surveyed repeatedly.[14]

3. *Artifacts.* The change may not be real, but only an expression of a change in methods of measurement—in diagnostic criteria or techniques, in the completeness of recording or notification, in laboratory procedures, etc.

4. *Regression towards the mean.*[15] Even if the methods have not altered, an artifact may arise if measurements are very unreliable or if the characteristics they measure are very unstable. If such measurements are repeated in the same subjects, the second value will tend to be lower than the first if the initial value was high, and vice versa. A study sample selected on the grounds of initially high values of blood pressure will tend to have lower blood pressures when examined a second time, and this may be interpreted as an effect of treatment. There are various ways of overcoming this problem, one of the simplest being to use a suitable control group that is selected in the same way as the intervention group.

Depending on circumstances and the detailed objectives of the study, a control group may be exposed to an alternative treatment or programme, to no intervention whatever, or to placebo treatment. In therapeutic trials the controls are commonly given the usual standard treatment for their disease.

The groups that are compared should be similar. A story is told of a sea captain who tested a seasickness remedy during a voyage, and was very enthusiastic about the results: 'Practically every one of the controls was ill, and not one of the subjects had any trouble. Really wonderful stuff'. A sceptic asked how he had chosen the controls and subjects. 'Oh, I gave the stuff to my seamen and used the passengers as controls'.[16] Similarly, trials in which a vaccine was administered to volunteers (who may be a very select group) and in which the subsequent incidence of the disease was compared with that in a general population have led to erroneous conclusions. Experiments of this sort are similar to surveys in which different populations are compared, in that all the possibly relevant characteristics of the groups should be studied, and a careful search made for differences that may explain the findings of the study.

Various experimental and quasi-experimental designs, and methods of allocating subjects to experimental and control groups, will be discussed in Chapters 30 and 31.

NOTES AND REFERENCES

1. Hill A B 1962 Statistical methods in clinical and preventive medicine. Livingstone, Edinburgh, p 365.
2. Doll R, Peto R 1976 Mortality in relation to smoking: 20 years' observations on male British doctors. British Medical Journal 2: 1525.
3. Knottnerus J A 1987 Subject selection in hospital-based case-control studies. Journal of Chronic Diseases 40: 183.
4. Armenian, H K, Lakkis N G, Sibai A M, Halabi S S 1988 (American Journal of Epidemiology 127: 404) used hospital visitors as convenient controls when civil war conditions in Beirut restricted access to community controls.
5. This question is considered by Gordis L 1982 (American Journal of Epidemiology 115: 1), who concludes that there does not seem to be strong justification for using dead controls for dead cases, and that this procedure may introduce its own biases. In a study in which both living and dead controls were used, McLaughlin J K, Blot W J, Mehl E S, Mandel, J S 1985 (American Journal of Epidemiology 121: 131; 122: 485) found that heavier smoking and drinking, and more diseases, were reported for dead than living controls: 'it appears that exposures associated with premature death are overrepresented in dead controls'; they give reasons for believing that the difference is real, and not attributable to the obtaining of information from next of kin.
6. These conclusions about *Berkson's bias* are based on algebraic analyses by Feinstein A R, Walter S D, Horwitz R I 1986 An analysis of Berkson's bias in case-control studies. Journal of Chronic Diseases 39: 495; Peritz E 1984 Berkon's bias revisited. Journal of Chronic Diseases 37: 909.
7. See Greenland S 1985 Control-initiated case-control studies. International Journal of Epidemiology 14: 130.
8. For statistical treatments of the effects of matching, see Breslow N 1982 Design and analysis of case-control studies. Annual Reviews of Public Health 3: 29; Cochran W G 1983 In: Moses L E, Mosteller F (eds) Planning and analysis of observational studies. Wiley, New York, Chapter 5; Kleinbaum D G, Kupper L L, Morgenstern H 1982 Epidemiologic research: principles and quantitative methods. Lifetime Learning Publications, Belmont, California, Chapter 18; Anderson S, Auquier A, Hauck W W, et al 1980 Statistical methods for comparative studies: techniques for bias reduction. Wiley, New York, Chapter 6.
9. As an example of the use of neighbourhood controls, in a study in Toronto 'five age-matched controls were obtained for each case. They were also matched by neighbourhood and by type of dwelling (house or apartment) in the expectation that this would lead to reasonably close socioeconomic matching. Controls were obtained by door-to-door calls, which started at the fourth door to the right of the case and proceeded systematically round the residential block or through the apartment building'. No one was found at home in two-thirds of the dwellings visited. To get an idea of whether this produced bias in the selection of controls and hence influenced the findings, a separate analysis was subsequently done, in which cases were compared with only 'those controls who were enrolled immediately after the case (or another control) had been interviewed—i.e., controls obtained without an intervening failure'. Clarke E A, Anderson T W 1979 Does screening by 'Pap' smears help prevent cervical cancer? A case-control study. Lancet ii: 1.

In urban areas of North Carolina, a door-to-door search for neighbourhood controls matched by sex, age and race and with no history of heart attack or angina pectoris, in which the interviewer proceeded in ever-widening circles around the home of the index case, required an average of 98 minutes (94 km of travel) for each successfully matched case: Ryu J E, Thompson C J, Crouse J R 1989 Selection of neighborhood controls for a study of coronary heart disease. American Journal of Epidemiology 129: 407.

10. There may be *more than one control per subject*. If there is a constraint on the number of subjects, this increases the efficiency of the study. This may be especially important in a clinical trial where treatment is inconvenient, costly or potentially hazardous. Enlarging the control group compensates for the small number of subjects. The additional benefit is small if the ratio is increased beyond three or four; but a higher ratio may be indicated on economic grounds if the treatment is very expensive. See note 8.

11. *Individual matching* requires the prior formulation of a set of matching criteria. For each variable, it may be decided that the control must be in the same category as the case (e.g. the same 5-year age group: 30–34, 35–39, etc.; this is sometimes called *category, within-class* or *stratified matching*), or must have a defined degree of similarity (e.g. an age within 2 years of the case's; this is caliper matching).

Matching may be made easier (and less exact) by reducing the number of matching variables or relaxing the requirements. For example, an age disparity of up to 10 years may be regarded as acceptable. Alternatively, it may be decided that a close match will be sought, but a less close match (using a less strict criterion) will be accepted if necessary. A method sometimes used is *'nearest available' matching*, i.e. selecting the potential control who is nearest (say, in age) to the case. This method has the advantage that matches can always be found, but it is less effective than other methods in the control of confounding.

Clear rules must be laid down, stating the procedures and priorities. If one potential control is closely matched in age and less closely in educational level, and another is closely matched in education and less closely in age, which will be chosen? Standard procedures should also be laid down to cover instances where there are two or more potential controls who satisfy the criteria equally. It may be decided to select the one who is closest to the case in respect of a given matching variable (age), or the one who best meets one or more additional matching criteria, which are applied only in such instances. Use may also be made of random numbers.

A computer can list potential controls in a convenient format, and can perform 'nearest available' and 'mean' matching. See Cochran (1983; see note 8) pp 82–83.

For a detailed discussion of the above and other matching methods, see Anderson S, Auquier A, Hauck W W et al 1980 Statistical methods for comparative studies: techniques for bias reduction. Wiley, New York, Chapter 6.

12. Illustrations of misleading conclusions yielded by uncontrolled trials are cited by Ederer F 1975 (American Journal of Ophthalmology 79: 758), who cites Professor Hugo Muench of Harvard University's second law: 'Results can always be improved by omitting controls'.

13. Roethlisberger F J, Dickson W J 1939 Management and the worker. Harvard University Press, Cambridge, Massachusetts.

14. Murray M, Swan A V, Kiryluk S, Clarke G C 1988 The Hawthorne effect in the measurement of adolescent smoking. Journal of Epidemiology and Community Health 42: 304.

15. The term *regression toward the mean* comes from a 19th century finding that although tall parents tended to have tall children, the children tended to be less tall than their parents; the children of short parents tended to be taller than their parents. The principle is that 'if all the flies in a closed room are on the ceiling at eight o'clock in the morning, more flies will be below the ceiling than above the ceiling at some time during the next 24-hr period'; Schor S 1969 Journal of the American Medical Association 207: 120.

Ways of preventing spurious conclusions, say in a study of the effect of treatment on people with high cholesterol levels, include (1) comparing the changes in treated and control groups that were selected in exactly the same way; (2) using two or more initial measurements (e.g. one when allocating the subject to the treatment group, and another for use as the baseline for measuring change;

or basing the allocation on a mean of two or more measurements); and (3) statistical solutions; see, e.g. Chinn S, Heller R F 1981 Some further results concerning regression to the mean. American Journal of Epidemiology 5: 277; Woolson R F, Lachenbruch P A 1982 Regression analysis of matched case-control data. American Journal of Epidemiology 115: 444; Anderson et al (1980; see note 8), Chapter 12.

16. Wilson E B Jr 1952 An introduction to scientific research. New York: McGraw-Hill, p 42.

8. Sampling

It is often decided to study only a part, or sample, of the study population (the 'sampled' or 'parent' population). Samples may be chosen of cases, people exposed to suspected causal factors, or potential controls. The decision to sample may be forced on the investigator by his lack of resources. The procedure may make for better use of available resources; because of the restricted number of individuals to be studied, it is possible to investigate each of them more fully than might otherwise have been possible, and to make greater efforts to ensure that information is in fact obtained from each individual. Frequently it is decided to have the best of both worlds, by obtaining easily acquired types of information about the total study population, but limiting certain parts of the study, which require more intensive investigations, to one or more samples.

Provided that certain conditions are met, there is no difficulty in applying the results yielded by a sample to the parent population from which it has been selected, with a degree of precision which meets the investigator's requirements. Statistical techniques are available which make it possible to state with what precision and confidence such inferences may be made. The conditions to be met are:

1. The sample must be *well chosen*, so as to be representative of the parent population.
2. The sample must be *sufficiently large*. If a number of representative samples drawn from the same parent population are investigated, it can be expected that, by chance, there will be differences between the findings in each sample; this problem of *sampling variation* is minimized if the sample is large.
3. There must be *adequate coverage* of the sample. Unless information is in fact obtained about all or almost all its members, the individuals studied may not be representative of the parent population; i.e. there may be *sample bias*.

Mere size is not enough. A sample that is badly chosen or in-
adequately covered remains a biased one, however big it may be.
This was strikingly shown by the notorious poll conducted by the
Literary Digest in 1936 which, although based on 2 000 000 ballots,
dismally failed to predict Roosevelt's landslide victory in the presi-
dential election. These ballots constituted 20% of the 10 000 000
that had been sent out to an unrepresentative sample comprising
Literary Digest and telephone subscribers.

SAMPLING METHODS

A sample chosen in a haphazard fashion, or because it is 'handy', is
unlikely to be a representative one. Such samples have been termed
'chunks' or 'accidental' or 'incidental' samples, or 'samples of
convenience'. Their use has no place in community medicine research,
except possibly in exploratory surveys where the investigator is
doing no more than obtaining a 'feel' of the situation.

The recommended method is *probability sampling*, the distinctive
feature of which is that each individual unit in the total population
(each *sampling unit*) has a known probability of being selected.
Generalizations can be made to the 'parent' population with a
measurable precision and confidence (see p 270). We will discuss
four types of probability sampling: random, systematic, cluster and
stratified sampling. Probability sampling may be performed in more
than one stage (two-stage and multi-stage sampling).

Use is sometimes made of *judgement samples*, i.e. quota and purposive samples. In *quota sampling* the general composition of the
sample, e.g. in terms of age, sex and social class, is decided in advance;
quotas, or required numbers, are determined for, say, men and
women of different ages and social classes, and the only requirement
is that the right number of people be somehow found to fill these
quotas. The disadvantage of this method is that the persons chosen
may not be representative of the total population in each category, and
generalizations made from the findings may be incorrect. *Purposive
samples* are those selected because the investigator believes them to be
typical of the population he wishes to study. In a study of general
practices, for example, he may select what he believes to be a representative cross-section of practices. Generalizations from the findings
may or may not be valid.

It is important to set up the sampling rules in advance and to avoid
any possibility that selection may be influenced by whim or convenience. The interviewers in a household survey, for example,

should be told in advance which homes to visit. If inclusion in the sample depends on information that is collected during the visit, the interviewer should be given precise instructions for making the choice.[1]

Random sampling

Random sampling (or 'simple random sampling') is a technique whereby each sampling unit has the same probability of being selected—the laws of chance alone decide which of the individual units in the parent (or 'target') population will be selected. To avoid confusion with the colloquial meaning of the word 'random', i.e. 'haphazard' or 'without a conscious bias', the term 'strict random sampling' is sometimes preferred.

The basic procedure is:

1. To prepare a *sampling frame*. This is usually a list showing all the units from which the sample is to be selected, arranged in any order. Its preparation may require considerable effort; it is seldom easy, for example, to obtain an up-to-date list of the elderly people living in a neighbourhood. In a country or city that maintains a population register, this may constitute a sampling frame; but such registers are often out-of-date, especially with regard to addresses; moreover, with the increase in concern for the individual's right to privacy, registers of this kind are becoming less accessible to investigators. The sampling frame for random-digit dialling (see p 85) is a list of telephone numbers. If the frame is an incomplete and biased representation of the study population, the sample too will inevitably be biased, however strictly the rules of random sampling are applied.
2. To decide on the size of the sample.
3. To select the required number of units at random, by drawing lots or using random numbers. The use of random numbers is explained on pages 87–89. When one matched control has to be chosen randomly from a small group of suitable candidates, it is often simplest to draw lots or (if there are up to six candidates) to throw a die.

The ratio 'number of units in sample/number of units in sampling frame' is referred to as the *sampling ratio* or *sampling fraction*. It is usually expressed either in the form '1 in *n*' (e.g. '1 in 3', '1 in 4', etc.) or as a percentage or proportion.

Random sampling does not ensure that the characteristics of the sample and the population will coincide exactly; chance differences will exist: but by the use of appropriate statistical methods[2] it is possible to calculate the probability that these divergences lie within given limits (see p 270).

Random sampling may be applied not only to the selection of subjects from a population, but to the selection of times or locations. In the latter instance, areas or the co-ordinates of points are used as the sampling units; the sampling frame may be a map rather than a list.

Systematic sampling

Instead of selecting randomly, a predetermined system may be used. The usual technique requires a list, not necessarily numbered, of all the sampling units. Having decided on the size of the required sample, the investigator calculates the sampling ratio, expressed as '1 in n', rounds n off to the nearest whole number, and uses this figure (k) as a *sampling interval*. He then selects every kth item in the list, starting with an item (from the first to the kth) selected at random. This technique is often easier than simple random sampling.

Such a sample can be considered as essentially equivalent to a random sample, provided that the list is not arranged according to some system or cyclical pattern. If a 1 in 30 systematic sample is selected from a list of persons arranged according to decreasing age, there may be an appreciable age difference between a sample where the first member selected was the first on the list, and one where the first person selected was the 30th. If the list is one of dwelling units, listed in such a way that ground-floor and upper-floor dwellings alternate, then a 1 in 2 systematic sample (or any systematic sample using an even number as the sampling interval) will contain either ground-floor dwellings only, or upper-floor dwellings only.

Other methods of systematic sampling may be used, not requiring prior listing of the sampling units. For example, it may be decided to select every third patient admitted to a hospital, or every patient whose personal identity number, social security number, hospital registration number, or birthdate (day of the month) ends with a predetermined and randomly selected digit or digits. These methods are usually chosen because of their convenience.

Systematic sampling is a convenient and objective way of selecting controls in a case–control study. The choice becomes automatic, e.g. the first patient, or the first eligible one, admitted after the study case; or the patient closest in age in the same hospital ward.

Cluster sampling

In cluster sampling, a simple random sample is selected not of individual subjects, but of groups or clusters of individuals. That is, the sampling units are clusters, and the sampling frame is a list of these clusters. The clusters may be villages, apartment buildings, classes of schoolchildren, housing units, households or families (note that these latter terms are not synonymous),[3] etc.

This is often a convenient method, especially when at the outset there is no sampling frame showing all the individual subjects; it is, of course, also more convenient to investigate people living in a relatively small number of households or villages, rather than the same number of persons, randomly selected, in more scattered places of residence.

The technique has the disadvantage, however, that if the clusters contain similar persons ('high intraclass correlation'), it is difficult to estimate the precision with which generalizations may be made to the parent population.[4] If attitudes to contraception are studied by questioning a simple random sample comprising 200 individuals, it is easy to state the precision with which the findings may be applied to the total population. On the other hand, if 40 families containing 200 individuals are selected, and if attitudes on contraception tend to 'run in families', then in effect only 40, not 200 entities have been studied. Moreover, if a quarter of these families each contain 10 or more individuals, these large families will contribute an undue proportion — at least half — of the individuals in the sample (and a relationship may be assumed between family size and views on contraception).

Other things being equal, a large number of small clusters is preferable to a small number of large clusters.

Stratified sampling

To use this method, the population (the sampling frame) is first divided into subgroups or *strata* according to one or more characteristics, e.g. sex and age groups, and random or systematic sampling is then performed independently in each stratum (*stratified random sampling, stratified systematic sampling*).

This procedure has the advantage that there is less sampling variation than with simple random or systematic sampling. It eliminates sampling variation with respect to the properties used in stratifying, and if the strata are more uniform than the total population with respect to other attributes, it reduces sampling variation with respect to other properties also. The greater the differences between the strata and the less the differences within the strata, the greater is the gain due to stratification.

The same sampling ratio may be used in all strata. This is called *proportional allocation*, since the number of individuals chosen in each stratum is proportional to the size of the stratum. Alternatively, different sampling ratios may be used in different strata. This permits heavier sampling in subgroups with few members, so as to provide acceptable estimates, not only for the population as a whole, but also for each of its subgroups.

Estimates for the total population are prepared by combining the data for the various strata. If varying sampling fractions were used, an appropriate weighting procedure is required. If a uniform sampling fraction was used, the sample is *self-weighting* and can for some purposes be treated as if it were a simple random or systematic sample. The use of varying sampling ratios greatly adds to the complexity of the analysis and should not be decided upon lightly. There is of course no objection to the use of different sampling ratios if the strata are to be kept separate throughout the analysis—e.g. if Scotsmen, Irishmen and Jews are to be studied as separate groups; but then what we have is three study populations, and not a stratified sample.

Two-stage sampling

In two-stage sampling, the population is divided into a set of first-stage sampling units ('primary sampling units'), and a sample of these units is selected by simple random, stratified or systematic sampling. Individuals are then chosen from each of these primary units, using any method of sampling. The sample may be biased if very few first-stage units are selected.

The first-stage units may be census tracts, villages, classes of schoolchildren, households, or other aggregations. They may be time periods, e.g. if samples are chosen of patients who attend a clinic on randomly chosen days. This method has the same advantages as cluster sampling—less travel by interviewers, fewer school teachers to negotiate with, no need for a sampling frame showing all individuals in the population, etc.

The analysis is simplified if 'self-weighting' procedures are used. These ensure that each individual has an equal chance of entering the sample.[5] *Two-stage cluster sampling* (i.e. choosing a cluster within each cluster) is especially convenient, and may be sufficiently precise for some purposes.[5]

Multi-stage sampling

This method is used in large-scale surveys. A sample of first-stage sampling units is chosen, each of the selected units is divided into second-stage units, samples of second-stage units are selected, and so on. Different methods (simple random, stratified, systematic or cluster sampling) may be used at any stage.

Random-digit dialling

In a region where nearly everyone has a telephone at home, *random-digit dialling* (i.e. phoning numbers selected at random) is a convenient way of selecting a sample, either for telephone interviews or for subsequent home interviews or other investigations. Phone numbers are kept in the sample only if they turn out to be for residential addresses. If there is no reply the call is repeated a number of times, at different times and on different weekdays. A two-stage procedure may be used, whereby a sample of households is first selected by random-digit dialling and information is then obtained about the members of the household, the subsequent selection of subjects being determined by age, sex, or other eligibility criteria. The detailed procedure[6] is designed in a way that reduces the proportion of wasted calls; unlisted numbers are not excluded.

High success rates have been reported; in some studies in the USA, information on household composition was obtained for over 90% of the residential numbers phoned, and over 80% of the eligible subjects were subsequently interviewed.[6] Samples selected by random-digit dialling have been reported to be reasonably representative of the general population.

SUBSTITUTIONS

It usually happens that after a sample has been selected it is found that some of the selected subjects cannot be investigated. Persons may have died or moved away, may refuse, or may be unavailable for a variety of other reasons. It is tempting to replace such subjects with other randomly selected subjects. This is an acceptable (although usually unnecessary) procedure, provided that it is remembered that if the omissions produce a sample bias, substitutions will not remove this bias. The outcome will merely be a large biased sample instead of a small biased sample. What is important, if there are more than a few omissions, is to examine the possible bias by determining the reasons for omission and, if possible, studying the demographic and other characteristics of the subjects omitted; the relevance of this bias to the study findings can then be appraised.

SAMPLE SIZE

If numbers are too small it may be impossible to make sufficiently precise and confident generalizations about the situation in the parent population, or to obtain statistical significance (see p 253) when associations are tested. It may thus be impossible to achieve the study's objectives. On the other hand, it is wasteful to study more subjects than these objectives require. Moreover, if numbers are large enough *any* difference, however small, will be statistically significant, and there may hence be a tendency to ascribe false importance to trivial differences. ('Samples which are too small can prove nothing; samples which are too large can prove anything.[7]')

'How big should my sample be?' has been likened to the question 'How much money should I take when I go on vacation?'[8] (How long a vacation? Doing what? Where? With whom?) Calculations of sample size require both decisions and surmises. An investigator who wants to learn the incidence rate of diabetes, for example, must know how precise he wants his estimate to be and what confidence level he requires, i.e. (simplistically stated) what 'margin of error' will he accept, and what risk is he willing to take that the actual error is larger than this acceptable margin? To calculate the requisite sample size he must also have some idea of what the rate is. If he wishes to compare the incidence rates in two groups (in a survey or trial) he must start with an idea of the rate in one of the groups, and must know the magnitude of the difference he wants to be able to detect, what significance level he will use, and what power he wants the significance test to have for detecting the difference.[9]

Calculations can be avoided by using ready-made tables or computer programs.[10]

Consideration must also be given to practical constraints. A large sample may be difficult or impossible to find, or there may be an insufficiency of resources or time. A balance may have to be struck between the cost and the usefulness of the sample. The larger the sample, the less the sampling variation, i.e. the less the likelihood that the sample will be a misleading one. (The size of the sampled population is relatively unimportant.)[11] As a very rough guide, the usefulness of a sample is proportional not to its absolute size but to the square root of its size. To double the usefulness of a sample, its size must be increased fourfold; above a sample size of about 200, the absolute size of the sample must be augmented considerably to make an appreciable difference to its usefulness. This means that it may be necessary to balance increased cost (largely determined by the size of the sample) against increased usefulness (largely determined by the square root of its size). A 'sensitivity analysis'[12] may be helpful—a series of calculations of sample size, based on different assumptions and requirements.

Samples that are to be compared with one another, e.g. in case-control studies and clinical trials, are usually kept approximately equal in size, since (for a given total sample size) this provides the most precise results (i.e. a measure of association that has a narrow confidence interval). But equal groups are by no means essential, and there may be good reasons for having unequal ones.[13] The relative size of the groups must be taken into account when calculating sample size.

In some therapeutic and prophylactic trials in which the subjects enter the investigation serially, as they become available, no initial decision is made about the sample size. Instead, rules are set up in advance whereby at any stage it can be decided, on the basis of the findings to date, whether enough subjects have been studied to give a sufficiently definite answer, so that the trial can be stopped. This procedure is termed *sequential analysis*.[14]

A basic difficulty in calculations of sample size, whether they are done in advance or by the sequential method, is that the result depends on the attribute that is to be measured or compared. Samples of very different sizes are needed to study differences between two groups in their blood lipid levels, in their incidence of coronary heart disease, or in their mortality rates. It is seldom that a study is conducted to investigate only a single characteristic, and the real question often becomes not 'How many subjects do I need?' but 'With such-and-such a sample size (determined by practical considerations), about what variables and about what associations can I expect to get useful findings?—and in these circumstances, is the study worth doing?'

RANDOM NUMBERS

To use a list of random numbers in selecting a sample, a number must first be allocated to each sampling unit (e.g. from 1 to the total number of sampling units). Successive random numbers are then read from the list, and the sampling units whose numbers coincide with these random numbers are chosen. This is continued until enough units have been selected.

Random numbers can be churned 'out by a computer; programs for doing this are easy to write.[15] Alternatively, use may be made of a printed table of digits arranged in a random order. A short specimen (provided as an illustration, and *not* for use) is shown here (Table 8.1), and a table for actual use is provided in the Appendix (p 327).

Table 8.1. Random numbers

Rows	Columns		
	1–4	5–8	9–12
1	96 22	74 70	80 46
2	82 14	73 36	41 54
3	21 47	59 93	48 40
4	89 31	62 79	45 73
5	63 29	90 61	86 39
6	71 68	93 94	08 72
7	05 06	96 63	58 24
8	06 32	57 11	81 59
9	91 15	38 54	73 30
10	54 60	28 35	32 94

The use of such tables is very simple, although sometimes tedious. Numbers are read off the table, beginning at any haphazardly chosen point and proceeding in any predetermined direction, until the required number of units has been selected. Numbers not appearing in the list of sampling units are ignored, and numbers that reappear after they have already been selected are generally also ignored.

As an example, if five units are to be chosen out of nine, numbered from 1 to 9, one could start say at the '8' in row 4 of Table 8.1, and read off numbers 8, 9, 3, 1 and 6 (moving horizontally). Or one could move vertically and select the units numbered 8, 6, 7, 9 and 5; the two zeros would be ignored, as there are no subjects numbered '0'. To choose a sample from 86 units, we would use pairs of digits. Moving horizontally from the same starting-point, we would select the units numbered 89 (ignored), 31, 62, etc. To choose a sample from between 100 and 999 sampling units, we would use sets of three digits (893, 162, 794, 573, 632, and so on). With between 1000 and 9999 sampling units, we would use sets of four digits (8931, 6279, etc.).

Sometimes many numbers have to be discarded and the process may become very tedious. For example, with 195 units to choose from, if we started from the same '8' in row 4 and moved horizontally, we would find only two helpful numbers among the first 16 we looked at: 162 in row 4 and 050 (or 50) in row 7. In such instances short-cut methods may be used.[16]

NOTES AND REFERENCES

1. Specimen instructions for interviewers: 'Ask if any children aged under 15 years live in the home. If 'yes', carry on with the interview if there is an 'A' in the sealed envelope'; this requires a prior allocation of the required proportion of As, in accordance with the sampling fraction; the envelopes should be well shuffled.
2. For a detailed exposition of the statistical aspects of sampling and the handling of sample data, see Cochran W G 1977 Sampling techniques, 3rd edn. John Wiley, New York. Formulae for calculating standard errors of means and proportions based on different sampling methods are listed by Kelsey J L, Thompson W D, Evans A S 1986 Methods in observational epidemiology. Oxford University Press, New York; pp 266–269.
3. One research institute used the following operational definitions: 'A *household unit* is a room or group of rooms occupied or vacant and intended for occupancy as separate living quarters. In practice, living quarters are considered separate and therefore a housing unit when the occupants live and eat apart from any other group in the building, and there is either direct access from the outside or through a common hall, or complete kitchen facilities for the exclusive use of the occupants, regardless of whether or not they are used'. (The definition then goes on to explain what is meant by 'living apart', 'eating apart', 'direct access', etc.) A *household* is everyone who resides in a housing unit at the time the interviewer speaks to a household member and learns who lives there, including those who have places of residence both there and elsewhere. The household also includes people absent at the time of contact, if a place of residence is held for them in the housing unit and 'no place of residence is held for them elsewhere'. 'A *family unit* consists of household members who are related to each other by blood, marriage, or adoption. A person unrelated to other occupants in the housing unit—or living alone—constitutes a family unit with only one member'. If there is more than one family unit in the household, the 'primary family unit' is the one that owns or rents the home. 'If families share ownership or rent equally, the one whose head is closest to age 45 is usually considered to be the primary family'. Survey Research Center, Institute for Social Research 1976 Interviewer's manual. University of Michigan, Ann Arbor, pp 39, 91, 94.
4. For statistical aspects of cluster samples, see Cochran W G 1983 in: Moses L E, Mosteller F, (eds) Planning and analysis of observational studies. Wiley, New York, pp 61–65.
5. To ensure that each individual has an equal chance of selection (the 'equal probability of selection method', or *epsem* sampling), primary units may be selected with a probability proportional to their size (*PPS*), and an equal number of individuals are then chosen from each primary unit. A technique that is convenient if there are not too many primary units in the sampling frame is described by Yeoman K A 1970 Statistics for the social scientist: 2. Applied statistics, Penguin Books, Harmondsworth, pp 131–132. If there are many primary units (e.g. households), it is easier to stratify them according to their size and use a sampling ratio that is proportional to their size. A simple method for

choosing a single member of each selected household is described by
Cochran W G 1977 (see note 2), pp 364–365. An alternative to the
'proportional-to-size' selection of primary units is a selection by simple random or
systematic sampling, and the use of a uniform sampling ratio in the second stage.

A *two-stage PPS cluster sampling* method has been used in many World Health
Organization surveys in developing countries: randomly select 30 or more
clusters, with probability proportionate to the size of the cluster, then randomly
choose a household in each cluster, and then select one person from this
household and each of the nearest households until a predetermined number has
been chosen. Frerichs (1989) explains how a microcomputer spreadsheet
program, operated by initially computer-illiterate health professionals, can be
used to estimate the required sample size, select the first-stage clusters, and
calculate confidence intervals. Frerichs R R 1989 Simple analytic procedures for
rapid microcomputer-assisted cluster surveys in developing countries. Public
Health Reports 104: 24.

6. *Random-digit dialling* is usually done by the procedure described by Waksberg J
   1978 Sampling methods for random digit dialing. Journal of the American Statistical Association 73: 40. Its use is described by (inter alia) Hartge P, Brinton
   L A, Rosenthal J F, Cahill J I, Hoover R N, Waksberg J 1984 Random digit
   dialing in selecting a population-based control group. American Journal of
   Epidemiology 120: 825; Wingo P A, Ory H W, Layde P M et al 1988 The
   evaluation of the data collection process for a multicenter, population-based,
   case-control design. American Journal of Epidemiology 128: 206. The logistics
   of alternative methods are described by Harlow B L, Davis S 1988 Two one-step
   methods for household screening and interviewing using random digit dialing.
   American Journal of Epidemiology 127: 857.

   In a study in Washington requiring blood tests, potential subjects were chosen
   by random digit dialling. The response rate was 83% in this phase, 81% in the
   next phase (a telephone interview) and 67% in the third phase (blood-taking).
   The overall rate was thus $(83 \times 81 \times 67)\%$, or only 45%, illustrating the effect of
   offering repeated opportunities for non-response. Brown L M, Tollerud D J,
   Pottern L M et al 1989 Biochemical epidemiology in community-based studies:
   practical lessons from a study of T-cell subsets. Journal of Clinical Epidemiology
   42: 561.

7. Sackett D L 1979 Bias in analytic research. Journal of Chronic Diseases 32: 51.

8. Moses L E 1985 Statistical concepts fundamental to investigations. New England
   Journal of Medicine 14: 890.

9. *Calculations of sample size.* Refer to a statistics text, e.g. Fleiss J L 1981
   Statistical methods for rates and proportions, 2nd edn. John Wiley, New York,
   pp 33–39 or Cochran (1977; see note 2) Chapter 4. Formulae for use with a wide
   variety of statistical tests are given by Lachin J M 1981 Introduction to sample
   size determination and power analysis for clinical trials. Controlled Clinical Trials
   2: 93. For sample sizes when comparing several groups in a trial, see Fleiss J L
   1986 The design and analysis of clinical experiments. Wiley, New York,
   pp 371–376. For matched-pair studies, see Fleiss J L Levin B 1988 Sample size
   determination in studies with matched pairs. 1988 Journal of Clinical
   Epidemiology 41: 727.

10. For tables showing the sample sizes required when comparing proportions (e.g.
    of therapeutic successes) in two equal groups, see Fleiss (1981; see note 9)
    Chapter 3 or Schlesselman J J 1982 Case-control studies: design, conduct,
    analysis. Oxford University Press, New York, Appendix A. For
    pocket-calculator programs for calculating sample sizes for estimating a
    proportion or mean or for detecting a difference between two proportions or
    means, see note 2, p 242. PC programs (see note 3, p 34) include Epistat and PC-
    Size.

11. The *finite population correction*, the factor introduced into the calculation to allow for the effect of the size of the parent population, is one minus the sampling fraction. If the sampling fraction is low this factor is close to unity, and the correction has a negligible influence and may be omitted. Cochrane (1977; see note 2), pp 24–25.

12. Laird N M, Weinstein M C, Stason W B 1979 Sample size estimation: a sensitivity analysis in the context of a clinical trial for treatment of mild hypertension. American Journal of Epidemiology 109: 408.

13. *Unequal groups* (see note 10, p 77): for the calculation of sample sizes, see Fleiss (1981; see note 9), pp 46–47.

14. See Armitage P 1975 Sequential medical trials 2nd edn. Blackwell, Oxford.

15. *Epistat* (see note 3, p 34) generates and prints *lists of random numbers*. So do the following simple programs (written in Basic and Turbo-Pascal respectively):

RANDNUM. BAS

```
10 INPUT "Largest random number required: ", X
20 INPUT "Number of random numbers required: ", N
30 RANDOMIZE TIMER
40 LPRINT N "RANDOM NUMBERS BETWEEN 1 AND" X
50 FOR I = 1 TO N
60 LPRINT, INT (RND*X) + 1
70 NEXT I
```

RANDNUM. PAS

```
program RANDNUM;
uses crt, printer; {Include for TurboPascal 4.0, not 3.0}
var X, N, I: integer;
begin
    write ('Largest random number required: ');
    readln (X);
    write ('Number of random numbers required: ');
    readln (N);
    randomize;
    writeln (1st, N, 'RANDOM NUMBERS BETWEEN 1 AND', X);
    for I: = 1 to N
    do writeln (1st,'                    ', trunc((random*x) + 1))
    end.
```

16. Short cuts can be taken when *using tables of random numbers to choose a sample.* For example, if there are between 101 and 200 sampling units to choose from, read the successive three-digit numbers, and subtract the largest possible multiple of 200 from every number above 200 (also, read 000 as 200). Using the example in the text (p 88), the sampling units selected would then be 93 (893 minus 800), 162, 194 (794 minus 600), 173 (573 minus 400), 32, 190, 18, 39, etc. If there are between 201 and 300 sampling units, subtract a multiple of 300 from numbers above 300, discarding numbers above 900. If there are between 301 and 400 sampling units, subtract 400 from numbers above 400, discarding numbers above 800. And if there are between 401 and 500, subtract 500 from numbers above 500 (take 000 as 500).

9. The variables

The characteristics that are measured are referred to as variables, whether they are measured numerically (e.g. age or height) or in terms of categories (e.g. sex or the presence or absence of a disease).

When an association between two variables is studied the variables may be referred to as *dependent* and *independent*. The variable we try to 'hang on' to another variable is termed the *dependent variable*. For example, in a study of prevalence of a disease in different age and sex groups, the presence of the disease may be referred to as the dependent variable, and age and sex as independent variables. On the other hand, if we study the frequency of a given symptom among persons with different diseases, the type of disease is the independent variable. If we want to know whether transcendental meditation affects the blood pressure, blood pressure is the dependent variable. Whenever we consider a causal association the outcome (the postulated effect) is the dependent variable.[1] In a therapeutic trial, the treatment is the independent variable and the measure of outcome is the dependent variable.

A variable based on two or more other variables may be termed a *composite variable*. Adiposity, for example, may be measured in terms of a 'body mass index' (Quetelet's index) calculated by dividing the person's weight by the square of his height, or a 'ponderal index' (height divided by the cube root of weight); the units used—grams and centimetres or pounds and inches—must of course be specified. Dental caries may be measured by a DMF index, calculated by adding the number of permanent teeth that are decayed (D), the number that are missing (M), and the number that have been filled (F).

Incidence and prevalence rates, sex ratios, and all other *rates*[2] and ratios are composite variables, since they are based on separate numerator and denominator information.

During the planning of the study it is necessary to select and clarify the variables which will be measured.

SELECTION OF VARIABLES

The variables to be studied are selected on the basis of their relevance to the objectives of the investigation. If the study objectives have been formulated in writing, as previously recommended (see p 41), the key variables will have been specifically mentioned in the objectives; the more specific the formulation of objectives, the greater the number of variables that will have been included.

There may also be variables that have not been mentioned but require to be measured if the study is to attain its aims. In selecting these additional variables, it is helpful to start with a list of all the characteristics (other than the independent variables that have already been specified) that are known or suspected to affect or cause the characteristics (dependent variables) that the investigator wants to study. Each of these variables can then be considered in turn, to decide whether it should be included in the study on any of the following five grounds:

1. It is important enough to warrant study as an *independent variable* in its own right. Its omission was an oversight.
2. It is a possible *confounding factor*, i.e. it may obscure the relationship between some other independent variable and the dependent variable, or have other deceptive effects on that relationship. It may produce an association that has little meaning in itself (see p 256). The variable confounds the picture because it is associated with the other independent variable as well as with the dependent one. In a study of the relationship between work accidents and age, we may decide to take the type of occupation into account, since older workers may have fewer accidents merely because they are in safer jobs. Confounding effects can arise only if the confounding variable (occupation) both influences the dependent variable (accidents) and is associated with the independent variable (age). It may be decided to eliminate the effect of possible confounders by using matching (see p 72); but this does not obviate the need to measure them. In a trial, subjects may be randomly allocated to experimental and control groups in order to neutralize the effect of possible confounders (see p 285); but these variables should still be measured, so that the effectiveness of the randomization procedure can be checked.
3. It may be a *modifier variable* (see p 255), i.e. it may modify the relationship between some other independent variable and the dependent variable (or, in a trial, it may modify the effect of the

treatment). It specifies the conditions for the relationship. Are older workers especially prone to accidents only in their first year of employment? Or does their special proneness (or immunity) vary in different departments of the factory? To know this, we must add 'length of employment' and 'department' to our list of variables.

4. It may be an *intervening cause* (see p 260) that will explain a causal mechanism. Can a difference in the use of protective equipment explain the relationship between age and accidents?

5. It has a strong enough *influence* on the dependent variable to warrant its inclusion. If variables that strongly affect the dependent variable are included in the statistical analysis of associations (even for this reason only), this may (under certain conditions) appreciably increase the precision with which the effects of other independent variables—i.e. those of interest to the investigator— can be estimated, and increase the statistical significance of these effects. In a study of the effects of smoking or a disease on pulmonary function, for example, it would probably be decided to include sex, age, height, and the presence of a cold or cough, all of which may affect the test results.

Apart from variables with an obvious relevance to the study objectives, consideration should be given to the following three types of variables:

1. *Universal* variables. These are variables which are so often of relevance in investigations of groups or populations, that their inclusion should always be considered. They should not be automatically included, but should be automatically considered for inclusion. A suggested basic list of these variables is:

> Sex
> Age
> Parity
> Ethnic group
> Religion
> Marital status
> Social class, and attributes that may be used as indicators of social class or as variables in their own right, e.g. occupation, education, income, and household crowding index
> Place of residence (e.g. region, urban/rural)
> Geographical mobility (e.g. nativity, date of immigration)

This list may of course require modification to suit the investigator's specific interests and the reality of the populations in which he works. In certain communities it may be necessary to replace social class, for example, by some other measure of social stratification, or to add 'race' (which refers primarily to a group's relative homogeneity with respect to biological inheritance, whereas 'ethnic group' refers primarily to its shared history, social and cultural tradition, and way of life).

2. Measures of *time*. Apart from obviously relevant measurements (such as the date of onset in any study of disease incidence), in a follow-up survey or clinical trial it may be necessary to record the dates on which the subject entered and left the study. This is essential information for both the analytic techniques commonly employed in studies with varying observation periods: the use of 'person-years of observation'[3] as a denominator for the calculation of rates, and the life table method.[4]

3. Variables that delineate the *study population* or populations. The characteristics of the study population may indicate the extent to which generalizations may be made from the findings. If groups are to be compared, their demographic and other similarities and dissimilarities should be known; if a sample is to be used, its characteristics should be compared with those of the parent population; if there are many non-respondents, they (or a sample of them) should be compared with respondents. Measures of the attributes of the study population or populations should be included for these purposes. These may be attributes with a bearing on the study topic, or may be quite unrelated ones, introduced solely as checks on the adequacy of the matching, sampling or allocation procedures.

NUMBER OF VARIABLES

How many variables should be studied? The only answer, and not a very helpful one, is 'as many as necessary and as few as possible'. One thing is clear: the initial list is usually too long, and will have to be pruned to facilitate the collection and processing of the data. Bradford Hill tells of a plan submitted to him for a proposed inquiry into the causes of prematurity:

> It ran to a trifle of 180 questions, which covered a catholic range. For instance, it seemed that the author was confident that some person or persons—undefined in the draft I saw—could accurately inform her for

each of the woman's previous confinements of the time interval between birth of the child and the placenta; the incidence of congenital malformations in her blood relations; whether she wore high- or low-heeled shoes; how often she took a hot bath; the state of health of the father at the time of conception; and the frequency of sexual intercourse, which was engagingly included under the sub-heading "social amenities". This, in my view, is not the scientific method; it is mere wishful thinking, mere hoping that *some* rabbit may come out if only the hat be made big enough.[5]

CLARIFYING THE VARIABLES

Once the variables have been selected, each of them should be clarified. There are two aspects to be considered. First, an operational definition must be formulated, clearly defining the variable in terms of objectively measurable facts, and stating, if necessary, how these facts are to be obtained (see Chs 10 and 11). Secondly, the scale of measurement to be used in data collection should be specified (Chs 12 and 13).

An example is given showing part of the list of variables to be measured in a survey of illnesses among infants (Table 9.1). Whether the record should take this or another format is a matter of taste; but the information it contains should certainly be recorded somewhere. It will be noted that the list contains two variables, age and social class, on which no direct data are obtained. In this study, age is a composite variable based on the date of birth and date of admission, and social class is inferred from the father's occupation. The construction of the list in this way serves as a reminder of the basic data that must be collected.

If the investigation is concerned with more than one study population, more than one list of variables may be needed; but the full details about each variable need not be obsessively inserted in each list.

COMPLEX VARIABLES

Some variables are too complex to be easily measured as single entities, and are best broken up into component aspects that can be regarded as separate variables and measured separately.

If we wish to investigate the 'attitude to abortions', for example, we would be well advised to obtain separate measures of the attitudes to abortions performed for medical, economic and psychological reasons, to those carried out by medical practitioners and by unqualified persons, to those performed on married and unmarried

Table 9.1 Selected variable in a survey of illnesses among infants

Variable	Definition	Scale
Age	Infant's age at admission to hospital, calculated from date of birth and date of admission	Month (0 to 11) (99 if unknown)
Date of birth	Infant's date of birth, as recorded in hospital records	Full date
Date of admission	Date of infant's admission to hospital, as recorded in hospital records	Full date
Mother's age	Age at birth of infant, as stated by mother	1. Under 20 years 2. 20–24 years 3. 25–29 years 4. 30–34 years 5. 35–39 years 6. 40 years or more 9. No information
Social class	Father's occupational grade, using British Registrar-General's grading scheme (see p 103)	1. Social class I 2. Social class II 3. Social class III 4. Social class IV 5. Social class V 9. Unclassifiable
Father's occupation	Father's usual occupation, as stated by mother	Detailed occupation
Reason for admission to hospital	Final diagnosis, according to hospital records; if two or more, the one stated by hospital physician to have been the principal reason for admission	Detailed categories in International Classification of Diseases (9th revision)
Haemoglobin	In capillary blood, measured by cyanmethaemoglobin method within 24 hours of admission	g per 100 ml, rounded off downwards to nearest g
Mother's satisfaction with hospital	Response to specific question put to mother within week after infant's discharge or death	1. Very satisfied 2. Satisfied on the whole 3. Somewhat dissatisfied 4. Very dissatisfied 9. Don't know, or no answer

women, etc. It may afterwards be possible to combine these separate measures into a single integrated measure of 'attitude to abortions' (now a composite variable).

Similarly, if we wish to study electrocardiogram (ECG) findings we may, instead of making a global and probably subjective appraisal of the ECG pattern, give separate consideration to a series of different measurable aspects, Q and QS patterns, S-T junction and segment depression, etc. This approach is the basis of the Minnesota code for the classification of ECG findings, which is widely used in epidemiological studies.[6] Different combinations of ECG findings may afterwards be used to provide electrocardiographic diagnoses of myocardial infarction and other disorders (composite variables).

NOTES AND REFERENCES

1. By the definition used in the text, chronic bronchitis is the dependent variable in a study of the effect of smoking on the occurrence of chronic bronchitis, even if a retrospective study design is used. The term may also be used differently: in a study that compares the smoking habits of cases (bronchitics) and controls, a statistician might regard smoking habits as the dependent variable in the statistical analysis, the postulated effect (disease) being the independent variable; if a regression analysis is used, the variable predicted by the regression equation is called the dependent variable.

2. A *rate* expresses the frequency of a characteristic per 100 (or per 1000, per million, etc.) persons in the population. To calculate a death rate the number of deaths (numerator) is divided by the number of persons in the population (denominator) and multiplied by 100, 1000, or another convenient figure.

   The importance of *denominator data* in community medicine studies cannot be overstressed. It has been said that in the same way as a clinician keeps a stethoscope handy, an epidemiologist should always carry a denominator in his back pocket. The denominator is the 'population at risk'.

   If the numerator is confined to a specific category, e.g. males, the denominator should be similarly restricted (sex-specific rates, age-specific rates, etc.).

   A *prevalence rate* tells what proportion of individuals have a disease or other attribute at a given time. It is a measure of what *exists*. An *incidence rate* is a measure of what *happens* (e.g. disease onsets) during a specified period. Incidence may be expressed as a *cumulative incidence rate* ('risk')—the proportion of initially disease-free individuals who develop the disease during a stated period—or as a *person-time incidence rate* ('average incidence density'). For clarification, see any recent epidemiology textbook.

   Standardized and other *adjusted rates* are estimates of what the rate would be under specified conditions, e.g. if the age or sex composition of the study population conformed with a specified standard, or if the groups under comparison were similar with respect to defined independent variables. *Crude rates* are rates (for a whole population) that have not been adjusted.

3. To calculate *person-years* (or person-months, etc.) of observation, it is necessary to know the length of each subject's period of observation, from the start of follow-up until its end (i.e. until occurrence of the 'endpoint' event under study: death, loss of contact, conclusion of the study, or withdrawal from follow-up for some other

reason). The sum total of these periods can be used as a person-time denominator for an incidence or mortality rate. Miettinen (1985) calls it 'candidate time'. Miettinen O S 1985 Theoretical epidemiology: principles of occurrence research in medicine. Wiley, New York, p 319.

4. For simple explanations of the life table method (with special reference to clinical trials) see Hill A B 1977 A short textbook of medical statistics. Hodder & Stoughton, London, pp 205–213; or Peto R, Pike M C, Armitage P et al 1977 Design and analysis of randomized clinical trials requiring prolonged observation of each patient: II. Analysis and examples. British Journal of Cancer 35: 1.

5. Hill A B 1962 Statistical methods in clinical and preventive medicine. Livingstone, Edinburgh, p 360.

6. Prineas R J, Crow R C, Blackburn H 1982 The Minnesota code manual of electrocardiographic findings: standards and procedures for measurement and classification. John Wright PSG, Boston.

10. Defining the variables

Each of the variables measured in a study should be clearly and explicitly defined. Unless this is done, there can be no assurance that, if the study were performed by a different investigator, or repeated by the same investigator, similar findings would be obtained.

The same term may have more than one meaning, even in day-to-day usage; there are no hard and fast, universally accepted, 'correct' definitions. The investigator must choose a definition that will be useful to him for the purposes of the study. Like Humpty Dumpty, he can say, 'when *I* use a word, it means just what I choose it to mean—neither more nor less'.

There are two kinds of definition—conceptual and operational.

The *conceptual definition* defines the variable as we conceive it. This definition is often akin to a dictionary definition. For example, 'obesity' may be variously defined as: 'excessive fatness'; or as 'overweight'; or as 'a bodily condition which is socially regarded as constituting excessive fatness'. In effect, the conceptual definition is a definition of the characteristic we would like to measure.

In contrast, the *operational definition* (or 'working definition') defines the characteristic we will actually measure. It is phrased in terms of objectively observable facts, and is sufficiently clear and explicit to avoid ambiguity. Where necessary, it states the method by which the facts are obtained. 'Obesity', for example, might be operationally defined in different surveys as:

a weight, based on weighing in underclothes and without shoes, which exceeds, by 10 per cent or more, the mean weight of persons of the subject's sex, age and height (in a specified population at a specified time)

or as

a skinfold thickness of 25 mm or more, measured with a Harpenden skinfold caliper at the back of the right upper arm, midway between the tip of the acromial process and the tip of the olecranon process (this level being located with the forearm flexed at 90°), with the arm hanging freely and the skinfold being lifted parallel to the long axis of the arm

or as

a positive response to the question 'Are you definitely over-weight?'

or as

a positive response to the question 'Does your husband/wife think you are too fat?'

It is often helpful, but it is not always essential, to formulate the conceptual definition of a variable. On the other hand, it is always necessary to formulate the operational definition.

In doing this, the investigator is heavily influenced by considerations of practicability. In most research on blood pressure, the characteristic in which the investigator is interested is the pressure within the arteries; as intra-arterial measurements are usually not feasible, blood pressure is usually defined in terms of measurements made externally with a sphygmomanometer. This operationally defined blood pressure may be markedly different from the intra-arterial pressure, particularly in fat subjects. Similarly, social class may be operationally defined in terms of the classification of occupations (Table 10.1) used by the British Registrar-General (in the case of children, the father's occupation is used, and in the case of married women, the husband's).

Social class, so defined, does not necessarily correspond with the researcher's conception of social class, which may have to do with prestige or wealth or living conditions or lifestyle.[1] But in a particular investigation this definition (or some other simple definition, such as educational level) may be a practical one to use, while the information the researcher really wants may be difficult or impossible to obtain.

In other words, the investigator is playing what has been called a 'substitution game'. He is substituting what he *can* measure—a *proxy variable*—for what he *would like* to measure. Discrepancies may be unavoidable, but the investigator should at least be aware of them. If they are perforce large, he may need to reconsider whether it is worth his while measuring the variable at all, and even whether his whole investigation is worthwhile.

Table 10.1 Classification of occupations

Social class	Occupations (selected list)
I. Upper and middle	Higher professional, e.g. medicine, engineering, architecture, authors, scientists Large employers Directors of business
II. Intermediate	Lower professional, e.g. teachers, pharmacists, social workers Owners of small businesses and managers Farmers
III. Skilled workers and clerical workers	Artisans, clerks, foremen, supervisors
IV. Intermediate	Semi-skilled workers, e.g. factory operatives Agricultural labourers
V. Unskilled workers	Labourers, etc. Domestic servants Casual workers

As an example, suppose we wish to perform a survey to test the hypothesis that drivers whose emotional health is disturbed have a higher risk of being involved in road accidents. Clearly, 'emotional health' will be difficult to define in operational terms. The defining of 'accidents', on the other hand, seems an easier nut to crack; after all, everyone knows what an accident is. In actual fact, the task is not so easy. Do we want to include all mishaps occurring on the road, including 'near misses', or only those which result in damage? If the latter, are we to include any damage, whether to vehicles, lamp-posts, cats, dogs, etc. or only injury to human beings? If we confine the study to accidents causing injuries to humans, will we include mild and transient injuries, such as temporary emotional shock, or only more severe ones?—and if the latter, what precisely do we mean by 'more severe'? Whatever definition of 'accident' we are considering, is it a practical one? Will we be able to get the required information? Maybe we will have to fall back on accidents reported to the police or insurance companies (which are not necessarily representative samples of accidents), or even confine ourselves to fatal accidents. In the latter instance our case ascertainment may be fairly complete, but we will be investigating only the tip of the iceberg, and ignoring the main bulk of accidents. Maybe accidents defined in different ways have different associations with emotional health.[2] Can we find a definition that meets our need, or should we give the whole thing up as a bad job?

In the light of what has been said above it is clearly impossible to suggest a list of 'recommended' definitions. Instead, we will draw attention to a number of questions which may arise when definitions are sought for certain frequently used variables.

1. *Occupation*—Present or usual occupation? Occupation for which subject was trained (profession or trade), or work actually performed? If retired or unemployed, will previous occupation be used?

2. *Education*—Number of years of education, or last grade attained, or type of educational institution last attended, or age at completion of full-time education?

3. *Income*—Personal income, family income, or average family income per member?

4. *Crowding index* (mean number of persons per room in housing unit)—What rooms are excluded (bathrooms, showers, toilets, kitchens, store-rooms, rooms used for business purposes, entrance halls)? Are children taken as wholes or halves in the computation?

5. *Social class*[1]—Based on occupation, education, crowding index, income, neighbourhood of residence, home amenities, or subject's self-perception? Based on one of these, or a combination? If based on occupation, will women be graded by their own or their husbands' occupations (Women's Lib!)? If the latter, how will unmarried women, widows and divorcees be graded? Will all members of the household be graded according to the occupation of the head of the household? And if so, how is 'head of the household'[3] defined? What occupational classification is suitable for use in the specific community being studied?

6. *Ethnic group*—In terms of 'race' (see p 96), country of birth, father's (or mother's) country of birth, 'extraction', tribe, religion, or subject's self-perception?

7. *Marital status*—In terms of legal status (single, married, widowed, divorced; and, in some communities, 'common law marriages' and 'separated'); or in terms of stability of union, e.g. stable union, casual union? Present status, or total marital experience ('second marriage', etc.)?

8. *Parity*—Total number of previous pregnancies, or only those terminating in still or live births, or number of children delivered?

9. *Date of onset of disease*—Date when first symptoms were noticed, or date when first diagnosed, or date of notification?

10. *Presence of chronic disease*[4]—Based on duration since onset? If so, what duration makes it chronic?—3 months, 6 months, a year? Based on presence of certain diseases that are defined as chronic whatever their duration? If so, what diseases? Do they include dental caries, myopia, obesity? Are chronic symptoms enough (cough, constipation)? What about conditions that come and go, e.g. frequently recurrent sore throats?

11. *Disability*—Capacity to function, or actual performance? Appraised by self, by family, or by examiner?[5] What functions are considered?—ability to get around alone, or ability to carry out major activity (work, housework, schoolwork—but what is a pensioner's 'major activity'?), or ability to see, hear, carry out activities of daily living? Emphasis on physical impairments, or on functional incapacity? Long-term disability only, or temporary disability also (days of work-loss or school absence, days in bed, days with restricted activity on account of illness or injury)? Measured as percentage disability, using rating scales established for entitlement to benefits (workmen's compensation, etc.)?

12. *Overall or general health*[6]—Appraised by physician or by self?— and if by self, appraisal in comparison with others of same age and sex? Physical, mental, social, or comprehensive health? Based only on presence or absence of specific diseases? Subjective well-being? Functional capacity? Positive aspects of health?

13. *Physician visit*—Including telephone consultations? What if the service was provided by a nurse or other person acting on the doctor's instructions? If a patient comes for a certificate or to collect a letter, is this a visit? Can a visit be paid absentia?—if a mother comes to consult a doctor about her child, is the visit ascribed to the mother or the child? If she consults the doctor about herself, and the doctor uses the opportunity to discuss her son's health, or to prescribe treatment for him, is the visit ascribed to the son also?

14. *Hospitalization*—Is hospitalization for childbirth included? Is the hospital stay of a well newborn baby included? Is overnight stay essential? Is overnight stay in a casualty ward included? What institutions qualify as hospitals?

If it is hoped to obtain information which can be directly compared with the findings of other studies, care must be taken to use the operational definitions used in the other studies. For a few variables, such as 'underlying cause of death'[7] and 'neonatal death', internationally recommended and generally accepted definitions are available.

Finally, it must be noted that there are certain variables for which, paradoxically, detailed operational definitions can be formulated only after the findings have been analysed. These are composite variables based on combinations of a number of separate items, using rules that are determined only after the actual inter-relationship between the items has been examined (see pp 127–129).

NOTES AND REFERENCES

1. For a brief discussion of measures of social class, see Susser M, Watson W, Hopper K 1985 Sociology in medicine, 3rd edn. Oxford University Press, New York. Also, see Abramson J H, Gofin R, Habib J, Pridan H, Gofin J 1982 Indicators of social class: a comparative appraisal of measures for use in epidemiological studies. Social Science and Medicine 16: 1739.

2. In a national study in Britain, the definition of 'childhood accident' was found to be a crucial factor in determining results. Accidents 'resulting in an injury for which the child was admitted to hospital' were associated with large family size, whereas accidents 'resulting in an injury which warranted medical attention' were not. Stewart-Brown S, Peters T J, Golding J, Bijur P 1986 Case definition in childhood accident studies: a vital factor in determining results. International Journal of Epidemiology 15: 352.

3. Identification of the *head of the household* usually presents no problem. In difficult cases, the members of the household may be asked whom they regard as the head. Alternatively, a detailed operational definition may be devised. One research institute defines the head of the household as the head of the family or, if there is more than one family in the household, as the head of the 'primary family unit' (see note 3, p 89). In the case of a married couple, with or without minor children, the husband is the head of the family even if the wife is supporting the family. In other instances, the head is the 'economic dominant' — i.e. the main breadwinner; in doubtful cases, it is the member who is economically most active, i.e. earning a living rather than getting a pension. If different members have equal economic power, the one closest to age 45 is selected. A mnemonic is suggested: 'HEAD', where H stands for 'Husband', 'E' for 'Economic dominant', 'A' for Age 45', and 'D' for 'Do not expect your informant to know our definition of a family head. Determine it yourself on the basis of these criteria'. Survey Research Center, Institute for Social Research 1976 Interviewer's manual, University of Michigan, Ann Arbor, pp 94–95. In some communities it would be absurd to use this definition.

4. In a well known survey of *chronic disease* in the USA, the initial working definition was: 'Chronic disease comprises all impairments or deviations from normal which have *one* or *more* of the following characteristics: are permanent, leave residual disability; are caused by nonreversible pathological alteration; require special training of the patient for rehabilitation; may be expected to require a long period of supervision, observation or care'. This was found to be too vague and to include too many trivial disorders. In practice the examining physicians recorded all chronic conditions they detected, but conditions were disregarded if they were not

'medically disabling', i.e. if it was thought they did not affect the patient's well-being or interfere with his activities and were unlikely to do so. The report states: 'It is difficult to state concisely and specifically what conditions are included in these data on "chronic diseases". In the final analysis, the definition is the list of 47 diagnostic categories, plus two "all other" groups, for which data are presented.' These hold-all 'other diagnoses' groups included a quarter of all cases. Commission on Chronic Illness 1959 Chronic Illness in the United States, Vol III. Chronic illness in a rural area: the Hunterdon study. pp 149–151; and 1957 Vol. IV. Chronic illness in a large city: the Baltimore study. pp 49–50; 513–520. Harvard University Press, Cambridge, Massachusetts.

In the United States Health Interview Survey a condition was considered chronic if it was reported to have been first noticed more than 3 months previously, or if it was in a list of 34 conditions that were always considered chronic. These were phrased in lay terms, e.g. 'heart trouble' and 'repeated trouble with back or spine'. National Center for Health Statistics 1975 Health interview survey procedure 1957–1974. Vital and Health Statistics series 1, no 11. Department of Health, Education, and Welfare, Washington, pp 127–128.

5. A Finnish study in which self-ratings of disability were compared with ratings by nurses who provided home care showed that the nurses reported much more performance of cooking and cleaning; ratings of the capacity for self-care with respect to dressing, eating and daily washing showed a very high concordance. Concordance was lower for 'bathing or sauna'. Kivela S L 1984 Measuring disability—do self-ratings and service provider ratings compare? Journal of Chronic Diseases 37: 115.

6. See recent symposia on measures of *overall health*, the *quality of life* and *functional status*: Lohr K N, Ware J E Jr, (eds) 1987 Advances in health assessment: conference proceedings. Journal of Chronic Diseases 40 (suppl 1); Katz S (ed) 1987 The Portugal conference: measuring quality of life and functional status. Journal of Chronic Diseases 40: 459. Also, see McDowell I, Newall C 1987 Measuring health: a guide to rating scales and questionnaires. Oxford University Press, New York.

7. World Health Organization 1977 Manual of the international statistical classification of diseases, injuries and causes of death, 1975 revision, vol 1. World Health Organization, Geneva, pp 763–764.

11. Definitions of diseases

It is as important to establish clear operational definitions for diseases as for other variables. This is a far from easy task. A clinician tends to establish his diagnosis by making a clinical judgement of the extent to which the picture presented by the patient conforms with his *concept* of a specific disease. In making this judgement he seldom uses rigid diagnostic rules. That is, his diagnosis tends to be based on a conceptual rather than on an explicit operational definition. Inevitably, doctors often disagree.

In a survey or trial, unless standard working definitions are used the findings will not be reproducible. If we have formulated and used an operational definition of rheumatic fever, we can report how many cases of rheumatic fever we have found, with the assurance that another investigator, using the same definition, would have obtained similar findings. This is the basis of good research. Our rigid rules may mean the inclusion of cases who some clinicians think do not have the disease, as well as the exclusion of patients who some clinicians think do have the disease, or who they believe should be given the benefit of the doubt and treated as if they had the disease, in order to prevent complications. Such discrepancies, although we should try to minimize them by choosing a satisfactory definition, need not concern us unduly. When we report our findings concerning rheumatic fever, we know and can explain exactly what we mean by the term.

Unfortunately, few diseases have satisfactory and widely accepted operational definitions. The definitions provided in medical text books are usually conceptual ones. Here is one example:[1]

> *The common cold.* Definition: The common cold is a symptom complex caused by viral infection of the upper respiratory passages. Most precisely, the term applies to afebrile, acute coryza of viral origin. In the broadest sense, the common cold refers to any undifferentiated or mild lower respiratory infection. The main difference between the common

cold and other infections of the respiratory tract is the absence of fever, nonexudative inflammation, and relatively mild constitutional symptoms.

It is obvious that this definition does not aim to provide rigid rules for the diagnosis of a cold. The statement that a cold is caused by viral infection does not mean that it cannot be diagnosed without a virological examination. The last sentence of the definition does not mean that every mildly ill patient with a respiratory infection who has no fever and non-exudative inflammation (how precisely is that diagnosed?) has a cold. Fever seems to rule out a cold; but the description of clinical manifestations (on the next page of the textbook) is more permissive, saying only that fever 'of any significant degree' is absent.

OPERATIONAL DEFINITIONS

By contrast, operational definitions of diseases, like those of other variables, would be phrased in terms of objectively observable facts, and would be sufficiently clear and explicit to avoid ambiguity. In an investigation based on questions put weekly to a population sample, for example, 'a common cold' might be defined as 'a report of a stuffy or running nose'. The diagnosis may not be completely valid, as some cases of allergic rhinitis may be included, and some persons with running noses may not report them, but the definition has the advantages that it is unequivocal and eminently practical. Similarly, in an investigation based on examinations by general practitioners, it might be decided to define 'influenza' as 'a reddened or sore throat or a running or stuffy nose, together with fever, muscular pains, and general malaise and/or prostration; to be diagnosed only in the absence of signs of suppuration in the throat, such as acute suppurative pharyngitis or acute follicular tonsillitis; not to be diagnosed unless influenza virus has been detected in material either from the patient or from other patients in the neighbourhood examined within the previous month (if influenza virus has not been found, the diagnosis is "influenza-like syndrome")'.

Operational definitions of this sort are formulated in terms of *diagnostic criteria*; that is, the definition constitutes a set of rules for the diagnosis of the disease, based on the presence of specified criteria. These criteria may be *manifestations* or *causal experiences*.[2] Manifestational criteria include physical signs, symptoms, behaviour, the course of the illness, the response to specific therapy, etc. 'Causal' criteria are types of experience begun at a time preceding the illness, and often loosely called 'the cause' of the illness, e.g. difficult birth, an accident, exposure to lead, or contact with a case of measles. For a specific disease, either manifestational or experiential criteria, or both, may be used.

The diagnostic criteria of a disease are chosen from those manifestations and experiences which are relatively frequent among persons whom clinicians diagnose as suffering from the disease, by comparison with their frequency among well persons and among patients with other diseases. Certain of these manifestations and experiences are selected as diagnostic criteria, and rules are established for the diagnosis of the disease. For example, the disease may be diagnosed:

1. only when all the criteria are present or
2. only when a sufficient number of them are present or
3. only when specific combinations of criteria are present or
4. only when certain specific criteria (or specific combinations) are present, and certain other additional conditions are met (e.g. a sufficient number of 'minor' criteria are present) or
5. only when a score, obtained by adding defined weights allocated to each of the criteria, reaches a specified level; such a weighting system makes it possible to attach more diagnostic importance to some criteria than to others or
6. only when one of the above conditions is met, and in addition the presence of certain defined other diseases can be excluded.

As an illustration, the following rules were suggested for the diagnosis of anxiety neurosis:[3]

A. The following manifestations must be present: (1) Age of onset prior to 40. (2) Chronic nervousness with recurrent anxiety attacks manifested by apprehension, fearfulness, or sense of impending doom, with at least four of the following symptoms present during the majority of attacks: (a) dyspnoea, (b) palpitations, (c) chest pain or discomfort, (d) choking or smothering sensation, (e) dizziness and (f) paraesthesiae.
B. The anxiety attacks are essential to the diagnosis and must occur at times other than marked physical exertion or life-threatening situations, and in the absence of medical illness that *could* account for symptoms of anxiety. There must have been at least six anxiety attacks, each separated by at least a week from the others.
C. In the presence of other psychiatric illness(es) this diagnosis is made *only* if the criteria described in A and B antedate the onset of the other psychiatric illness by at least two years.

The rules may sometimes be validated by a comparison with diagnoses established by a 'better' set of criteria, i.e. an operational definition which, prima facie or because it incorporates more sophisticated or accurate tests, appears to approach closer to the conceptual definition of the disease. Usually, the decision on the usefulness of the rules is based solely on the degree to which the diagnoses they establish conform with those made on the basis of clinical judgements. Despite the obvious limitations of this method it is frequently the only practicable one.

Depending on the purpose of the study, a more or less specific definition may be used. If the aim is to identify persons who almost certainly have the disease, a highly specific definition is required, using criteria that may fail to identify many people who clinicians say have the disease. On the other hand, if the aim is to detect all persons who have the disease, even at the expense of falsely including many who do not have it, less stringent criteria are required.

The operational definition should not only distinguish the disease from other diseases, but should also serve to delimit it along its own biological gradient. If the disease is poliomyelitis, it may be wished to include only the relatively few persons with persistent paralysis, or the larger number with transient paralysis, or the considerably larger number who take ill but have no paralysis, or the even larger number who have subclinical infections.

The choice of the criteria to be used is heavily influenced by the methods by which the data are to be collected. Very different criteria may be used in a study based solely on interviews, one in which clinical examinations are performed, and one utilizing biochemical, microbiological, radiological and other diagnostic tests. Taking chronic bronchitis as an illustration, a definition specifying 'chronic inflammatory, fibrotic and atrophic changes in the bronchial structures' is obviously of limited applicability outside the autopsy room; most patients would be reluctant to donate their lungs or portions of their lungs for the purpose of this diagnostic test. At the other extreme, no medical training is required to diagnose chronic bronchitis if it is defined as 'the production of phlegm from the chest at least twice a day on most days for a least three months each year for two or more years',[4] the data being obtained by the use of a standard questionnaire.

The use of standard definitions is especially important in multicentre trials and other studies conducted in a number of co-operating general practices or other health services.

We have stated that few diseases have satisfactory and widely accepted working definitions. Paradoxically, difficulties frequently arise not because of a lack, but because of a surfeit of operational definitions. Different investigators use different definitions, and their findings are difficult to compare. If it is wished to produce comparable findings, the criteria selected should therefore conform with those used elsewhere.

For some diseases, standardized criteria have been proposed by expert committees. Use of these criteria facilitates comparisons. Even then there may be difficulties, since there may be differences in the way the criteria are understood or applied. Moreover, experts tend to change their recommendations from time to time: a comparison of 'old' and 'new' World Health Organization criteria for definite myocardial infarction, for example, showed that only 82% of the cases who met the old criteria also met the new criteria; the new definition required Minnesota coding of the ECGs (see p 99) rather than subjective appraisal.[5]

SIDE-STEPPING THE ISSUE

In many (or even most) investigations, the need to formulate diagnostic criteria is side-stepped, and diseases are operationally defined in terms of reports of their presence. That is, the process of diagnosis is left to someone else (usually a doctor, sometimes the patient, a relative, teacher, etc.), and a report of the disease is taken as evidence of its presence; e.g. 'haemorrhoids' may be operationally defined as:

a recorded diagnosis of 'haemorrhoids' or 'piles' (in a specified clinical record)

or as

a positive response to the question 'Did a doctor ever tell you you had haemorrhoids or piles?'

or as

a positive response to the question 'Do you have piles?'

The use of second-hand diagnostic information of this sort, not based on defined criteria, has obvious limitations. It is often the only practicable approach, however, and should by no means be rejected, particularly if the information is obtained from well equipped clinical services with a high standard of medical practice. If this 'imperfect' method is the only practical method, it should be used, provided that consideration is given to the effects this 'imperfection' may have on the findings, and that (if necessary) caution is used in interpreting the findings.

NOTES AND REFERENCES

1. Jackson G G 1982 In: Wyngaarden J B, Smith L H Jr (eds) Cecil text book of Medicine 16th edn. Saunders, Philadelphia, pp 1624–1626.
2. MacMahon B, Pugh T F 1970 Epidemiology: principles and methods. Little, Brown, Boston, Massachusetts, pp 47–54.
3. Feighner J P, Robins E, Guze S B, et al 1972 Diagnostic criteria for use in psychiatric research. Archives of General Psychiatry 26: 57.
4. Fletcher C M 1963 Some problems of diagnostic standardization using clinical methods, with special reference to chronic bronchitis. In: Pemberton J (ed) Epidemiology: reports on research and teaching. Oxford University Press, Oxford, p 253.
5. Beaglehole R, Stewart A W, Butler M 1987 Comparability of old and new World Health Organization criteria for definite myocardial infarction. International Journal of Epidemiology 16: 373.

12. Scales of measurement

As part of the process of clarifying each of the variables to be studied, its scale of measurement should be specified.

TYPES OF SCALE

The scale of measurement may be *categorical* (consisting of two or more mutually exclusive categories) or *metric*.

A categorical scale consists of mutually exclusive categories (classes). If these do not fall into a natural order, the scale is *nominal*. Numbers may be used to identify the categories, but these are 'code numbers' with no quantitative significance. Examples are:

1. *Marital status*: single, married, widowed, divorced.
2. *Religion*: Christian, Jewish, Muslim, Buddhist, freethinker, other.
3. *Type of anaemia*: 1, iron deficiency anaemia; 2, other deficiency anaemias; 3, hereditary haemolytic anaemias; 4, acquired haemolytic anaemias; 5, aplastic anaemia; 6, other anaemias.

If the categories fall into what is regarded as a natural order, the scale is *ordinal*. The scale shows ranks, or positions on a ladder; each class shows the same situational relationship to the class that follows it. If numbers are used, they indicate the positions of the categories in the series. Examples are:

1. *Social class*: I, II, III, IV, V.
2. *Years of education*: 0, 1–5, 6–9, 10–12, more than 12.
3. *Severity of a disease*: mild, moderate, severe.
4. *Limitation of activity*: 0, none; 1, limited activity but not home-bound; 2, home-bound but not bed-bound; 3, bed-bound.

An ordinal scale is 'stronger' than a nominal one, in the sense that it provides more information. Where there is a choice, use of an ordinal scale is preferable.

A scale may be a mixed nominal and ordinal one, i.e. some but not all of the categories may be ranked. A scale including a number of ranked categories and also a category of 'unclassifiable' is of this sort—the scale as a whole is nominal, but it is ordinal if the 'unclassifiable' class is excluded. An example is Katz's Index of Independence in Daily Living, which includes seven graded categories ranging from independence in feeding, continence and four other functions, through dependence in various defined combinations of functions, to dependence in all six functions, and then has a category for persons not fitting into the previous classes.[1]

A scale with only two categories is a *dichotomy* (or *binary scale*).[2] Many statistical procedures are applicable to dichotomies but not to scales with three or more categories. Numbers may be used as code numbers, or to indicate the presence or absence of an attribute (1 and 0 respectively). Examples are:

1. *Agreement with a statement*: agree, disagree.
2. *Sex*: 1, male; 2, female.
3. *Presence of a disease*: 0, absent; 1, present.
4. *Occurrence of headaches*: 0, no; 1, yes.

Metric (dimensional) scales use numbers that indicate the quantity of what is being measured. They have two features: firstly, equal differences between any pairs of numbers in the scale mean equal differences in the attribute being measured, i.e. the difference between any two values reflects the magnitude of the difference in the attribute—the difference in temperature between 22 and 26°C is the same as that between 32 and 36°C; this makes the scale an *interval scale*. Secondly, in some metric scales, zero indicates absence of the attribute, as a consequence of which the ratio between any two values indicates the ratio between the amounts of the attribute—an income of $1000 is twice as high as an income of $500; this additional feature makes the scale a *ratio scale*. Most metric scales have both these features; exceptional ones, like the Centigrade scale for temperature, are interval but not ratio scales—0° does not mean 'absence of heat', and 20° is therefore not 'twice as hot' as 10°. Examples of ratio scales are:

1. *Weight*: measured in kilograms or pounds.

2. *Mortality rate*: number of deaths per 1000 persons at risk.
3. *Feminine beauty*: measured in milli-helens.[3]

A metric scale provides more information than an ordinal one, and is to be preferred when there is a choice.

Metric scales may be *continuous* or *discrete*. The scale is continuous if an infinite number of values is possible along a continuum, e.g. when measuring height or cholesterol concentration. It is discrete if only certain values along the scale are possible—a woman's parity, for example, cannot be 2.35.

A metric scale may be 'collapsed' into broader categories by grouping values together, e.g.

Income (in monetary units): 0–49, 50–99, 100–149, etc.

If equal *class intervals* are used, as in this example, the scale can still often be treated as metric. Strictly speaking, however, it may now be an ordinal scale, since the individual values may not be uniformly spread within the classes, and the intervals between the average incomes of people in adjacent classes may hence not be equal. The scale is degraded to an ordinal scale if an 'open-ended' category is used (for instance, a top income group of '500 or more'). An accurate mean value cannot be calculated from such a scale. Similarly, the scale becomes an ordinal one if the class intervals vary, e.g. 0–49, 50–199, 200–399, etc.

The selection of a scale for measuring a variable is partly determined by the variable itself and the methods available for measuring it. Marital status, type of work, and type of anaemia cannot be measured by metric scales. For most variables, however, alternative methods of measurement are available.

Clearly, decisions concerning scales of measurement may influence the methods by which data will be collected. If it is decided to measure the frequency or severity of headaches (ordinal scales) instead of merely determining whether the subject suffers from headaches (using a 'yes–no' nominal scale), different questions are required. Scales of measurement are often printed in questionnaires in the form of alternative responses to questions, and also on examination schedules and other record forms, where the appropriate categories are indicated by checking, ringing, or underlining (see pp 211–215).

Different statistical procedures are appropriate for different kinds of scale. The scale used when the data are collected, however, is not necessarily the one that will be used throughout the analysis. Observations concerning a variable measured by one kind of scale may be analysed by a procedure suited to another kind of scale, in accordance with the research hypothesis and the purpose of the analysis. Age (measured by an interval scale) may indeed be treated as an interval scale variable, e.g. when calculating a mean age or examining a correlation between age and some other variable. But for some purposes it may be appropriate to use a nominal scale, merely dividing the subjects into different age groups, and not assuming a monotonic relationship (i.e. a consistent increase or decrease in the other variable when people in younger and older categories are compared). Ethnic group is measured by a nominal scale; but it may be treated as an ordinal scale variable by arranging the categories in a specific sequence, in an analysis designed to see whether its categories have an ordered relationship with another variable.

During the planning phase, thought should be given to the scales that will be used when the data are analysed. At this stage it is often helpful to construct *skeleton* or *dummy tables*, i.e. tables without figures or containing fictional figures respectively, incorporating the variables under consideration. If there are categories, they should be specified in the column or row headings. At this stage it is not essential to decide precisely how the finer categories will be 'collapsed' into broader categories for the purposes of analysis. It is often desirable to defer such decisions, since they may be difficult to make without knowing the actual distribution of the values. If doubt exists about the way a variable will be treated in the analysis, care should be taken to collect data in such a way as to leave the options open.

CRITERIA OF A SATISFACTORY SCALE

A satisfactory scale of measurement is one that meets the following seven requirements (the last four apply only to categorical scales).

1. Appropriate
2. Practicable
3. Sufficiently powerful
4. Clearly defined categories
5. Sufficient categories
6. Comprehensive
7. Mutually exclusive

1. It is *appropriate* for use in the study, keeping in mind the conceptual definition of the variable and the objectives of the study. Occupations, for instance, may be classified in different ways, depending on whether the purpose is to use occupation as a measure of social class, of habitual physical activity, or of exposure to specific physical and chemical hazards. Similarly, different classifications may be used for the region of birth of immigrants, depending on whether the variable is to be used as an indicator of environmental conditions in childhood, of ethnic group, or of genetic attributes. In measuring birth weights, it may be decided to use categories extending evenly along the whole weight spectrum, or, if the specific subject of inquiry is the effect of low birth weight, to use narrow categories for babies of low birth weight and broad categories for heavier babies.

2. It is a *practicable* scale—one that is geared to the methods that will be used in collecting the information. For example, if the data are to be obtained from records that list marital status as 'single', 'married', 'widowed' and 'divorced', there is no point in deciding upon a more elaborate scale of measurement, e.g. including 'married once', 'married more than once', etc. Account should be taken of the precision of the methods to be used in collecting the data. Can accurate ages be obtained in terms of years and months, or only in terms of years? If people tend to 'round off' their ages ('I am 40 years old', '50 years old', etc.), a scale showing each year separately will have only spurious precision (see p 153). Will it be possible to get detailed data on income or the number of cigarettes smoked per day, or is it only possible to use broad categories? Is the balance to be used for weighing sufficiently discriminatory to warrant measurements in tenths of kilograms, or should whole kilograms be used? Is there any point in recording liver enlargement in centimetres, if tests have shown a negligible correlation between measurements made by different physicians on the same patients?

3. The scale is *powerful* enough to satisfy the objectives of the study. If there is a choice, an ordinal scale should be used rather than a nominal one, and a metric scale rather than a categorical one. An analysis using the whole spectrum of haemoglobin levels is likely to be more informative than one using a dichotomy, such as 'below 12 g per 100 ml' and '12 or more g per 100 ml'. In measuring an attitude an ordinal scale should be used, based on

the provision of graded alternative responses to a question or on a score derived from the responses to a series of questions, rather than a simple dichotomy such as 'agree–disagree' or 'important–unimportant'.

4. The categories are *clearly defined*. Wherever necessary, operational definitions should be formulated not only for the variable, but for the categories. This applies especially to nominal and ordinal scales. If cases of a disease are to be classified as 'active' and 'healed', or patients with a malignant neoplasm according to the stage of the disorder, these categories need careful definition. In the case of numerical measurements decisions may be needed on the number of decimal places to be used, and on how values are to be rounded off—downwards, or to the nearest number. It is usually preferable to round off downwards, so that the category '73 kg', for example, includes all weights between 73.0 and 73.9 kg; if this is done it must be remembered that the average value of the weights in this category will be 73.5 kg.

5. The scale contains *sufficient categories*. While the number of categories should not be multiplied unnecessarily, the compression of data into too few categories may lead to a loss of useful information. For example, if immigrants from North Africa have a particularly high rate of mortality from cerebrovascular disease, this fact may become less obvious or may be completely masked if they are included in a broader category of 'immigrants from Africa and Asia'. Often 'articulated' scales are used—scales containing categories that 'branch', like the bones of the limbs—i.e. categories which are divided into subcategories and, if necessary, sub-subcategories; the use of such a scale leaves the options open for a later decision as to the use of broad or narrow categories. With numerical data it is often similarly advisable to collect the information in a detailed form and to decide later whether to use the full scale or a 'collapsed' one (or both). With numerical data the use of too few categories may prevent the calculation of an accurate mean.

6. The scale is *collectively exhaustive (comprehensive)*. It provides a niche for the classification of every subject. This may necessitate the inclusion of one or more of the following categories:

Other

Not applicable, e.g. information on the duration of marriage may be collected only from persons who are at present married;

in this case the scale used may be 'under 5 years', '5–9.9 years', '10–19.9 years', '20–29.9 years', '30–39.9 years', '40 years and more', and 'not applicable'.

Unknown (it may sometimes be desirable to subdivide this category, e.g. to distinguish between subjects who did not know the answer to a question and those with information lacking for other reasons: the question was not asked, the response was illegible, a page of the completed questionnaire was mislaid, etc.)

7. The categories are *mutually exclusive*. Each item of information should fit into only one place along the scale. For example, a scale including both '70 to 80' and '80 to 90' is generally unacceptable, as '80' could fit into either of these categories. Similarly, if a scale includes 'married' and 'remarried', a remarried person could fit into either category. If a scale for measuring the conditions producing disability includes the categories 'blindness' and 'deafness', either a clear rule should be formulated whereby persons who are both blind and deaf are assigned to one of these categories, or the scale should include the categories 'blind, not deaf', 'deaf, not blind' and 'blind and deaf'. In the Minnesota code for ECG findings (see p 99), where different codable items may coexist in the same scale of measurement (e.g. that for T wave items), only one is coded, the order of precedence being clearly stated.

INTERNATIONAL CLASSIFICATION OF DISEASES

The International Classification of Diseases (ICD), published by WHO[4] and now in its ninth revision (ICD-9), is widely used as a nominal scale for the categorization of diseases. Each disease category is given a three-digit code number, and almost all categories are further divided into subcategories with four-digit numbers. There are also some optional fifth-digit subclassifications.

Since our principles of nosology are far from rational the arrangement of the ICD is arbitrary. Some diseases are classified by their aetiology ('infectious and parasitic diseases'), some by their site ('diseases of the respiratory system'), some by a pathological feature ('neoplasms'), some by age at onset ('certain conditions originating in the perinatal period'), etc. Neoplasms are subclassified by their sites, but an optional supplementary histological classification is provided. Injuries are subclassified by their nature, but there is a supplementary code for external causes; the use of this 'E code' for injuries is mandatory for the preparation of statistics on underlying causes of death. Special short lists are provided for the tabulation of mortality and morbidity.

An innovation in the ninth revision is the provision of dual codes for some diseases—a dagger code (marked with a †) for classifying the disease according to its aetiology, and an optional asterisk code (*) for classifying it according to its manifestation. Tuberculous meningitis can be coded 013.0† (which appears in the section devoted to tuberculosis), 320.4* (in the section for meningitis), or both. The new asterisk codes would, it was thought, add to the value of the ICD in the planning and evaluation of medical care. If one uses the asterisk coding it is important to say so. If *both* codes are used, the categories of the classification are not mutually exclusive.

A further innovation is the incorporation of 'glossary descriptions' of mental disorders, in order 'to assist the person making the diagnosis, who should do so on the basis of the descriptions rather than the category titles, which may differ in meaning from place to place'. These descriptions fall far short of ideal operational definitions.[5]

There is also a classification of conditions or circumstances that are *not* diseases. This is the 'V code', which lists a variety of reasons, other than illness, that may bring a person into contact with a health service. It includes immunization, contraceptive management, antenatal care, etc.

Coding is best left to experienced coders. One can do it oneself, but care must be taken. To code a disease, it is first looked up in the index, which is published as a separate volume. The index includes many diagnostic terms which are not specifically stated in the classification itself. After using the index, reference should be made to the appropriate item in the classification, since this may contain a note leading to a modification of the code number. The conventions used in the classification must be clearly understood if the book is to be used effectively.[6] Before drawing inferences from tabulations based on the ICD it is wise to examine the details of the classification, so as to be sure of what is and what is not included in the various categories.

Adaptations of the ICD include an American 'clinical modification' (ICD-9-CM),[7] which is more detailed than the ICD; it divides the ICD's four-digit categories into more specific five-digit categories.

CLASSIFICATIONS FOR USE IN PRIMARY CARE

The International Classification of Health Problems in Primary Care (ICHPPC) is a classification designed primarily to permit a general or family practitioner to code diagnoses or other problems at the time of the patient encounter.[8] It includes diseases (classified more simply than in the ICD), important signs and symptoms, social and family problems, forms of preventive care, and administrative procedures.

A newer version (ICHPPC-2-Defined), which is an adaptation of the ninth revision of the ICD, contains definitions of most of the rubrics. These were designed as 'the briefest possible definitions which would reduce variability in coding', and stipulate criteria that *must* be fulfilled if miscoding is to be avoided. As examples, a diagnosis is coded as 'acute upper respiratory infection' (a category that includes colds, nasopharyngitis, pharyngitis and rhinitis) only if two criteria are met: (1) evidence of acute inflammation of the nasal or pharyngeal mucosa and (2) absence of criteria for more specifically defined acute respiratory infections listed in the classification. A diagnosis of 'anxiety disorder, anxiety state' requires both of the following: (1) 'generalized and persistent anxiety or anxious mood, which cannot be associated with, or is disproportionately large in response to, a specific psycho-social stressor, stimulus, or event' and (2) 'no evidence of other psychological disorders'. For the rubric 'problems with aged parents or in-laws' the criterion (surprise! surprise!) is 'a problem experienced by an adult (age 18 or over) with his parents or in-laws'.

The authors stress that the definitions are not intended to serve as a guide to diagnosis. Their purpose is to reduce chances of miscoding *after* a diagnosis has been made, and not to reduce diagnostic error.

The International Classification of Primary Care (ICPC)[9] permits patients' encounters to be classified not only according to the physician's diagnosis or assessment of the health problem (using the ICHPPC codes), but also according to the reason for the encounter as expressed by the patient, and the nature of the diagnostic and therapeutic interventions undertaken in the process of care. One or more of these axes may be used. The patient's reason for encounter (which may need clarification by the care provider) may be a symptom, a disease, getting a prescription, test result or certificate, etc. The 'process' components include various diagnostic, preventive, therapeutic and administrative procedures, and referrals. The ICPC is consistent with the use of problem-oriented clinical records, which use the SOAP acronym: S = subjective (the patient's reason for the encounter), O = objective signs, A = assessment (diagnosis) and P = plan (the process of care or intervention); but objective signs are not classified by the ICPC. The authors suggest use of the ICPC as a basis for an information system based on disease episodes (from onset to resolution) for which there may be more than one encounter.

NOTES AND REFERENCES

1. Katz S, Ford A B, Moskowitz R W, Jackson B A, Jaffe M W 1963 Studies of illness in the aged: the index of ADL: a standardized measure of biological and psychosocial function. Journal of the American Medical Association 185: 914.
2. *Dichotomies* can be treated not only as nominal, but also as ordinal, interval, or (in some instances) ratio scales. Many statistical procedures are applicable to dichotomies but not to nominal scales that have three or more categories. Dichotomies and other nominal scales can usefully be regarded as different types of scales.
3. A milli-helen is 'the quantity of beauty required to launch exactly one ship'. Dickinson R E 1958 The Observer (letter, Feb. 23rd).
4. World Health Organization 1977 Manual of the international statistical classification of diseases, injuries, and causes of death, 1975 revision, vol 1. WHO, Geneva. Also ibid. (1978) vol 2.
5. The following definition of 'anxiety states', a rubric which includes 'anxiety neurosis', 'anxiety reaction' and 'panic disorder', may be compared with the definition shown on p 777. 'Various combinations of physical and mental manifestations of anxiety, not attributable to real danger and occurring either in attacks or as a persisting state. The anxiety is usually diffuse and may extend to panic. Other neurotic features such as obsessional or hysterical symptoms may be present but do not dominate the clinical picture.'
6. The ICD uses round brackets (. . .)to enclose words or phrases whose presence or absence does not matter. Square brackets [. . .] enclose alternative wordings or explanatory phrases. Terms preceding a colon are incomplete, and must be completed by one of the modifiers that follow the colon. 'NOS' stands for 'not otherwise specified'. As an example, part of the specification of 464.0 Acute laryngitis reads:

   Laryngitis (acute):
   NOS
   Haemophilus influenzae [H. influenzae]
   Ulcerative

   This means that diagnoses of 'laryngitis' and 'acute laryngitis' are coded 464.0 if they stand alone or are accompanied by the modifiers 'Haemophilus influenzae' (of which 'H. influenzae' is an alternative wording) or 'ulcerative'. 'Streptococcal laryngitis' would not be coded 464.0, since it is not included in the above extract or in the remainder of the specification. Some exclusions are specifically stated; e.g. 'Excludes: influenzal laryngitis (487.1)'.
7. The International Classification of Diseases, 9th Revision, Clinical Modification. ICD-9-CM. Commission on Professional and Hospital Activities, Ann Arbor, Michigan.
8. World Organization of National Colleges, Academies and Academic Associations of General Practitioners/Family Physicians (WONCA). Classification Committee (1983) ICHPPC-2-Defined, 3rd edn. Oxford University Press, Oxford.
9. Lamberts H, Wood M (eds) 1987 ICPC: International Classification of Primary Care. Oxford University Press, Oxford.

13. Composite scales

Variables based on two or more other variables may be termed 'composite variables'. Examples are: (1) caloric intake, which is calculated from the intake of a variety of foodstuffs, (2) the stage of a disease, which may be based on a set of symptoms and clinical signs, and (3) an attitude, when measured by the responses to a series of separate questions. The scales used for measuring composite variables may be termed 'composite scales'.

The manner in which the component data are brought together into a composite scale is usually decided upon in advance, using rules that enter into the operational definition of the composite variable. There are also techniques that require the collection and analysis of the component data before deciding how to combine them.

The scale may be based upon *combinations of categories*. For instance, hypertension may be defined as a systolic blood pressure of 160 mmHg or more together with a diastolic pressure of 95 mmHg or more, and the absence of hypertension as a systolic pressure below 140 mmHg together with a diastolic pressure below 90 mmHg.[1] If other combinations of systolic and diastolic pressures are placed in an intermediate or 'borderline' group, this provides a composite scale of the ordinal type. The scale might be elaborated by adding 'and/or receiving specific treatment for hypertension' to the definition of hypertension, and adding 'and not under treatment' to the definitions of the other categories. A composite scale of the nominal type is sometimes referred to as a *typology*.

Composite scales may also be based upon the use of *formulae*. Examples are: the length of gestation, which is usually estimated from the date of onset of the last menstrual period and the date at which pregnancy ended; average family income per head; adiposity indices based on weight and height; and all rates.

Use may also be made of *composite scores*, arrived at by adding together separate scores allotted to the component items. There are two types of composite score, depending on how the scores are allotted to the individual items; raw and weighted scores.

The simplest kind of *raw score* is based upon items each given alternative scores of 0 or 1. This method is often used for scoring questionnaires like the Cornell Medical Index (CMI),[2] which contains 195 'yes–no' questions about the presence of symptoms, illnesses, etc. The score is the total number of positive responses (taking every 'yes' as 1 and every 'no' as 0). Similarly, the diagnosis of rheumatoid arthritis may be based on a score expressing the total number of specified diagnostic criteria that are fulfilled.[3]

'Likert-type' scales,[4] which are often used in studies of attitudes, are raw scores based on graded alternative responses to each of a series of questions. For example, the subject may be asked to indicate his degree of agreement with each of a series of statements relevant to the attitude. A score is attached to each possible response, e.g. '1, strongly approve; 2, approve; 3, undecided; 4, disapprove; 5, strongly disapprove', and the sum of these scores is used as the composite score. The 'undecided' category is sometimes omitted in such scales, to force the respondent to take a stand. A commonly used Likert-type scale is the *Apgar score* used to appraise the status of newborn infants. This is the sum of the points (0, 1 or 2) allotted for each of five items: heart rate (over 100 beats per minute, 2 points; slower, 1 point; no beat, 0), respiratory effort, muscle tone, response to stimulation by a catheter in the nostril, and skin colour.

Weighted scores are based upon the allocation of different weights to the component items. These weights may be determined arbitrarily, on the basis of the apparent respective importance of the items. For instance, in a study of the quality of medical care, scores were given for the quality of records, the quality of diagnostic management and the quality of treatment and follow-up. These scores were then combined into a composite score, using the following weights: records, 30%; diagnostic management, 40%; treatment and follow-up, 30%.[5] The weighting of items may be based on the relative importance attributed to them by a set of experts (see Ch. 19). It may also be determined by a careful analysis of data collected in a previous investigation. For example, following a detailed examination of patients in a metabolic laboratory a 'clinical diagnostic index of thyrotoxicosis' was developed: scores were allocated to various complaints and simple clinical signs (preference for cold, +5; palpable thyroid, +3; increase in weight, −13; etc.) and it was proposed that if the sum total of these scores was 20 or more, this could be taken to indicate the presence of thyrotoxicosis.[6]

Composite scales may also be based on the use of a *gradated set of items*. This method is often used in the study of attitudes. The subject is asked, for example, whether he agrees or disagrees with a series of statements, which have been so selected that each has a defined relative position along the continuum of the attitude being measured. The subject's attitude may thus be measured by determining with which statements he indicates agreement. The statements may be so selected that each respondent may be expected to agree with only one or two statements and disagree with all the others (*Thurstone-type scale*[7]) or they may be so selected that he may be expected to agree with all statements up to or after a particular point in the series (cumulative scale).[7]

Any composite score based on arbitrary decisions about the inclusion and weighting of items is open to criticism unless its validity can be demonstrated (see Ch. 16). If tests of validity are not feasible, the minimal requirement is an examination of the findings to see whether they are consistent with the assumption that the various items are measures of a single attribute. Of course this in itself cannot guarantee that the scale does in fact measure a single dimension, or that what the scale measures is indeed what the investigator wants to measure.

For an additive scale, one way of examining internal consistency is to calculate the correlation between each item and the total score of the other items; poorly correlated items can then be excluded from the scale. Another useful measure of 'consistency–reliability' is *Cronbach's alpha coefficient*; a value of 0.7 or higher is generally regarded as satisfactory, indicating that the items may be measures of much the same attribute.[8] Since correlations may occur by chance in any sample, it is generally wise to do these analyses in different parts of the study population (say, men and women, or randomly selected groups). Internal consistency is sometimes measured by the 'split-half' method, in which a questionnaire designed to measure a single attribute is divided, purposively or randomly, into two halves; the whole questionnaire is administered, and then the findings yielded by the two halves are compared; if there is little variation, this is taken as evidence of consistency.

Sometimes the method of combining the items into a composite scale is decided by hindsight, by waiting until the data have been collected and then analysing the results to see how the separate items 'hang together'. One way of doing this is *factor analysis*, a complicated procedure that examines data for a group of variables, reports the fundamental dimensions that underlie the data (calling them 'factor 1', 'factor 2', etc.), and states what weights should be attached to the items in order to measure each dimension. The investigator then generally sees whether he can 'give a name to' the characteristic measured by each factor. This kind of analysis too is most convincing if it is replicated in different samples. The measurement of *health locus-of-control* can be cited to illustrate the use of factor analysis. Sets of questions were devised in order to grade people according to their belief that their health was under their own control (internal locus-of-control) or determined by external factors. But factor analysis revealed several dimensions, not just one: there were correlated but distinct beliefs, including belief in personal control of health, belief in control by health providers and others, and belief in the role of chance.[9]

Complicated computations can sometimes be avoided by using a *Guttman scale* (or *scalogram*).[10] As an example of such a scale, consider the following three 'yes-no' questions: 1. 'Do you weigh more than 50 kg?' 2. 'Do you weigh more than 75 kg?' 3. 'Do you weigh more than 100 kg?' The only four possible combinations of correct replies (to questions 1, 2, and 3 respectively) are 'no-no-no', 'yes-no-no', 'yes-yes-no' and 'yes-yes-yes'. Question 2 cannot be answered 'yes' unless question 1 is also answered 'yes', and question 3 cannot be answered 'yes' unless both questions 1 and 2 are also answered 'yes'. If the questions are answered correctly all the responses will conform with the above four combinations ('scale types') and there will be no deviant combinations of responses. There are four scale types ('no-no-no' = scale type 0, 'yes-no-no' = scale type 1, 'yes-yes-no' = scale type 2, and 'yes-yes-yes' = scale type 3), comprising an ordinal scale, and each individual's position along the continuum (in this case, of weight) can be inferred from his responses.

The advantage of the technique is that we do not need to be certain in advance that the items will make up a Guttman scale. In a questionnaire we can include a number of items that appear relevant to the variable we wish to measure, and that we think represent different points along the continuum of variation. Then, after collecting the data we see whether the questions, or some of them, are 'scalable'; that is, is there a set of questions with responses that all, or almost all, fall into the 'scale types' of a Guttman scale? If there are such questions, this not only provides a simple way of combining responses into a composite scale, but it also supports the probability that the items do in fact 'hang together' to represent a single dimension. The main criteria of 'scalability' are (1) that the 'coefficient of reproducibility' (the proportion of responses that fit into 'scale types') must be at least 90%,[11] and (2) that the frequency of no single deviant ('non-scale') type should exceed 5% of the sample size. If a few responses do not fall into scale types, they can be assigned to scale types by the use of arbitrary rules. Guttman scales may be used for attitudes, dietary habits, clinical manifestations, or any other attribute.

The construction of a good composite scale is never easy. However, it is comforting that *how* a number of items are brought together into a composite scale may not be of great consequence, if the items have a clear-cut ranking of their categories and do in fact measure a single dimension. This was shown in a survey of disability in London, where information was obtained about the capacity to perform a number of activities. Four separate composite scales were developed, including a Guttman scale (which gave a coefficient of reproducibility of 94%) and an additive scale in which each activity, and the degree of difficulty in performing it, was given an arbitrary score based on the criteria used by local social workers for defining handicap. The scores yielded by the different methods turned out to be highly correlated with each other.[12]

NOTES AND REFERENCES

1. Expert Committee on Cardiovascular Disease and Hypertension 1959 Hypertension and coronary heart disease: classification and criteria for epidemiological studies. WHO Technical Report Series No. 168. WHO, Geneva.

2. Brodman K, Erdman A J Jr, Wolff H G 1956 Cornell Medical Index Health Questionnaire (Manual). Cornell University Medical College, New York; Abramson J H 1966 The Cornell Medical Index as an epidemiological tool. American Journal of Public Health 56: 287.

3. Ropes M W, Bennett G A, Cobb S, Jacox R, Jessar R A 1957 Proposed diagnostic criteria for rheumatoid arthritis. Annals of the Rheumatic Diseases 16: 118.

4. For futher details of Likert-type scales, see Selltiz C, Wrightsman L S, Cook S W 1976 Research methods in social relations, 3rd edn. Holt, Rinehart & Winston, New York, pp 418–421.

5. Morehead M A 1967 The medical audit as an operational tool. American Journal of Public Health 57: 1643.

6. Crooks J, Murray I P C, Wayne E J 1959 Statistical methods applied to the clinical diagnosis of thyrotoxicosis. Quarterly Journal of Medicine 28: 211.

7. For further details on Thurstone-type and cumulative scales, see Selltiz et al, (1976; see note 4) pp 413–417 and 421–422. See papers on the construction of a Thurstone-type scale for the seriousness of sleep problems (showing that the task is not as simple as it seems): McKenna S P, Hunt S M, McEwen J 1981 Weighting the seriousness of perceived health problems using Thurstone's method of paired comparisons. International Journal of Epidemiology 10: 93; Kind P 1982 A comparison of two models for scaling health indicators. International Journal of Epidemiology 11: 271. For examples, see Shaw W E, Wright J M 1967 Scales for the measurement of attitudes. McGraw-Hill, New York; Miller D C 1977 Handbook of research design and social

measurement, 2nd edn. Part 4. David McKay, New York. Scales that may be treated as interval scales (*Thurstone-type equal-appearing interval scales*) can be constructed by asking a number of judges to rate the degree to which each item reflects the characteristics being studied; this is a popular technique among sociologists.

8. Tests for the internal consistency of a scale are described by Guilford J P, Fruchter B 1978 Fundamental statistics in psychology and education, 6th edn. McGraw-Hill, Singapore, pp 327–430, 461–467; also, see SPSS-x User's Guide, 3rd edn, 1989. SPSS, Chicago, Chapter 46. For pocket calculator programs, see Abramson J H, Peritz E 1983 Calculator Programs for the Health Sciences. Oxford University Press, New York.

9. Lau R R, Ware J E Jr 1981 Refinements in the measurement of health-specific locus-of-control beliefs. Medical Care 19: 1147; Ware J E Jr 1984 Methodological considerations in the selection of health status assessment procedures. In: Wenger N K, Mattson M E, Furberg C D, Elinson J (eds) Assessment of Quality of Life in Clinical Trials of Cardiovascular Therapies. LeJacq Publishing (Way market-Doyma, New York), pp 87–111.

10. The *scalogram (Guttman scale) technique* is described in detail by Stoufter S A, Guttman L, Suchman E A, Lazarsfeld P F, Star S A, Clausen J A 1966 Measurement and prediction. Wiley, New York; and briefly by Goode W J, Hatt P K 1952 Methods of Social Research. McGraw-Hill, New York, pp 285–295; and Riley M W 1963 Sociological Research, vol 1, pp 470–478; vol 2, pp 97–99. Harcourt, Brace and World, New York.

11. A high coefficient of reproducibility is not sufficient evidence that there is a Guttman scale, since a proportion of the responses will inevitably fall into scale types even if there is no true patterning. This proportion is determined by the marginal frequencies of the items (i.e. the numbers of 'yes' and 'no' responses to each question), and it may be over 90%. To overcome this, a *coefficient of scalability* can be calculated, based upon a comparison of the coefficient of reproducibility with the '*minimum marginal reproducibility*' or the '*coefficient of reproducibility by chance*' (Riley 1963 vol 1; see note 10) calculated from the marginal frequencies. For pocket-calculator programs, see Abramson & Peritz (1983; see note 8).

12. Bebbington A C 1977 British Journal of Preventive and Social Medicine 31: 122.

14. Methods of collecting data

During the planning phase of the study it is necessary to decide upon the method to be used for collecting information concerning each of the variables listed for investigation. If there are two or more study groups or populations, separate consideration may have to be given to the methods to be used in each. Preferably these methods should not differ, but differences are sometimes unavoidable.

The methods of collecting information may be broadly classified as follows:

1. *Observation,* i.e. the use of techniques varying from simple visual observation to those requiring special skills, e.g. clinical examinations, or sophisticated equipment or facilities, such as radiographic, biochemical and microbiological examinations.
2. *Interviews and self-administered questionnaires* (see Chs 17 to 19).
3. *The use of documentary sources* — clinical records and other personal records, death certificates, published mortality statistics, census publications, etc. (see Ch 20). Data derived from these sources are called *secondary*, as opposed to the *primary data* (based on observation, interviews or questionnaires) first recorded by the investigators.

There are usually alternative methods of collecting the desired data. Information about hypertension, for example, may be obtained by measuring blood pressure (observation), by asking the subjects whether a doctor has ever told them they have 'high blood pressure' (interview), or by referring to medical records (documents). Furthermore, observational measurements of blood pressure may be made sitting or lying, with or without a prior rest period, by intra-arterial pressure measurements, ordinary indirect sphygmomanometry, an electronic gadget, etc. Diet may be studied by weighing the food eaten, by asking questions, or by using written records in which the subject has noted the amounts and types of foodstuffs eaten. If questions are asked, they may refer to the food eaten in the last 24 hours or in the last 48 hours, or the frequency with which different food items are usually consumed, etc. Exposure to tobacco smoke can be studied by asking questions about the smoking habits of the subjects or the people with whom they live or work. It can also be studied by measuring the concentration of carbon monoxide in expired air or of thiocyanate or cotinine in the saliva or other body fluids. If attitudes, feelings, values or motivations are to be measured, they will usually be inferred from the responses to questions, a large variety of which can be devised; sometimes they may be inferred from observations or documentary records of actions, or from the responses to projective tests (in which the subject is required to react to a picture or other stimulus).

Different methods may yield very different information. The prevalence of chronic diseases, for example, may be studied by interviews, or by conducting examinations or using existing clinical records. Most comparisons have shown very little correspondence between information obtained from interview surveys and that obtained by medical examinations. There is usually considerable under-reporting of chronic diseases in interviews. Laymen are not physicians, and cannot be expected to supply the same information. They differ in what they know, and they differ in their language and concepts ('kidney trouble' is by no means the same thing as 'renal disease'). On the other hand, neither are physicians laymen, and interviews are preferable to medical sources when information is sought on symptoms or degree of disability, or on mild short-term diseases that are unlikely to bring the patient to a doctor or to be present at the time of an examination conducted in the course of a survey. As far as 'general health' is concerned, it has been said that 'the bulk of the research evidence can be interpreted as indicating that a clinical assessment of general health and the responses to survey questions about health are only slightly correlated phenomena'.[1] Which of these methods gives more useful information is open to question. Mortality has been found to be higher for elderly people who rate their health as unfavourable than for those who rate their health as favourable, independently of the physician's rating of their health. In at least one study, mortality was more closely related to the subjective rating than to an objective rating.[2]

Different medical sources may also yield differing information. Death certificates or autopsies will not reveal cases who have survived; official notifications of disease may not cover all cases; clinical records will tell us nothing about patients who have not attended for care or have attended and been misdiagnosed; and cross-sectional surveys will reveal only what is present at the time of the examination—they will not reveal myocardial infarcts that have healed, leaving no symptoms or electrocardiographic traces, although ample evidence of the disease may be found in previous clinical records, and they will not reveal cases who have died. In fact, any morbidity survey using information from only one source is likely to be incomplete.

The choice of methods of data collection is largely based on the accuracy of the information they will yield. In this context, 'accuracy' refers not only to correspondence between the information and objective reality—although this certainly enters into the concept — but also to the information's relevance. The issue is the extent to which the method will provide a precise measure of the variable the investigator wishes to study. Two aspects of accuracy, reliability and validity, will be discussed in Chapters 15 and 16.

The selection of a method is also based on practical considerations, such as:

1. The need for personnel, skills, equipment, etc. in relation to what is available, and the urgency with which results are needed.
2. The acceptability of the procedures to the subjects—the absence of inconvenience, unpleasantness, or untoward consequences.
3. The probability that the method will provide a good coverage, i.e. will supply the required information about all or almost all members of the population or sample. If many people will not know the answer to a question, the question is not an appropriate one. If many of the clinical records of a factory health service do not show blood pressure, the use of these records is not a very practicable way of studying blood pressure. If determinations of triglycerides in the blood serum can only be usefully performed on subjects who are fasting, this may be a difficult condition to meet in many members of a healthy population living at home, although the test may be a practicable one in a hospital situation.
4. The investigator's familiarity with a study procedure may be a valid consideration, but keep the 'Law of the Hammer' in mind: 'Give a small boy a hammer, and he will find that everything he encounters needs pounding. It comes as no particular surprise to discover that a scientist formulates problems in a way which requires for their solution just those techniques in which he himself is especially skilled'.[3]

These practical aspects should be considered not only in relation to the measurement of each separate variable, but also in relation to the methods of data collection as a whole. Each of a long series of questions or clinical tests may itself be a 'practicable' one; but put together, they may make up a 3-hour interview or examination, which may be impracticable in terms of the time available to the study personnel, or unacceptable to the subjects.

Accuracy and 'practicability' are often inversely correlated. A method providing more satisfactory information will often be more elaborate, expensive or inconvenient. Clinical examinations provide more accurate information on chronic diseases than do interviews, but they are more expensive, require medical or paramedical personnel, and are less acceptable to the subjects and hence associated with a higher refusal rate. Accuracy must be balanced against practical considerations, and that method chosen which will provide the maximal accuracy within the bounds of the investigator's resources and other practical limitations. In making this choice, account must be taken of the importance of the data, in the light of the purposes and objectives of the study. If the information is not very important, a simple although less accurate method may suffice; if more accurate information is essential, an elaborate or inconvenient method may be unavoidable. The aim is not 100% accuracy, but the maximal accuracy required for the purposes of the study and consistent with practical possibilities.

Information on the accuracy and practicability of the proposed methods can often be obtained from previous methodological studies or from experiences in other investigations. In reading the literature on his study topic, the investigator should pay especial attention to methodological aspects.

Usually, however, it is found that there is a need to test at least some of the projected methods. It may be necessary to determine, for example, how long an interview or examination will take, how acceptable it is, whether questions are clearly intelligible and unambiguous, or whether the requisite data are available in clinical records. (Such 'pretests' are discussed in Ch. 23.) Specific tests of reliability and validity may be required, as discussed later.

QUALITATIVE RESEARCH

Some study methods are qualitative rather than quantitative, i.e. they are not based on measures of quantity or frequency; their findings are described in words rather than numbers. Qualitative methods are often used in exploratory studies (see p 23) and as part of the process by which a practitioner of community medicine gets to know the community for which he provides health care—finding out about the community's interests and concerns, its formal and informal leaders, its services and how they function and are used, and so on (see p 313). Qualitative methods are widely used by anthropologists, e.g. to study concepts of health and disease or other cultural factors affecting health and health care.

Qualitative methods[4] include 'field studies' (observations of 'ongoing social life in its natural setting',[5] *participant observation*[6] (involving the researcher's participation in the action he is observing), unstructured interviews with key informants, group discussions, in-depth interviews in which people describe their attitudes, perceptions, motivations, feelings and behaviour, and the study of case histories.

The need for accuracy and the importance of reaching conclusions that a repeated study (were it feasible) would replicate are as important for qualitative as for quantitative research. The value of the distinction between these two kinds of research has been queried, on the grounds that even the most 'qualitative' of research attempts rough measurement,[7] and in health studies the two approaches should in any case complement one another.[8]

NOTES AND REFERENCES

1. Feldman J 1960 The household interview survey as a technique for the collection of morbidity data. Journal of Chronic Diseases 11: 535
2. Suchman E A, Phillips B S, Streib G S 1958 An analysis of the validity of health questionnaires. Social Forces 36: 223. Mossey J M, Shapiro E 1982 Self-rated health: a predictor of mortality among the elderly. American Journal of Public Health 72: 800.
3. Kaplan A 1964 The conduct of inquiry. Harper and Row, New York.
4. Smith R B, Manning P K (eds) 1982 A handbook of social science methods, vol 2: Qualitative methods. Ballinger, Cambridge, Massachusetts. Burgess R G (ed) 1982 Field research: a sourcebook and field manual. George Allen & Unwin, London.
5. Arnold D O 1982 Qualitative field methods. In Smith & Manning (1982; see note 4).
6. *Participant observation*, involving the researcher's participation in the action he is observing, is a technique widely used in anthropology but little used in public health research. An example would be a study of doctor-patient relationships, carried out by the physician participating in the relationships. The hazards of this method are that the observer may himself influence the action he is observing, and that his own involvement may give him a biased viewpoint.
7. Goode W J, Hatt P K 1952 Methods in social research. McGraw-Hill, New York, p 314.
8. Kroeger A 1983 Anthropological and socio-medical health care research in developing countries. Social Science and Medicine 17: 147; Health interview surveys in developing countries: a review of the methods and results. International Journal of Epidemiology 12: 465.

15. Reliability

The concept of 'reliability' is best explained by case illustrations.[1]

1. In a study in rural India, in which the incidence of accidental injuries was studied by paying periodic home visits and asking about injuries occurring since the last home visit, the incidence was doubled when inquiries were made at intervals of 2 weeks instead of a month.[2]

2. In the USA, a comparison of death certificates with census records completed shortly before death showed that only 72% of white persons recorded as divorced on their census records were also recorded as divorced on their death certificates; 17% were recorded as widowed, 5% as single, and 6% as married.[3]

3. A film was prepared, portraying the measuring of the blood pressures of seven subjects; it showed the mercury column in the sphygmomanometer, while the sound track played the accompanying sounds. When nurses were shown the film and asked to read the subjects' blood pressures, there was much variation between the pressures recorded by different nurses. The same film was later used to test physicians, with similar results ('some of the best results have been achieved by statisticians who had never taken a blood pressure before but who had been trained in objective and accurate recording of data').[4]

4. In a study of the utilization of hospital beds, panels of four physicians made appraisals of whether randomly selected beds were being appropriately used, i.e. whether the patient required hospital care on the day of observation. All four agreed in only 75% of cases.[5]

5. In Taiwan, two highly skilled ophthalmologists examined the same population sample, seeking evidence of trachoma, an infective disease of the eye often leading to disfigurement and sometimes to blindness. They used the same criteria (physical

signs) and the same examination procedure; both had exceptionally keen vision. One found 122 cases of active trachoma, and the other found 136; but these included only 75% who were diagnosed by both experts; the other 108 were diagnosed by only one or other of them.[6]

6. The same chest X-ray films were examined independently by five experts in order to determine the presence of tuberculosis. Of 131 films which were recorded as positive by at least one reader, there were only 27 where all five observers agreed; in 17 cases, four observers gave a 'positive' verdict; in another 17, three said 'positive' and two said 'negative'; in 23, two said 'positive'; and in 47, one said 'positive' and four said 'negative'. The films were later reread by the same observers, and there were many reversals of verdict. For instance, one radiologist, who had found 59 positive cases the first time, found 78 the second time, comprising 55 who had been positive the first time, and 23 new cases.[7]

7. Material with a known concentration of haemoglobin (9.8 g per 100 ml) was sent to a number of hospital laboratories, and a separate determination of haemoglobin was performed in each laboratory; the results ranged from 8 to 15.5 g per 100 ml.[8]

8. A standard suspension of red blood cells was examined in a number of laboratories; when visual counting was performed the red blood cell counts ranged from 2.2 to 4.5 million cells per mm^3; when electronic cell counters were used the range was from 0.7 to 4.7 million.[9]

9. In a study of the medications taken by patients with congestive heart failure who were treated by a sample of general practitioners and internists in private practice in a city in the USA, information was obtained both from patients and from their physicians. Medications that could be obtained without prescription were not included. Discrepancies were found in 73% of cases: 22% of the patients were not taking drugs their doctors thought they were, another 22% were taking drugs without their doctors' knowledge, and both these discrepancies occurred together in another 29%.[10]

10. A number of studies have shown that if children are measured during the morning they are on average taller, by half a centimetre or more, than if they are measured in the afternoon.[11]

These examples all provide evidence of inconsistent or unstable information. 'Reliability' (also termed 'reproducibility' or 'repeatability') refers to the stability or consistency of information, i.e. the extent to which similar information is supplied when a measurement is performed more than once. The reliability of a procedure of measurement is equivalent to a marksman's capacity to hit the same spot each time he fires, irrespective of how close he comes to the bull's-eye.

High reliability does not necessarily mean that a procedure is a satisfactory one; measurements that are 'far from the bull's-eye' may not provide the investigator with helpful information (what is more reliable—or less useful—than a broken watch?). On the other hand it is obvious that the less reliable the procedure the less useful it will be. The problem of reliability is especially acute in longitudinal studies where an attempt is being made to assess change, since the findings may express variability in the measurements rather than a real change in the attribute which is being measured (see p 75). In a study designed to measure the incidence rate of new cases of a chronic disease, performed by repeating a diagnostic procedure after a period of time, unreliability of the procedure will tend to produce an unduly high estimate of incidence. This is because persons who are falsely diagnosed as new cases on the second occasion, and ill persons falsely diagnosed as being healthy on the first occasion, will usually outnumber new cases that are missed, while well persons misdiagnosed as ill at the first examination will be excluded from the population at risk of developing the disease, thus further increasing the incidence rate.

The term 'error' should not be used to describe variation (although it often is), unless there is definite knowledge that a certain value is correct.

When the variation between measurements tends to be in a single direction, e.g. if one laboratory consistently yields lower readings that another, this is *systematic variation* or *bias*. If the variations in the two directions cancel each other out, this is *non-systematic variation*. In a large study in England and Wales, for example, it was found that in only 65% of the cases where death was ascribed to arteriosclerotic heart disease by the treating physician, was the assignment to this cause confirmed by autopsy. However, there were other cases that were diagnosed on autopsy only, so that the total numbers of deaths ascribed to this disease by clinicians and pathologists were fairly similar.[12]

The fact that variation is non-systematic offers no guarantee against erroneous conclusions. If we use an unreliable measure—bias or no bias—we are likely to *misclassify* individuals (as sick or well, smokers or non-smokers, etc.) and hence to obtain deceptive information about relationships between characteristics (see page 159). Moreover, it is never easy to be sure that bias is not present in some part of the study population, since the balance between the opposing tendencies may differ in different strata. In the above study, for example, the findings varied in different age groups. Among people aged 45–64 years, slightly *more* deaths were ascribed to arteriosclerotic heart disease by clinicians than by pathologists; whereas among people aged 75 and more, 22% *fewer* cases were ascribed to this cause by clinicians. If the information about a specific group is biased, we may reach wrong conclusions about the characteristics of that group.

SOURCES OF VARIATION

Variation between measurements may have its source in (1) changes in the *characteristics* being measured (a lack of 'constancy'[13]); (2) the *measuring instrument*, i.e. variation between readings (a lack of 'precision'[13], or between instruments (a lack of 'congruency'[13]); and (3) the *person* collecting the information (a lack of 'objectivity'[13]). For example, if two clinicians measure the same subject's blood pressure and record different readings, the possible explanations are (1) that the blood pressure altered between the two measurements; (2) that the sphygmomanometer or the measuring procedure as a whole provides variable results or, if different sphygmomanometers or procedures were used, that these provide different results; and (3) that the clinicians differ in the way they read or record blood pressure measurements.

1. *Variation in the characteristic being measured* may be caused by variation in any of the whole complex of factors which determine the characteristic. These factors include the measuring procedure itself. For example, blood pressure may be affected by the conditions under which the measurement is performed—the subject's posture and emotional state, the clinician's sex and pulchritude, etc. The response to a question may be affected (and 'response instability' thus produced) by the respondent's motivations, his state of fatigue or boredom, the circumstances of the interview (at home or in hospital, the presence of other persons, etc.), the interviewer's sex, appearance and manner, etc. Behaviour may be changed by the subject's awareness that he is being studied; he may modify his diet if he is aware that what and how much he eats are being observed and measured. In a clinical trial the subject's condition may be influenced by his awareness of whether he is

receiving the treatment under test or is a member of a control group.

2. *The measuring instruments* (a term that may be extended to include not only mechanical devices, but biochemical and other tests, questions, questionnaires, and the measuring procedure as an entity) may not yield consistent results, or different instruments may give different results.

3. *The persons collecting the information* (observers, interviewers, or persons extracting data from documentary sources) may vary in what they perceive, in their skill, integrity, propensity to make mistakes, etc. They may be influenced, consciously or unconsciously, by their preconceptions and motivations; in a clinical trial, an investigator's awareness of whether he is dealing with an experimental or control subject may bias his observations. Observers tend to find what they expect to find. This (the 'Rosenthal effect') has been demonstrated repeatedly; for example, experimenters who compared groups of rats that they had been told came from 'clever' and 'stupid' strains found that the 'clever' rats were much better at learning to negotiate mazes—although in fact the two groups were genetically identical.[14] In a reliability study in which auscultatory measurements of the fetal heart rate were compared with the electronically recorded rate, it was found that when the true rate was under 130 beats per minute the hospital staff tended to overestimate it, and when it was over 150 they tended to underestimate it.[15]

Observer Variation

'Observer variation' is a term which, strictly speaking, refers to variation arising from the persons making the observations, and not from changes in the characteristic being measured or from the measuring instrument. In practice, it is often extremely difficult to separate these aspects completely, and the term is therefore used to indicate any differences between observations by different observers (interobserver variation) or by the same observer on different occasions (intraobserver variation). Interobserver variation in blood pressure measurements may be caused not only by the way in which the measurements are read and recorded, but by the effect of the clinicians' demeanour on the subjects' blood pressure or by differences in the procedure of measurement (the rate at which the cuff is deflated, the level at which the sphygmomanometer is placed, etc.). Inter-

interviewer variation may be due not only to the way in which the interviewers perceive, interpret and record what the respondents say, but to the way they ask questions and their influence on the respondent.

In clinical examinations, observer variation is often due to the fact that different clinicians use different definitions of what they are measuring. This is one reason for the unreliability of diagnosis which besets studies in psychiatric epidemiology.[16] Clinicians may also be influenced by what they have come to regard as 'normal'. A physician working in a malnourished population may regard as well nourished a child who, if seen by a physician accustomed to a better nourished population, would be appraised as malnourished. There may also be a tendency for the examiner to find what he thinks he ought fo find.

MEASURING RELIABILITY

Although efforts should obviously be made to collect reliable information, it must be stressed that complete reliability is not essential. The measurement of a phenomenon should not be given up simply because there is some degree of unreliability. 'There is a danger in studies of reliability of permitting the perfect to become the enemy of the good or committing the error of errorlessness.'[17] It is important, however, to know *how much* unreliability there is, particularly with regard to the variables that play an important part in the investigation—how much variation arises from the method of measurement, as compared with the variation between the individuals or groups being studied? Unless this is known it may be difficult to avoid reaching unwarranted conclusions. Sometimes previous methodological studies may provide a sufficient guide. However, it is often necessary to measure reliability, either before embarking on the study, i.e. by performing a pretest (see Ch. 23), or by building reliability tests into the study itself.

Reliability is measured by performing two or more independent measurements and comparing the findings, using an appropriate statistical index.[18] The comparison may be based on observations by different observers or interviews by different observers, on repeated measurements or interviews using the same instrument or questionnaire (the *test–retest* method), or on measurements with different instruments. Replicate tests may be made on the same blood specimens. A question may be repeated in the same questionnaire, or differently worded questions asking for the same information may be included.

The results of a test–retest comparison depend on the interval between the tests. A questionnaire-based measure of overall health, for example, was found to have a test–retest reliability of about 0.85 (this was the proportion of variance not attributable to random variation) over a 1-month period, but only about 0.56 over a 3-year interval.[19] The purpose of the measurement should be kept in mind when reliability is tested. Long-term reliability is appropriate if the aim is to measure a fairly stable attribute, such as a personality trait, but not if the aim is to measure transient or changeable characteristics. Tests of an 'anxiety inventory' demonstrated that test–retest reliability (for intervals of 1 hour to 104 days) was much higher for questions designed to measure 'anxiety-trait' ('how you feel in general') than for those designed to measure 'anxiety-state' ('how you feel right now'); the figures (for women) were 0.76–0.77 and 0.16–0.31 respectively.[20]

It is often advisable to appraise reliability in different subgroups of the sample. The test–retest reliability of the anxiety-state questionnaire, for example, was much higher for men (0.33–0.55) than for women (0.16–0.31). The Minnesota Leisure Time Physical Activity Questionnaire has a high test–retest reliability (5-week interval), but reliability is somewhat lower among people who report more activity.[21] For investigators who wish to use a set of questions on the frequency of consumption of various foods, it may be important to know that test–retest reliability (over a 9-month period) was unaffected by age or relative weight.[22]

Reliability may of course differ for different items in an examination or interview. Repeated questioning of a sample of post-menopausal women, for example, revealed a high degree of concordance for a history of hysterectomy and a family history of breast cancer, but many disagreements with respect to a history of hot flushes.[23]

Sometimes it is impracticable or inadvisable to make repeated measurements of the same persons. In a test of an interview schedule, for instance, the two sets of responses may not be independent. The first interview may lead the respondent to give more thought to the survey topic, and change his mind; or he may try to be consistent in his two sets of replies, be less careful to give accurate answers the second time of asking, etc. Under such conditions, reliability may be tested by randomly dividing the subjects among a number of observers or interviewers, in order to see whether the differences between the groups are greater than are likely to be produced by the random allocation itself. If repeated measurements are made on the same subjects although there is reason to believe that their sequence may affect the findings, the order in which subjects are examined by different observers or interviewers or with different instruments should be determined by random allocation (see p 286) or a satisfactory equivalent method.

Intraobserver variation may be particulary difficult to study in instances where the measurements are made by direct observations on human subjects, since the observer may remember the subjects and attempt (consciously or unconsciously) to be consistent in his two sets of observations. This difficulty is possibly less acute when the observations are based on X-ray plates, electrocardiogram tracings, etc. which may be less distinctive than faces and personalities.

If reliability is low, the possible role of each possible source of variation should in principle be measured, by testing each source separately. For example, in studying the reliability of haemoglobin determinations, one factor at a time may be varied, while the rest of the procedure is kept constant. In this way, separate attention can be given to the effect of the time of day that blood is sampled, the effect of using capillary or venous blood, the effect of using a tourniquet, the effect of delay in examining the specimen, the differences between biochemical methods, instruments, or technicians, the variation of results from a single photometer or technician, etc. Such tests can provide a rational basis for solutions; that is, they may indicate methods of correcting or allowing for the variation produced by each source. It may be difficult and sometimes impossible, however, to separate the different sources of error; moreover, this kind of methodological study is a formidable undertaking. In small-scale investigations, what is usually done instead is to make assumptions concerning the probable major sources of variation, and to take arbitrary steps aimed at counteracting them.

ENHANCING RELIABILITY

Measures should be taken, not to attain complete reliability, but to reduce variation to reasonable limits.

To this end, clearly defined standardized procedures are required. The variables should have clear operational definitions, a standard procedure of examination should be used, and standard questions should be asked in a standard way. There should be detailed step-by-step descriptions of the methods (but remember that 'a carefully detailed manual of methods, however massive, is not good for much, if ignored by the field workers').[24]

The instrument should be one that supplies relatively consistent measurements. In particular, the variation associated with the instrument should be small in relation to the total range of variation of the attribute being measured; a ruler with coarse calibrations is sufficient if a large expanse is to be measured, but one with finer calibrations is needed if a short length is to be measured (an instrument or test meeting this requirement may be called *precise* or of high *discrimination*). If more than one measuring device is used, they should be of the same model and/or standardized against each other. Equipment should be tested from time to time. Quality control procedures should be undertaken, e.g. chemical tests on a standard reference solution and comparisons of replicate tests of the same specimens.

The use of composite scales of measurement, based on a number of related items (e.g. questions) generally increases reliability. In this context it may be noted that disease diagnoses based on a combination of manifestations are often of higher reliability than the data on the separate items. The use of repeated measures may also increase reliability: with quantitative measurements that show appreciable variation, the mean of two or more readings may be used; this is the recommended method for certain tests of lung function.[25]

If the procedure is one requiring special skill, the necessary training should be provided. If there is more than one observer, they should attune their methods, possibly by working together for a while. Where necessary, they should have standard reference pictures, such as colour photographs of different stages of a skin disorder, or X-ray plates or photographs showing radiological abnormalities.

If it is not possible to use a single observer and much interobserver variation is expected, each individual should if possible be independently examined by more than one examiner. An advantage of this is that the disagreements can be exploited to produce a more discriminatory scale of measurement.[26] For example, if the severity of a disease is graded as 1 (mild), 2 (moderate) or 3 (severe), it may be assumed that subjects allocated to grade 1 by one clinician and to grade 2 by another lie close to the borderline between grades 1 and 2; such cases could be placed in an intermediate category, 1½, lying between grades 1 and 2 in the ordinal scale. Alternatively, when there is disagreement the cases may be re-examined and discussed until agreement is reached, or a referee may be called in for a casting vote; these latter procedures have been criticized, however, on the grounds that 'forced' agreement may not mean a correct decision, but submission to the more experienced or forceful of the observers. Parallel observations of this kind are facilitated if there are permanent records of the observations, such as electrocardiogram tracings or retinal photographs.

BLIND METHODS

Use is often made of 'blind' methods, i.e. the concealment of facts from observers, interviewers, the study subjects, or anyone else who may influence the results, where such concealment may reduce bias. This applies both to trials and to non-experimental studies.

A *single-blind* experiment (or a *single-masked* one, to use a term preferred by researchers on eye diseases)[27] may be one in which the researcher makes his observations without knowing whether the subject is in the treatment or control group, or one where this information is kept from the subjects. A *double-blind*[28] experiment is one where neither observers nor subjects know to which group the subjects belong; in a double-blind experiment to test the efficacy of prayer, some patients were prayed for and others not; the patients were not told of the prayers, and the physicians appraising their clinical progress did not know for which cases divine intercession had been requested.[29] If the processing and analysis or monitoring of data are also done 'blind', an experiment may be called *triple-blind.*

Keeping subjects blind to their treatment generally requires a placebo or alternative treatment that cannot be identified by its appearance, taste, smell or effects. Elaborate stratagems may be needed to maintain the secret, such as the production of special pharmaceutical preparations and the use of containers identified only by symbols or numbers. Even then, the truth will often out. To test for breakdowns of secrecy it is helpful to ask subjects or physicians to guess the treatments, so as to see whether correct guesses outnumber what might be expected by chance. In a double-blind trial of the prevention and treatment of colds by vitamin C, half the subjects said they knew whether they were getting vitamin C or placebo—and were generally right (many admitted opening and tasting the capsules); colds were reported to be milder and of shorter duration in the vitamin C treatment group, but only among subjects who thought they knew what capsules they were having—there was no apparent effect among other subjects.[30]

If it is essential for the doctors who treat the subjects of a clinical trial to know what their patients are receiving, or if there is no way of hiding this information, it may be decided to base the evaluation on appraisals made by independent 'blinded' investigators. This reduces the chance of biased assessments, but does not control any effects the physician may have on the patient's progress as a result of his awareness of the treatment.

In non-experimental studies, 'blind' methods may prevent bias caused by the observer's or interviewer's knowledge that the subject is a case or a control (*exposure suspicion bias*, p 248) or that there has or has not been exposure to the causal factor under study (*diagnostic suspicion bias*), or in other situations where the findings may be influenced by a 'halo effect' due to the observer's prior impression of the individual he is studying. In a methodological study of the validity of wives' reports of their husbands' circumcision status, foreskins should be sought without knowledge of the wives' tales. The effect of prior knowledge may be especially troublesome in a longitudinal study in which subjects are examined repeatedly. In such a study it may be advisable to plan a record system that ensures that the examiner will not see the previous findings when he makes his observations.

A double-blind method may be used in non-experimental studies. This was done in a case-control study of the relationship of childhood leukaemia to parents' exposure to diagnostic X-rays (the mother before or during pregnancy, the father before conception).[31] The interviewer was not told whether a leukaemic patient's or control's household was being visited, and the questions that might reveal this were left to the end of the schedule. The person interviewed was told that this was a health survey, but did not know it had to do with leukaemia. Efforts are often made to conceal the specific hypotheses from both interviewers and subjects, in so far as this is feasible and ethical.

NOTES AND REFERENCES

1. A bibliography of over 400 publications on observer variation with respect to information from patients, clinical examinations, clinical decisions and paraclinical tests and procedures is provided by Feinstein A R 1985 A bibliography of publications on observer variability. Journal of Chronic Diseases 38: 619.
2. Gordon J E, Gulati P V, Wyon J B 1962 Archives of Environmental Health 4: 575.
3. National Center for Health Statistics 1969 Comparability of marital status, race, nativity, and country of origin on the death certificate and matching census record, United States, May–August, 1960. Vital and Health Statistics, series 2, no. 34. Public Health Service, Washington D C.
4. Wilcox J 1962 Observer factors in the measurement of blood pressure. Journal of the American Medical Association 179: 53; Rose G A, Holland W W, Crowley E A 1964 A sphygmomanometer for epidemiologists. Lancet i: 296.

5. Zimmer J G 1967 An evaluation of observer variability in a hospital bed utilization study. Medical Care 5: 221.
6. Assaad F A, Maxwell-Lyons F 1967 Systematic observer variation in trachoma studies. Bulletin of the World Health Organization 36: 885.
7. Birkelo C C, Chamberlain W E, Phelps P S, Schools P E, Zacks D, Yerushalmy J 1947 Tuberculosis case finding: a comparison of the effectiveness of various roentgenographic and photofluorographic methods. Journal of the American Medical Association 133: 359.
8. Belk W P, Sunderman F W 1947 A survey of the accuracy of chemical analyses in clinical laboratories. American Journal of Clinical Pathology 17: 853.
9. Lewis S M, Burgess B J 1969 Quality control in haematology: report of interlaboratory trials in Britain. British Medical Journal iv: 253.
10. Hulka B S, Kupper L L, Cassel J C, Efird R L, Burdette J A 1975 Medication use and misuse: physician–patient discrepancies. Journal of Chronic Diseases 28: 7.
11. Baker I A, Hughes J, Jones M 1978 Temporal variation in the height of children during the day. Lancet 1: 1320.
12. Heasman L A, Lipworth L 1966 Accuracy of certification of causes of death. General Register Officer, Studies on Medical and Population Subjects no. 20. HMSO, London, pp 84, 118.
13. Zetterberg H L 1963 On theory and verification in sociology, Bedminster Press, Totowa, N J, pp 50–51.
14. Rosenthal R 1976 Experimenter effects in behavioural research. Irvington, New York.
15. Day E, Maddern L, Wood C 1968 Auscultation of foetal heart rate: an assessment of its error and significance. British Medical Journal ii: 422.
16. Blum R H 1962 Case identification in psychiatric epidemiology: methods and problems. Milbank Memorial Fund Quarterly 40: 253.
17. Elison J 1972 In: Handbook of Medical Sociology, 2nd edn. Levine S, Reeder L G (eds) Freeman H E, Prentice Hall, Englewood Cliffs, N J, p 493.
18. A variety of statistical indices may be used to express the results of reliability tests. The simple 'reliability coefficient' or 'per cent agreement' (the proportion of cases placed in identical categories by two independent determinations) may be misleading, since agreement may occur by chance. *Kappa* is a better index for categorical measures, since it makes allowance for the contribution of chance agreement (estimated from the proportions of cases allocated to each category by the separate determinations); kappa can also be used for ordered categories; see Fleiss J L 1981 Statistical methods for rates and proportions, 2nd edn. Wiley, New York, pp 212–236. A kappa of 75% or more may be taken to represent excellent agreement, and values of 40–74% indicate fair to good agreement; most comparisons of clinical examinations, as well as interpretations of X-rays, electro-cardiograms and microscopic specimens yield values of 40–74%; see Sackett D L, Haynes R B, Tugwell P 1985 Clinical epidemiology: a basic science for clinical medicine. Little, Brown, Boston, Chapter 2. Indices for use with metric variables include the correlation coefficient, the intraclass correlation coefficient, the components of variation according to one-way analysis of variance, regression coefficients, and the mean, frequency distribution and quantiles of discrepancies.

Different indices may be appropriate, depending on the purpose for which the attribute is measured—for example, is the intention a comparison of different individuals or groups, or is it the measurement of change? See Kirshner B, Guyatt G (1985), who discuss the appraisal of reliability, validity, and responsiveness ('power of the test to detect a clinically important difference,') and the requirements for different purposes: discrimination between subjects, prediction of prognosis or the results of another test, and assessment of change with time (A methodological framework for assessing health indices. Journal of Chronic Diseases 38: 27). Also see Healy M J R (1989), who considers measures of measurement error and the acceptable level of measurement error in different contexts (Measuring measurement errors. Statistics in Medicine 8: 893).

19. Ware J E Jr 1984 Methodological considerations in the selection of health status assessment procedures. In: Wenger N K, Mattson M E, Furberg C D, Elinson J (eds) Assessment of quality of life in clinical trials of cardiovascular therapies. LeJacq Publishing, pp 87–111.

20. Spielberger C D, Gorsuch R I, Lushene R E 1970 Manual for the state–trait anxiety inventory. Consulting Psychologists Press, Palo Alto, California. Cited by Siegel J M, Feinstein L G, Stone A J 1985 Personality and cardiovascular disease: measurement of personality variables. In: Ostfeld A M, Eaker E D (eds) Measuring psychosocial variables in epidemiologic studies of cardiovascular disease. NIH publication no. 85–2270. National Institutes of Health, US Department of Health and Human Services, pp 367–401.

21. Folsom A R, Jacobs D R Jr, Caspersen C J, Gomez-Martin O, Knudsen J 1986 Test–retest reliability of the Minnesota Leisure Time Physical Activity Questionnaire. Journal of Chronic Diseases 39: 505.

22. Colditz G A, Willett W C, Stampfer M J et al 1987 The influence of age, relative weight, smoking and alcohol intake on the reproducibility of a dietary questionnaire. Internatioal Journal of Epidemiology 16: 392.

23. Horwitz R I, Yu E C 1985 Problems and proposals for interview data in epidemiological research. International Journal of Epidemiology 14: 463.

24. Anderson D W, Mantel N 1983 On epidemiologic surveys. American Journal of Epidemiology 118: 613.

25. Medical Research Council's Committee on the Aetiology of Chronic Bronchitis 1965. Definition and classification of chronic bronchitis for clinical and epidemiological purposes. Lancet i: 775.

26. Fletcher C K, Oldham P D 1964 Diagnosis in group research. In: Witts L J (ed) Medical surveys and clinical trials, 2nd edn. Oxford University Press, London, pp 25–49.

27. The term 'double-masked' is recommended by Ederer F 1975 (Practical problems in collaborative trials. American Journal of Epidemiology 102: 111), who goes on to say: 'Carrying out masking successfully is usually more easily said than done... One ophthalmologist measured patients' visual acuity with their bodies draped with a cloth and their heads covered with a hood'. Ingelfinger F J 1973 (Blind as a clinical investigator. New England Journal of Medicine 288: 1299) criticizes the term 'blind' ('The sections were read blindly under high–powered magnification'), especially if it supersedes a detailed account of the precautions taken to prevent bias (in such instances, he suggests that 'double-purblind' might be a good term!).

28. 'A fascinating instance of the blind leading the blind. With this, neither the physician nor the patient knows whether a drug or a placebo is being given—until, that is, the patient either recovers or expires. Some think this technique was borrowed from Russian roulette'—Armour R 1971 It all started with Hippocrates. Bantam Books, New York, p 132.

29. Joyce C R B, Welldon R M C 1965 The objective efficacy of prayer: a double-blind clinical trial. Journal of Chronic Diseases 18: 367.

30. Lewis T L, Karlowski T R, Kapikian A Z, Lynch J M, Shaffer G W, George D A 1975 A controlled clinical trial of ascorbic acid for the common cold. Annals of the New York Academy of Sciences 258: 505.

31. The Tri-State Leukaemia Survey provided evidence suggesting that diagnostic X-rays can produce severe genetic damage in a small minority of exposed persons, resulting in an increased risk of leukaemia in the progeny. Bross I D J, Natajaran N 1977 Genetic damage from diagnostic radiation. Journal of the American Medical Association 237: 2399. The controversy about the interpretation of the findings is discussed in an absorbing book by Bross I D J 1981 Scientific strategies to save your life: a statistical approach to primary prevention. Marcel Dekker, New York.

16. Validity

This chapter deals with the validity of *measures*. Later chapters will consider the validity of *studies*, i.e. their capacity to produce sound conclusions.

The *validity of a measure* refers to the adequacy with which the method of measurement does its job—how well does it measure the characteristic that the investigator actually wants to measure? It is equivalent to a marksman's capacity to hit the bull's-eye.

If we wish to know how much sugar a person consumes, we may obtain more valid information by asking how many spoons of sugar he puts in his tea or coffee and how many cups he drinks a day, than by merely asking him whether he has a 'sweet tooth'. The data will be still more valid if we obtain information about everything he eats or drinks, and calculate his sugar intake by using tables showing the average sugar content of various foodstuffs; and they will be even more valid if, instead of using these tables, we perform laboratory analyses of samples of the foods and drinks he actually consumes.

Clearly, if a measure is not reliable (see Ch. 15) this must reduce its validity; if the shots are scattered they cannot all hit the bull's-eye. If reliability is high the measure is not necessarily valid—the shots may all hit an innocent bystander. ('Just because it's reliable doesn't mean that you can use it').[1] But if reliability is low the measure cannot be valid. Similarly, a composite scale measure with little internal consistency (see p 127) cannot be valid.

There is little point in considering whether a measurement is valid in relation to the operational definition of the variable being measured. If the operational definition is a good one, it will be phrased in terms of observable facts. These facts are hence automatically ('by definition') valid as a measure of the variable, as operationally defined. If prematurity is defined in terms of birth weight, as recorded in hospital records, then information on birth weight must constitute a valid measure of prematurity, so defined. If intelligence is defined as 'what is measured by an intelligence test', then an intelligence test must be a valid measure of intelligence.

It is more meaningful to consider validity in relation to the conceptual definition of the variable, i.e. in relation to what the investigator would like to measure. In planning the methods of data collection, the investigator should satisfy himself that the measures he chooses, particularly for variables that play an important part in his study, have as close a relevance as possible to what he actually wants to measure, taking account of his resources and other practical limitations. There are various ways of appraising validity.

APPRAISING VALIDITY

1. Face validity
2. Content validity
3. Consensual validity
4. Criterion validity
5. Predictive validity
6. Construct validity

Face validity

The relevance of a measurement may appear obvious to the investigator. This is referred to as *face validity* (or *logical validity*). It may be obvious, for instance, that the dates of birth recorded on birth certificates provide a valid measure of age. In choosing between different measures, common sense may indicate that some are more valid than others. It may be self-evident that the records kept in an obstetrics ward will provide a more valid indication of birth weights than information obtained by questioning mothers, or that an appraisal of the neurological status of neonates will provide a more valid measure of prematurity (as the investigator conceives it) than information on birth weights.

In formulating the questions to be included in a questionnaire, a prime consideration is whether they have face validity—do they seem likely to yield information of real relevance to what the investigator wants to measure? It must be remembered, however, that face validity may be deceptive. The question 'Do you have frequent headaches?', for example, may not necessarily provide a valid measure of the occurrence of frequent headaches. A positive response may reflect a general propensity to complain, or a state of emotional ill health, and have little relevance to headaches per se.

Sometimes the findings (of a pretest or the study itself) point to poor face validity. If there are many 'don't know' answers to a question, this is ipso facto evidence that the question does not supply the information the investigator needs. 'Unreasonable' findings—their non-conformity with expectations—may be evidence of poor validity: if the prevalence of acne in adolescents turns out to be only 1%, the measure is probably invalid. *Digit preference* points to impaired validity. For instance, if the question 'How old are you?' yields an undue number of replies of '20', '30', '40', etc. compared with the number of replies ending in digits other than zero, this may be taken as evidence of low face validity; in this instance it would probably be decided to use grouped ages, rather than single years, as the scale of measurement, and not to use ages ending in zero in defining the categories (i.e. to use '25–34', '35–44', etc. rather than '20–29', '30–39', etc.). Similarly, a question on the date of the first day of the last menstrual period, put to pregnant women, has been found to yield unduly high numbers of certain dates—the 1st, 10th, 15th, 20th, and 25th days of the month.[2] A question concerning the number of days since the onset of symptoms, put to patients seeking care for infectious diseases, may yield high numbers of replies of 1, 2, 3, 4, 7, 10 and 14 days. In the measurement of blood pressures, digit preference—usually a high proportion of readings ending in zero—is a well known phenomenon, and one that makes it more difficult to assess associations between blood pressure and other variables.[3]

Content validity

If the variable to be measured is a composite one, one way of appraising validity is to see whether all the component elements of the variable (as conceived) are measured. This is *content validity*. A composite scale for measuring satisfaction with medical care should include attitudes to all features the investigator regards as important, such as professional competence, the personal qualities of doctors and nurses, the cost and convenience of medical care, and so on.[4] Thyrotoxicosis, which is conceptually defined in terms of specific metabolic and biochemical processes as well as symptoms and physical signs, will be more validly measured if metabolic and biochemical tests are used as well as symptoms and signs.

Consensual validity

When a number of experts agree that a measure is valid, this is *consensual validity*. Many experts agree, for example, that the British

Registrar-General's classification (p 103) is a valid measure of social class, or that a specific index based on the presence, frequency and duration of cough and phlegm is a valid indicator of chronic bronchitis. It must be remembered, however, that different groups of experts may differ in their consensus of opinion, and that a consensus may change—expert committees frequently recommend changes in diagnostic criteria (see p 113).

Criterion validity

The best and most obvious way of appraising validity is to find a *criterion* (or, in epidemiological jargon, a 'gold standard') that is known or believed to be close to the truth, and to compare the results of the measure with this criterion (*criterion validity*, sometimes called *concurrent validity*).

The ideal criterion is the 'true value' of the attribute that is being measured. A perfectly valid measure is one that correlates completely with 'God's opinion' concerning the attribute.[5] As 'God's opinion' is difficult to determine, the best criterion is a measure that has higher face validity than the measure being tested, or that has been tested previously and found to be of high criterion validity. As examples, questionnaire data on birth weights may be checked against the weights recorded in obstetric records, and blood pressure measurements (made by indirect sphygmomanometry) against direct intra-arterial pressure measurements; the causes of death recorded on death certificates may be compared with those inferred from post-mortem examinations, and readings of electrocardiogram tracings with the appraisals made by a panel of experts; biochemical results may be checked by using standard solutions whose composition has been measured by tests of established accuracy. The responses to a 'yes–no' question on stiffness in the joints or muscles on waking in the morning (one of the diagnostic criteria of rheumatoid arthritis) may be validated by comparing them with the responses elicited by a skilled interviewer who asks additional questions to ensure that the sensation is really one of stiffness, and not of 'pins and needles', general lassitude, etc. Similarly, the validity of a simple dietary questionnaire may be tested by a comparison with the findings obtained by a Burke research dietary history, a method involving very detailed questioning, with built-in cross-checks, by an experienced interviewer.[6] The validity of a new blood test for the diagnosis of rheumatoid arthritis may be tested by examining its correlation with diagnoses established by clinicians after comprehensive examinations, using their own individual diagnostic criteria (which have face validity), generally accepted diagnostic criteria (which have consensual validity), or diagnostic criteria that have themselves been tested against some criterion.

If an unquestionably 'more valid' measure of the characteristic is available for use as a criterion, the comparison can provide convincing evidence of validity. It must be kept in mind, however, that validity measured in this way may not be quite as well founded as it appears, since (like face validity) it is in the last resort based on judgement—if only the judgement that the criterion is of higher validity than the measure that is being tested.

It is often—in fact, usually—impossible to use the above approach. For one thing, there may be no measure which can be unequivocally regarded as a more valid one. If we wish to test the validity of a composite measure of social class, based on occupation, education and income, what unquestionably 'more valid' measure can we find? If we wish to test the validity of information on an attitude—a man's attitude to his work or his wife or whether he approves of contraceptive practices—how can we come close to the 'true value' of the attitude, to obtain a criterion of validity? Furthermore, even when a 'more valid' measure is theoretically available, the information required may not be available in practice. For example, the histopathological features of the bronchi constitute a suitable but not very practicable criterion for testing the validity of an index of chronic bronchitis based on the occurrence of cough and phlegm.

Predictive validity

In the absence of a suitable criterion, validity can sometimes be appraised by seeing whether a follow-up study shows an association between the measurements and a subsequent event that is believed to be an outcome of what was measured. The prophetic value of the measure is examined; this is *predictive validity*. For example, the validity of measures of prematurity (birth weight, gestation period, neurological maturity, etc.) may be tested by examining their association with death or survival during the first month of life, on the assumption that since prematurity is associated with neonatal mortality, the more strongly the measure is associated with neonatal mortality, the more valid it is. The validity of various minor electrocardiographic abnormalities as measures of coronary heart disease may be tested by examining their relationship to the subsequent occurrence of myocardial infarction. The validity of measures of social support may be appraised by examining their capacity to predict mortality, psychiatric symptoms, and other adverse health outcomes,[7] and the validity of clinical appraisals of disease severity by their capacity to predict a fatal outcome.[8]

Construct validity

Another way of appraising validity is to see whether there are associations with other variables that there is reason to believe should be linked with the characteristic under study. This is *construct validity*: — 'the extent to which a particular measure relates to other measures consistent with theoretically derived hypotheses concerning the concepts (or constructs) that are being measured.'[9] A measure of attitudes to work, for example, might be compared with information on what the subjects actually do (absenteeism, frequency of disputes at work, etc.), since it is reasonable to predicate some degree of association—although certainly not a one-to-one relationship— between these activities and the 'true' attitude to work. A scale measuring reported satisfaction with medical care might be validated in a similar way, using such criteria as the changing of doctors, the abandonment of health insurance, or the submission of formal complaints about the care received. If there are theoretical reasons for believing that satisfaction with medical care is correlated with income or ethnic group or emotional health, evidence of such correlations might be taken as indirect evidence of validity. Tests of physical fitness might be used to validate a questionnaire on habitual physical activity. A new measure of mental health would be expected to show a stronger correlation with other mental health measures than with measures of physical health; validity appraised by a comparison with another measure of the characteristic is sometimes termed *convergent validity*.

The value of this approach depends on the relevance (again a function of judgement) and reliability of the measurements used as criteria.

DIFFERENTIAL VALIDITY

A measure may be of different validity in different groups or populations. Low birth weight, for example, may be a particularly unsatisfactory index of prematurity in a population where neonates, like adults, are small for genetic reasons. A measure of chronic bronchitis based on the presence of cough and phlegm may be of high validity in one population, but less so in another, where there is a low prevalence of chronic bronchitis and a very high prevalence of other disorders (such as pulmonary tuberculosis) which may cause cough and phlegm. Indirect sphygmomanometer readings are a better index of intra-arterial blood pressure among leaner than among fatter persons. The validity of a set of questions used as an index of emotional ill health may vary according to educational level,[10] and the validity of simple questionnaires and tests for identifying people with presenile or senile dementia is seriously impaired by the effect of educational level on the responses.[11] In surveys in the USA, more under-reporting of hospitalization was found among non-whites than among whites.[12] In Boston, mothers tended to under-report their children's attendances at outpatient clinics if there had been many such attendances, and to over-report them if there had been few.[13]

If we contemplate the use of a study method that others have developed and validated, we should satisfy ourselves of its validity in our own study population. The fact that the method has been 'validated' is not enough. Do we think that our study population is so similar that the method will be valid here too? Is it a valid measure of what *we* want to measure? Or is a special test of validity required? Whatever study methods we use, we should be aware of the possibility that their validity may not be uniform within our study population. As we shall see later, this may have important implications when we come to look at associations between variables.

TESTING VALIDITY

A reasonable degree of face validity is a sine qua non for the choice of a measure; so, for composite variables, is content validity. Sometimes the results of previous tests of criterion, predictive or construct validity are available. If the validity of a measure is uncertain and the variable is of more than peripheral interest in the study, a test of validity should be considered. Information about validity may influence the choice of study methods and, at a later stage, the interpretation of the findings.

Validity is most convincingly tested by comparing the findings with a suitable 'gold standard'. If no 'more valid' measure is available for use as a criterion, associations with expected outcomes (predictive validity) or other expected correlates (construct validity) may be explored. Validity may be measured either in a pretest, or during the study proper—which may require the collection of extra information (concerning the criterion) for a sample of the study population—or even (if doubts arise only later) by collecting new data during the analysis phase. It is often advisable to test validity in different subgroups of the study population, in order to see whether it varies. In some instances a simple tryout may be enough to raise or dispel doubts about the capacity of the measure to yield reasonable and full responses.

Criterion validity may be measured by the correlation between observed and 'true' measurements, the size and direction of the discrepancies between them, or other statistical indices. Where there is a 'yes–no' measure of a 'yes–no' attribute (e.g. the presence of a disease), *sensitivity* and *specificity* are used. In such instances the findings may be shown in a simple table (Table 16.1), where TP represents the 'true positives', FP the 'false positives', FN the 'false negatives, and TN the 'true negatives'. The measure's *sensitivity* is the proportion with a positive result, among people who 'truly' have the attribute (e.g. the disease), i.e. $TP/(TP + FN)$. The *specificity* of the measure is the proportion with a negative result, among people who 'truly' do not have the attribute, i.e. $TN/(FP + TN)$.

Table 16.1   Results of a 'yes–no' measure of a 'yes–no' attribute

	Attribute present	Attribute absent
Positive finding	TP	FP
Negative finding	FN	TN

See text for details.

If both sensitivity and specificity are high, the measure is of high validity. Sensitivity and specificity must be considered together; separately, neither is very meaningful; the presence of a nose is a highly sensitive measure of kwashiorkor (100% of cases have noses) but its specificity is 0% (no individuals free of kwashiorkor are noseless); conversely, a bright green coloration of the ears is a highly specific index of kwashiorkor (100%), but its sensitivity is 0%.

It must again be stressed that the validity of a measure may vary in different situations. A combination of signs and symptoms, used as an index of a disease, may have a higher sensitivity in a hospital population (where persons have more advanced disease) than among diseased persons found in a household survey. On the other hand, its specificity may be lower in the hospital population, where the persons free of this disease are more likely to have other diseases producing the same manifestations. Validity may also vary with the prevalence of the disease in the study population. In a population with a low prevalence, for instance, the people who have the disease may tend to have it in a mild form, which may mean that there are many 'false negatives', and hence a low sensitivity.

INFORMATION BIAS

A measure that has low validity is a poor proxy for the characteristic that we want to measure. Serum triglyceride estimations based on blood samples taken from people who have recently had a meal may be a reflection of what they ate rather than of the metabolic pattern that interests us. If the presence of a hernia is reported by only 54% of men who turn out to have obvious bulging inguinal hernias, and if hernias are reported by men who have none,[14] the *misclassification* of study subjects by interview data is likely to produce a biased picture of the prevalence of this disorder, the direction of the bias depending on the balance between false negatives and false positives. This is an example of *information bias* (bias attributable to shortcomings in the way information is obtained or handled).

Low validity may produce deceptive information not only about the occurrence of an attribute, but also about its associations with other variables. Suppose we want to compare the prevalence of a disease in two groups, using a measure that makes errors when classifying people as well or ill. Patients will be 'diluted' with healthy people, and/or healthy people will be 'contaminated' by patients. It has been shown that if the measure has the same validity (sensitivity and specificity) in the two groups we are comparing ('non-differential validity'), the misclassification will tend to reduce any true difference between the prevalence in the two groups, or may even make it dwindle to vanishing point.[15] If the measure is of different validity in the two groups—i.e. if there is a difference in sensitivity, specificity or both—the difference may be lessened, obscured or increased, or its direction may change; also, a difference may be seen when really there is none. The possibility of a spurious association exists whenever differential validity is suspected; if women who have borne deformed babies are for this reason especially prone to recall and report minor injuries that occurred during early pregnancy, a retrospective comparison with mothers of normal babies may produce deceptive evidence of an association between deformities and these injuries.[16] The direction of information bias is especially difficult to predict if both the variables involved in an association (e.g. disease and personality type) are subject to misclassification—anything may happen. This is not an uncommon situation.

EVALUATION OF SCREENING AND DIAGNOSTIC TESTS

The testing of validity plays a central role in the evaluation of tests used for the detection of diseases. This applies both to *screening tests,* which are simple tests aimed at the identification of people who merit fuller examination for the presence of diseases, and to *diagnostic tests,* which establish the presence or absence of diseases more definitively.

The key indices are the test's sensitivity (its capacity to identify cases of the disease) and its specificity (its capacity to exclude people who are free of the disease). If both sensitivity and specificity are high, the test is a valid indicator of the disease (it has a high *discriminatory capacity*). Frequently, however, sensitivity and specificity are inversely related. A positive sputum culture, for example, is a very specific test for respiratory tuberculosis, but one of low sensitivity; radiological examination is more sensitive, but less specific. Similarly, a blood glucose value exceeding 180 mg/100 ml 2 hours after a meal is a very specific test for diabetes, but 50% of diabetics will not have such high values. If a lower critical level is used, say 120 mg/100 ml, only 11% of diabetics will be missed, but the test will not be very specific.[17]

The purpose or purposes for which a test is used should be kept in mind when validity is appraised. Tests have at least three different purposes:[18] discovery of a disease, confirmation of its suspected presence, and exclusion of its presence. Some tests are used for only one of these purposes, some for two, and some for all three. Consideration should also be given to the circumstances in which the test will be used — is it to be used in a mass programme for the examination of apparently healthy people, or as a component of periodic health examinations, or as a routine test for all patients who seek medical care, or for patients in a defined high-risk group, or is it for use only when there are symptoms or when there is a positive screening test or other evidence suggesting the presence of the disease?

A *discovery test* is one used when there is no special reason to suspect the presence of the disease. It may be a screening test, like self-examination of the breast for the detection of breast cancer, or it may be a diagnostic one, like examination of the scrotum in order to detect undescended testes. The aim is usually to find as many of the cases as possible. High sensitivity is therefore of special importance. If it is a screening test, however, specificity cannot be ignored, since if this is low there will be an unduly large number of 'false positive' cases requiring further investigation. The sensitivity and specificity of a discovery test should, if possible, be measured in the kind of population in which the test is to be used. For the measurement of sensitivity, there is often little choice—a sufficiently large sample of people with the disease has to be found for this purpose, by whatever means available. Specificity, however, should be measured in an appropriate sample of people free of the disease—selected from the general population, or from people who seek medical care, or from a defined high-risk group, in accordance with the way the test will be used.

It is often helpful to estimate the *predictive value*[19] of a discovery test, using indices that express the probable findings when it is used in a population or group of patients with a known or assumed prevalence of the disease—what proportion of people with positive tests will be ill, and what proportion of those with negative tests will be well? The data required for these estimates are the sensitivity and specificity of the test and the prevalence rate of the disease in the population or group in which the test will be used.

A *confirmation test* is one used when the presence of disease is suspected. Its purpose is to verify this suspicion. The presence of tubercle bacilli in the sputum, for example, will confirm a diagnosis of tuberculosis (but their absence does not exclude the diagnosis). For this purpose, specificity must be high; sensitivity is less important. The specificity of the test should be measured in patients in whom the disease is suspected, but who turn out to be free of the disease.

An *exclusion test* has the purpose of 'ruling out' the presence of a suspected disease. If an appropriate tuberculin skin test is done, for example, a negative result will virtually exclude a diagnosis of active tuberculosis (except in moribund patients); a positive result, however, does not necessarily confirm the diagnosis. Most exclusion tests are elaborate procedures, and they can often be used as confirmation tests also. Their essential feature is an extremely high sensitivity; there must be very few false negative results.

Validity is not the only consideration when evaluating a screening procedure. Using the basic evaluative scheme shown on page 48, the following are the kinds of questions that are usually asked.[20]

1. *Requisiteness.* Is the test needed? Are other satisfactory tests not available? How important is it to detect the disease? What is the impact of the disease on the individual (shortening his life, disability, pain and discomfort, cost of care), on the individual's family, and on the community (mortality, morbidity rate, reduced productivity, cost of care)? Is effective intervention possible, and

how good is the evidence for this? Does early detection make treatment easier? Does it make it more effective?

2. *Quality.* How well does the test achieve its desired effects—i.e. how valid is it (sensitivity, specificity, predictive value)? Are there untoward side-effects? May the 'labelling' of symptom-free people as 'diseased' have undesirable effects? What is the impact of false positive results (false 'labelling')?

3. *Efficiency.* What is the cost per test and per case found, in comparison with other tests? What is the cost compared with the cost of *not* detecting the disease? What resources are needed—are highly-trained personnel required? What is the cost-effectiveness of the test, using sensitivity and specificity as measures of effectiveness?

4. *Satisfaction.* How acceptable is the test? Is there a demand—is there dissatisfaction if the test is *not* done?

5. *Differential value.* How do the size of the problem, the need for the test, and the acceptability of the test vary in different groups or populations? Is the validity of the test consistent in different groups?

EVALUATION OF RISK MARKERS

The same questions should be asked in the evaluation of a risk marker, which aims to identify individuals or groups who are especially likely to develop a given disorder in the future (see p 39). A high level of predictive validity is not enough. There must also be good reason to think that the detection of vulnerability is likely to be beneficial—i.e. that techniques and resources are available for reducing the risk, and that the expected benefit outweighs any harm that may be done by 'labelling' and intervention. The use of the marker must also be practical in terms of cost, resources, acceptability and convenience. The most useful risk markers are probably those whose presence can be determined by questions, or simple procedures that can be built into ordinary clinical care.

With respect to validity, the primary requirement is a high sensitivity, since the usual aim is to find as many of the vulnerable individuals as possible. Account must also be taken of false positives; if these are numerous the predictive value of a positive test will be low, and the more intensive care recommended for vulnerable people will often be given unnecessarily.

An important consideration is the prevalence of the risk marker. This may be high either because the disorder it predicts is a very common one, or (if the disorder is less common) because the risk marker has a low specificity. If over half the children under care fall into a high-risk group needing special attention, it may be decided that the risk marker is of little value, since modification of the care programme so as to give extra care to *all* children may be a more efficient and effective solution.

NOTES AND REFERENCES

1. Baer D M 1977 Reviewer's comment: 'Just because it's reliable doesn't mean that you can use it'. Journal of Applied Behavior Analysis 10: 117.
2. Frazier T M 1959 Error in reported date of last menstrual period. American Journal of Obstetrics and Gynecology 77: 915.
3. Hessel P A 1986 Terminal digit preference in blood pressure measurements: effects on epidemiological associations. International Journal of Epidemiology 15: 122.
4. For an example of how a composite scale to measure satisfaction with medical care was developed, see Hulka B S, Zyzanski S J, Cassel J C, Thompson S J 1970 Scale for the measurement of attitudes toward physicians and primary medical care. Medical Care 8: 429; Zyzanski S J, Hulka B S, Cassel J C 1974 Scale for the measurement of 'satisfaction' with medical care: modifications in content, format and scoring. Medical Care 12: 611.
5. A concept ascribed to A L Cochrane.
6. Burke B S 1947 The dietary history as a tool in research. Journal of the American Dietetic Association 23: 1041.
   Methods used in dietary studies, and their reliability and validity, are reviewed by Lee-Han H, McGuire V, Boyd N F 1989 A review of the methods used by studies of dietary measurement. Journal of Clinical Epidemiology 42: 269. The uses of survey data for assessing dietary and nutrition-related health states are described in Life Sciences Research Office, Federation of American Societies for Experimental Biology 1989 Nutrition monitoring in the United States: an update report on nutrition monitoring. DHHS publication no. (PHS) 89–1255. US Department of Health and Human Services, Hyattsville, Maryland, pp 13–29.
7. Orth-Gomer K, Unden A-L 1987 The measurement of social support in population surveys. Social Science and Medicine 24: 83.
8. Charlson M, Sax F L, MacKenzie R, Fields S D, Braham R L, Douglas R G Jr 1987 Journal of Chronic Diseases 39: 439.
9. Carmines E G, Zeller R A 1979 Reliability and validity assessment. Sage Publications, Beverley Hills, pp 22–26.
10. Abramson J H, Epstein L M, Flug D, Jarus A 1973 Validity of simple indicators of emotional ill-health for use in epidemiological surveys. Methods of Information in Medicine 12: 97.
11. The results of tests for dementia can be statistically manipulated so as to remove the effect of education; but this makes it difficult to study the possible role of education or education-related factors in the aetiology of dementia. See Kittner S J, White L R, Farmer M E et al 1986 Methodologic issues in screening for dementia: the problem of education adjustment. Journal of Chronic Diseases 39: 163, and Berkman L F 1986 The association between educational attainment and mental status examinations: of etiological significance for senile dementias or not? Journal of Chronic Diseases 39: 171.
12. National Center for Health Statistics 1965 Reporting of hospitalization in the health interview survey, and comparison of hospitalization reporting in three

survey procedures. Vital and Health Statistics, series 2, nos 6, 8. Public Health Service, Washington, DC.

13. Kosa J, Alpert J J, Haggerty R J 1967 On the reliability of family health information: a comparative study of mothers' reports on illness and related behavior. Social Science and Medicine 1: 165.

14. Abramson J H, Gofin J, Hopp C, Makler A, Epstein L M 1978 Epidemiology of inguinal hernia: a survey in Western Jerusalem. Journal of Epidemiology and Community Health 32: 59.

15. If a measure is wrong more often than it is right (false positive rate plus false negative rate exceeds 100%) spurious associations may be produced even if misclassification is non-differential. Validity as low as this is unusual. The effects of *misclassification* are described by Fleiss J L 1981 Statistical methods for rates and proportions, 2nd edn. Wiley, New York, pp 188–200; Kleinbaum D G, Kupper L L, Morgenstern H 1982 Epidemiologic research: principles and quantitative methods. Lifetime Learning Publications, Belmont, California, Chapter 12; see also Abramson J H 1988 Making sense of data: a self-instruction manual on the interpretation of epidemiological data. Oxford University Press, New York, Units C3–C6.

16. A study in Boston of the reporting of events during pregnancy, based on a comparison with antenatal records, showed that the mothers of malformed infants reported urinary tract and yeast infections, and the use of birth control after conception, much more fully than the mothers of normal children. There were slight or no differences in the completeness of reports of other events Werler M M, Pober B R, Nelson K, Holmes L B 1989 Reporting accuracy among mothers of malformed and nonmalformed infants. American Journal of Epidemiology 129: 415.

17. United States Public Health Service 1960 Diabetes program guide. Division of Special Health Services, PHS publ. no. 506. United States Government Printing Office, Washington DC.

18. Feinstein A R 1977 Clinical Biostatistics. C V Mosby, St Louis, Chapter 15.

19. The *predictive value of a positive test* expresses the proportion of persons with positive tests who will be found to have the disease, when the test is applied to a population with a specified prevalence of the disease; the *predictive value of a negative test* expresses the proportion of those with negative tests who will be found to be disease-free.

20. As well as asking whether the *screening* test is suitable, one should ask whether the disease is one for which screening is an appropriate procedure, and whether suitable treatment is available: Burr M L, Elwood P C 1985 Research and development of health promotion services—screening. In: Holland W W, Detels R, Knox G (eds) Oxford textbook of public health, vol 3: Investigative methods in public health. Oxford University Press, Oxford, pp 373–384. For a comprehensive evaluation of procedures that might be done in periodic health examinations, see Canadian Task Force on the Periodic Health Examination 1979 Canadian Medical Association Journal 121: 1193.

17. Interviews and self-administered questionnaires

Interviews may be less or more structured. A clinician uses a relatively unstructured interview—his approach is flexible, he follows leads as they arise, and the content, wording and order of the questions vary from interview to interview. In the same way, a public health worker conducting interviews as part of the investigation of a local outbreak of disease has an idea of what he wants to learn—the nature and time of onset of the symptoms, the patients' prior movements, their contacts with other ill persons, their recent meals, their milk and water supply, and so on—but does not decide in advance exactly what questions will be asked, or in what order.

In other situations a more standardized technique may be used, the wording and order of the questions being decided in advance. This may take the form of a *highly structured interview*, in which the questions are asked orally, or a *self-administered questionnaire*, in which case the respondent reads the questions and fills in the answers by himself (sometimes in the presence of an interviewer who 'stands by' to give assistance if necessary). For simplicity, we will use the term 'questionnaire' to indicate the list of questions prepared for either of these purposes. (In the behavioural sciences, a 'questionnaire' usually means a self-administered questionnaire, and the term is not applied to the interview schedule used by an interviewer.)

Standardized methods of asking questions are usually preferred in community medicine research, since they provide more assurance that the data will be reproducible. Less structured interviews may be useful in a preliminary survey, where the purpose is to obtain information to help in the subsequent planning of a study rather than facts for analysis, and in intensive studies of perceptions, attitudes, motivations and affective reactions. Unstructured interviews are characteristic of qualitative (non-quantitative) research (see p 134).

MODE OF ADMINISTRATION

The choice between a self-administered questionnaire and a highly structured interview may not be an easy one. The use of self-administered questionnaires is simpler and cheaper; such questionnaires can be administered to many persons simultaneously (e.g. to a class of schoolchildren), and unlike interviews, can be sent by post. On the other hand, they demand a certain level of education and skill on the part of the respondent; people of a low socioeconomic status are less likely to respond to a mailed questionnaire.

Face-to-face or phone interviews have many advantages. A good interviewer can stimulate and maintain the respondent's interest, and can create a rapport and atmosphere conducive to the answering of questions.[1] If anxiety is aroused (e.g. 'Why am *I* being asked these questions?—Have I an illness they haven't told me about?'), the interviewer can allay it. If a question is not understood an interviewer can repeat it and if necessary (and in accordance with guidelines decided in advance) provide an explanation or alternative wording. Optional follow-up or probing questions that are to be asked only if prior responses are inconclusive or inconsistent cannot easily be built into self-administered questionnaires. A self-administered questionnaire is perforce restricted to simple questions with simple instructions, designed to elicit simple data. In a face-to-face interview, observations can be made as well; the so-called 'coronary-prone behaviour pattern', for example, was originally detected in interviews during which note was taken not only of what the subject said but of how he said it, whether he clenched his fists and his teeth, etc.[2] Furthermore, the interviewer can use visual aids; cups and saucers of various sizes and models of food servings can be an invaluable aid in a quantitative dietary interview.

In general, apart from their expense, interviews are preferable to self-administered questionnaires, with the important proviso that they are conducted by skilled interviewers. Otherwise, there is much truth in the statement that 'to gain information by interview resembles the use of questionnaires, except that questionnaires only contain errors caused by the patient, but interviews include errors caused by the interviewer as well'.[3] Self-administered questionnaires have, however, been successfully used in many studies.[4] A decision on the use of a self-administered questionnaire may require a pretest to obtain information on the response rate, rates of unanswered items, and the quality of responses.

The main problems with postal questionnaires are that response rates tend to be relatively low, and that there may be under-representation of less literate subjects. The questionnaires often find their way to wastepaper baskets, even if they are simple, attractively designed, accompanied by a persuasive covering letter and a stamped return envelope, and followed by one or more reminders. Response rates may be high, however, in surveys where subjects have a special motivation, as in the instance of questionnaires sent to patients or ex-patients by their own physicians or treating agencies, enquiring about their progress. If the questions are formulated suitably the replies are in general similar to those obtained in interviews.[5]

Phone interviews are sometimes preferred to mailed questionnaires and face-to-face interviews. Selection of a method depends on feasibility (e.g. the prevalence of telephones), costs (which vary in different circumstances) and the nature and purpose of the study. Comparisons yield inconsistent findings; one recent study showed little difference in cost or data quality between phone and personal home interviews; the mailed questionnaires were cheaper, but more answers were missing, more medical conditions were unreported, and questions about exposure to hazardous chemicals and activities yielded less reliable responses; another study showed more under-reporting of doctor visits in phone interviews than in mailed or home interviews.[6] Some questions are easier to ask on the telephone, and others are easier to ask face-to-face; but the differences between these two interview modes do not appear to be important or consistent—one expert jubilates that 'it seems almost too good to be true that telephone interviewing produces results that are practically no different from face-to-face interviewing, and I continue to be surprised at our good fortune'.[7]

There is sometimes less concealment of socially undesirable behaviour when a more impersonal mode is used. In a study of the use of seat restraints for children in cars, non-use of a restraint on the last trip was reported by 30% of parents in phone interviews and 26% in postal questionnaires, but by only 18% in face-to-face interviews.[8] In another comparative study the proportion of respondents who admitted to 'nervousness, worry or depression or trouble sleeping' (symptoms that might be considered embarrassing) was somewhat higher for mailed questionnaires than for phone interviews.[9]

Mixed strategies are often used—for example, trying mail or telephone first, and using home interviews only for persistent non-respondents.[9]

COMPUTER-ASSISTED INTERVIEWS

Computer-aided interviewing is likely to increase in popularity. The interviewer reads the question from a computer screen instead of a printed page, and uses the keyboard to enter the answer. Skip patterns (i.e. 'if so-and-so, go to Question such-and-such') are built into the program, so that the screen automatically displays the appropriate question. Checks can be built in and an immediate warning given if a reply lies outside an acceptable range or is inconsistent with previous replies; revision of previous replies is permitted, with automatic return to the current question. The responses are entered directly on to the computer record, avoiding the need for subsequent coding and data entry. The program can make an automatic selection of subjects who require additional procedures, such as special tests, supplementary questionnaires, or follow-up visits.

This procedure can be used both for phone interviews (*computer-assisted telephone interviewing* or *CATI*) and for personal interviews. Its use in home interviews requires a portable (lap-top) computer.

The advantages of the procedure are obvious. Consideration should also be given, however, to its drawbacks. The main disadvantages are its cost (which is, however, counterweighed by the savings in coding and data entry expenses), the need for programming skills, and the time required for writing and testing the program. There is also a possibility of error, mainly due to typing slips when entering the answers. In one careful comparison it was found that 2.0% of recorded responses were erroneous, as compared with 1.1% when a paper-and-pencil technique was used.[10] This too is counterbalanced by the avoidance of errors that may occur during the transfer and entry of ordinary interview data. The automatic skip patterns can, however, lead to other and irremediable errors. Suppose that subjects are asked if they smoke and, if they say 'yes', are then asked about the number and kind of cigarettes smoked. In an ordinary interview, if the response to the first question is 'yes' but is erroneously entered as 'no', and the subsequent questions are (correctly) asked and answered, the inconsistency can be detected when the data are checked, and the reply to the first question can be corrected. In a computer-aided interview, if 'no' is entered by mistake the other questions will not be asked at all. Also, if the interviewer has to code responses before keying them in, there is later no way of detecting coding errors, since there is no record of the actual responses. Other drawbacks are that the use of a computer lengthens the interview slightly, and that interviewers may find their work boring. Printed questionnaires must be available for emergency use; in one study using computer-aided personal interviews, printed forms were needed in 5% of instances.[10]

If the right software is available, computer-assisted interviewing presents no technical problems—it is just necessary to type a questionnaire.[11] Ready-made programs for computer-assisted interviews on health topics are already available,[11] and there will probably soon be many more.

There is as yet little experience with self-administered computer interviews. In a randomized trial in a study of drinking habits in Edinburgh, men who entered their own responses into the computer reported the consumption of 30% more alcohol than men asked the same questions in face-to-face interviews. The subjects were required to respond by pressing a single key (for 'yes' or 'no'), or a number and the 'Return' key. The computer interviews took twice as long as the face-to-face interviews.[12]

VALIDITY

Information obtained by interviewing and questioning is often referred to as 'soft' data, as opposed to the presumably 'hard' data[13] derived from observations. A man who says he has heart disease may have a non-cardiac disease, or none at all. In a study of questionnaire responses by registered nurses in the USA, an examination of the medical records of women who reported cancer of the uterus confirmed the diagnosis in only 74% of cases.[14] In a Californian study, the proportions of various chronic diseases (recorded in medical records) that were not reported in interviews ranged from 15 to 79%, and the over-reporting rate from 1 to 83%.[15] A person who says he does not have a disease may be unaware that he has it, or may have forgotten, or may be unwilling (on a conscious or unconscious level) to admit its presence—particularly if the disease carries a stigma (this has been called 'unacceptable disease bias'). In a survey in which comparisons were made with cancer-registry data, it was found that only 51% of men with a previous diagnosis of cancer of the lip reported this condition when asked about previous illnesses, and only another 13% reported it when they were specifically asked about cancer.[16]

People may be reluctant to admit to induced abortions, drug abuse, overindulgence in alcohol or tobacco, or other socially unacceptable behaviour—a study in Holland showed that a question-based survey of alcoholism would miss over half the known problem drinkers.[17]

Self-reported weight may tend to be an underestimate, and self-reported height an overestimate; in one study the prevalence of obesity (using a definition based on weight and height) was 50% higher when based on actual measurements than when based on reported weights and heights.[18] A mother reporting that her children have an abundance of milk, fruit, vegetables and meat may be saying this only to put herself into a favourable light, whereas a mother reporting that her children have none of these foodstuffs may be trying to elicit sympathy or welfare assistance.

Interviews conducted at home and in a clinic may elicit different information, and the responses may depend on who else is present. Suspicions about the interviewers' motives may influence responses. Different answers may be given to an interviewer who is older than, younger than, or the same age as the respondent, or who is of the same, a higher or lower social class, or of the same or a different ethnic group. Doctors and lay interviewers may obtain different responses to the same questions—the easiest way to ensure a high degree of satisfaction with medical care is to base the appraisal on interviews conducted by the treating physicians themselves.

A tactic sometimes used is to have the interviewer make an appraisal of the respondent's 'reliability' (trustworthiness), based on impressions gained during the interview; this appraisal may be aided by asking additional informal questions (preferably after the structured part of the interview) that plumb consistency and accuracy. These appraisals can be taken into account when the data are analysed, e.g. by comparing the results for 'reliable' and 'unreliable' informants.

The interviewer, as well as the respondent, may be a source of bias—his expectations or preferences may influence the answers or the way they are interpreted and recorded. An interviewer who knows what hypothesis the study is testing may tend to get responses that fit in with his view of the validity of the hypothesis. Bias of this sort is least likely to occur in cohort studies in which the interviewer is unaware of the subject's prior exposure to the causal factors under study, and is most likely to occur in a case-control study in which the interviewer knows whether the subject is a case or a control.

Answers may also be influenced by the wording of the questions (see Ch 18). A greater number of surgical procedures may be reported in reply to a question about 'stitches' than to one about 'operations'. In one study 'How old were you when you had your first child?' was found to be a much more reliable question (*kappa* = 88%) than 'How old is your eldest child?' (*kappa* = 66%).[19] The sequence of the questions may also affect the responses.

Memory is fallible, and *recall bias* often occurs. Mild injuries and illnesses, brief stays in hospital, and other past episodes and experiences that made little impact on the respondent may be forgotten and not reported, especially if the time lapse is long. On the other hand, if the question refers to the recent past (say the last month), episodes that occurred longer ago may also be reported (*telescoping bias*). As a compromise, questions about acute illnesses and injuries are usually confined to the previous 2 weeks. Test–retest reliability of interview data on 'simple' events (such as hysterectomy) is high, but it is lower for more complicated data, such as age at occurrence of menopause or other events, or the reasons for starting or stopping drug treatment.[20]

Cues may be needed to tickle the memory. When mothers were asked about the taking of prescription drugs during pregnancy, for example, specific mention of headache, nausea, and various other symptoms increased the number of reports of having taken drugs by 32–58%, and mentioning the drugs by name increased the reports by an extra 6–40%.[21] The number of chronic diseases reported can be doubled if a check-list (phrased in lay terms) is shown or read to the respondents,[22] and can be further increased by using an extensive questionnaire that provides multiple cues and includes probing questions.[23] Reporting of symptoms may be doubled if a check-list is shown to the respondents.[24] Responses become more accurate in studies in which respondents can use memory aids, such as health diaries or wall calendars maintained for this purpose (see p 203); in a randomized controlled study, 50% more symptom episodes were reported by subjects who had been given wall calendars for the recording of symptoms.[25]

'Simple memory failure' of this sort can produce biased estimates of prevalence or incidence and (if groups are being compared) can make it more difficult to detect differences that actually exist. Other effects may occur if there is 'differential memory failure', i.e. where the validity of what is recalled varies in the groups that are compared (see *differential validity*, p 156). True differences between the groups may then be diminished, magnified or masked, and spurious differences may be produced. Precautions can be taken to detect and deal with this form of recall bias.[26] For example, in a case-control study where an association with a specific drug is postulated and it is believed that taking of the drug may be over-reported by cases and/or under-reported by controls, questions may be asked about other drugs (or other factors) known to be unrelated to the disease, to see whether they are reported more frequently by cases than by controls;

these results will provide an indication of the degree of recall bias, and can be taken into account when analysing or interpreting the study findings. Also, at the end of the interview the subjects may be asked about their beliefs concerning the cause of the disorder; recall bias is especially likely if the respondents suspect the drug under study to be a cause.

The replies to questions also depend on who is asked. Husbands and wives tend to report more illness for themselves than for their spouses ('the health of the nation improves markedly when proxy respondents are used; differences are even more noticeable when the respondent for a family is Uncle Joe').[27] Respondents may be unaware of most of the diseases suffered by their brothers and sisters, may not correctly report the causes of their relatives' deaths, and may be more likely to report that family members have a given disease if they themselves have the disease.[28] The frequency with which a man drinks beer may be reported differently by himself and his wife.

Whatever the variable we are trying to measure, we are dealing with statements, and not with direct measurements. This applies as much to attitudes, for which there are no more direct methods of measurement, as to any other variable. If a respondent says he feels well, we have not necessarily learnt his self-perception of his health, but only his reported self-perception of his health—which, however useful it may be as a datum in its own right, is not quite the same thing.

The validity of responses may be appraised by the methods described in Chapter 16. Many studies have compared interview responses with presumably accurate medical records. These found that only 30–53% of documented diagnoses were reported; most hospital admissions and operations were reported, but diagnostic X-ray examinations and many medications were poorly reported.[29] Comparisons with old records may permit tests of the validity of interview data about long past events or experiences; the validity of such data is sometimes surprisingly high.[30] Observational data that can be used as criteria are sometimes available. A comparison with angiographic findings, for example, showed that the sensitivity of the WHO questionnaire on intermittent claudication, as an indicator of severe grades of peripheral arterial disease, was 50%, and its specificity was over 98%.[31] Where suitable criteria are not available, construct validity (see p 156) may be examined. A questionnaire on habitual physical activity, for example, was validated by finding the expected associations with age, sex, kind of job, self-appraisals of physical activity, caloric intake, maximal oxygen intake, body fatness, and exposure to health promotion programmes.[32] When possible, differential validity in different subgroups of the study population should be examined.

INTERVIEW TECHNIQUE

The accuracy of interview data can be boosted not only by the choice of an appropriate mode of administration, the use of memory aids, and careful attention to the construction of the questionnaire and the selection and wording of questions, but by proper interview technique.[1] The main requirement is that the interviewer should beware of influencing the responses. Questions should be asked precisely as they were written, and re-worded or supplemented by explanations only when this is absolutely necessary. The questions should be asked in a neutral manner, without showing (by words, inflection or expression) a preference for any particular response. Agreement, disagreement or surprise should not be shown, and the precise answers should be recorded, without sifting or interpreting them. This, like the ability to encourage the respondents' participation and other necessary skills, demands training and practical experience. Good interviewers are made, not born (although some people are congenitally incapable of becoming good interviewers).

It may be noted that physicians, nurses and social workers often make poor interviewers in a research setting. They have been trained to see their role as the provision of help to patients or clients, and often have difficulty in accepting or fulfilling the different role of collecting standardized data. They may be incapable of merely reading out questions, but insist on rephrasing them or altering their order. They are often skilled interviewers, but have been trained to conduct interviews of a different type, in which selective information is sought to clarify a specific case problem, and efforts are made to exert influence by providing advice, directions, information or reassurance; these habits are not easily unlearned.

NOTES AND REFERENCES

1. For useful practical advice on the art of interviewing, see Survey Research Center, Institute for Social Research 1976 Interviewer's manual. University of Michigan, Ann Arbor, pp 7–34; or Kornhauser A, Sheatsley P B 1976 Questionnaire construction and interview procedure. In: Selltiz C, Wrightsman L S, Cook S W (eds) Research methods in social relations, 3rd edn. Holt Rinehart & Winston, New York, pp 541–573.
2. Rosenman R H, Friedman M, Straus R et al 1964 A predictive study of coronary

heart disease: the Western Collaborative Group Study. Journal of the American Medical Association 189: 15 (appendix; included in reprints only).

3. Glaser E M 1964 Volunteers, controls, placebos and questionaries in clinical trials. In: Witts L J (ed) Medical surveys and clinical trials. Oxford University Press, Oxford, pp 115-129.

4. In Rand's Health Insurance Study (a large-scale trial of methods of financing health care) extensive use was made of self-administered questionnaires to measure health status. Response rates were over 90%, the rate of missing data was below 1%, and the data were of adequate quality. When asked their preferences, 70% of participants opted for self-administered questionnaires and 12% for personal interviews; 18% stated no preference. Ware J E Jr 1984 In: Wenger N K, Mattson M E, Furberg C D, Elinson J (eds) Assessment of quality of life in clinical trials of cardiovascular therapies. LeJacq Publishing (Haymarket-Doyma, New York), pp 87-111.

5. In a survey of women's experiences with childbearing, a randomized comparison showed a lower response for *postal interviews* (75%) than for home interviews (92%). Replies on painful and delicate subjects were similar for the two methods; there were differences in reports of attitudes and of doing the 'right' or 'wrong' thing, but some were in one direction and some in the other. Cartwright A 1988 Interviews or postal questionnaires? Comparisons of data about women's experiences with maternity services. Milbank Quarterly 66: 172.

6. For comparisons of different *modes of interview*, see O'Toole B I, Battistutta D, Long A, Crouch K 1986 A comparison of costs and data quality of three health survey methods: mail, telephone and personal home interview. American Journal of Epidemiology 124: 317; Brambilla D J, McKinlay S M 1987 A comparison of responses to mailed questionnaires and telephone interviews in a mixed mode health survey. American Journal of Epidemiology 126: 962; Siemiatycki J 1979 A comparison of mail, telephone, and home interview strategies for household health surveys. American Journal of Public Health 69: 238.

7. Bradburn N M 1984 Discussion: telephone service methodology. In: Cannell C F, Groves R M (eds) Health survey research methods DHHS publication no. (PHS) 84-3346. National Center for Health Services Research, Washington, DC, pp 146-148.

8. Pless I B, Miller J R 1979 Apparent validity of alternative survey methods. Journal of Community Health 5: 22.

9. Siemiatycki (1979; see note 6).

10. Birkett N J 1988 Computer-aided personal interviewing: a new technique for data collection in epidemiologic surveys. American Journal of Epidemiology 127: 684.

11. *Epi Info* is a public domain program that can prepare questionnaires for *computer-assisted interviews* (see note 5, p 242).

Ready-made public-domain programs include *DIETQL* and *DIETQS* (Smucker R, Block G, Coyle L, Harvin A, Kessler L 1989 A dietary and risk factor questionnaire and analysis system for personal computers. American Journal of Epidemiology 129: 445). These are detailed frequency-type dietary questionnaires, with questions on demographic data, smoking, social networks, family history of cancer, and other topics. The programs are flexible—the sequence can be changed, and questions can be omitted or added. There are inbuilt checks for errors, and automatic branching to the next relevant question. The programs provide instant standardized coding into computer data files. A companion program, *DIETANAL*, estimates each respondent's average daily intake of about 30 nutrients. (Programs available from Dr Gladys Block, Division of Cancer Prevention and Control, National Cancer Institute, Bethesda, MD, USA.) *Sociopolitical Surveys* permits the user to write questions with five response levels, and creates a data file. *Survey System* and *Social Surveys* are similar.

12. Waterton J, Duffy J C 1984 A comparison of computer interviewing techniques and traditional methods in the collection of self-report alcohol consumption data in a field survey. International Statistical Review 52: 173.

13. In a review of what *hard data* means, Feinstein (1983) considers five attributes— preservability, objectivity, dimensionality, accuracy (criterion validity) and consistency—and, after citing examples of data that are not regarded as 'soft' although they are ephemeral, subjective, non-dimensional, or inaccurate, concludes that the fundamental quality of 'hard' data is their consistency—they are 'repeatable by the same observer and reproducible by another'. Feinstein A R 1983 An additional basic science for clinical medicine: IV. The development of clinimetrics. Annals of Internal Medicine 99: 843.

14. Colditz G A, Martin P, Stampfer M J et al Validation of questionnaire information on risk factors and disease outcomes in a prospective cohort study of women. American Journal of Epidemiology 123: 894.

15. Madow W G 1973 Net differences in interview data on chronic conditions and information derived from medical records. Vital and Health Statistics series 2: 57.

16. Chambers L W, Spitzer W O, Hill G B, Helliwell B E 1976 Underreporting of cancer in medical surveys: a source of systematic error in cancer research. American Journal of Epidemiology 104: 41.

17. Mulder P G H, Garretsen H F L 1983 Are epidemiological and sociological surveys a proper instrument for detecting true problem drinkers? International Journal of Epidemiology 12: 442.

18. Stewart A W, Jackson R T, Ford M A, Beaglehole R 1987 Underestimation of relative weight by use of self-reported height and weight. American Journal of Epidemiology 125: 122.

19. Yorkshire Breast Cancer Group 1977 Observer variation in recording clinical data from women presenting with breast lesions. British Medical Journal 2: 1196.

20. When interviews of post-menopausal women were repeated after 2–22 months, kappa values were 0.89–0.93 for data on hysterectomy, a family history of breast cancer, hot flushes, and other 'simple' variables; in 22% there were discrepancies of over 2 years in reported age at menopause. Horwitz R I, Yu E C 1985 Problems and proposals for interview data in epidemiological research. International Journal of Epidemiology 14: 463. In studies of menarcheal and menopausal age in population groups, calculations based on the current status of females of different ages are to be preferred to historical information.

21. Mitchell A A, Cottler L B, Shapiro S 1986 Effect of questionnaire design on recall of drug exposure in pregnancy. American Journal of Epidemiology 123: 670.

22. Linder F E 1965 National health interview surveys. In: Trends in the study of morbidity and mortality. Public Health Papers 27. WHO, Geneva, p 78.

23. National Center for Health Statistics 1972 Reporting health events in household interviews: effects of an extensive questionnaire and a diary procedure. Vital and Health Statistics, series 2, no. 49. Public Health Service, Washington, D C.

24. Spilker A, Kessler J 1987 Comparison of symptoms elicited by checklist and fill-in-the-blank questionnaires. Pharmaco-Epidemiology Newsletter 3: 8.

25. Marcus A C 1982 Memory aids in longitudinal health surveys: results from a field experiment. American Journal of Public Health 72: 567.

26. Raphael K 1987 Recall bias: a proposal for assessment and control. International Journal of Epidemiology 16: 167. Also, see Coughlin S S 1990, Recall bias in epidemiologic studies. Journal of Clinical Epidemiology 43: 87.

27. Kirscht J P 1971 Social and psychological problems of surveys in health and illness. Social Science and Medicine 5: 519.

28. *Family histories of disease* should be used with caution. Many false negative and some false positive reports of diseases in siblings were obtained in a study in the USA, and reported causes of death of relatives often differed from the certified

causes: Napier J A, Metzner H, Johnson B C 1972 Limitations of morbidity and mortality data obtained from family histories—a report from the Tecumseh Community Health Study. American Journal of Public Health 62: 30. Better conformity between reported and certified causes of death was found in a study in Sweden: Waern U, Hedstrand H, Aberg H 1976 What middle-aged men know of their parents' cause of death and age at death: a comparison between history and death certificate. Scandinavian Journal of Social Medicine 4: 123.

When people with rheumatoid arthritis were questioned, 27% reported that their parents were free of arthritis; but when their unaffected siblings were questioned, 50% reported that the same parents were free of arthritis; Schull W J, Cobb S 1969 The intrafamilial transmission of rheumatoid arthritis: III. The lack of support for a genetic hypothesis. Journal of Chronic Diseases 22: 217.

Marshall J, Priore R, Haughey B, Rzepka T, Graham S 1980 (Spouse-subject interviews and the reliability of diet studies. American Journal of Epidemiology 112: 675) found that in about 60% of couples there was exact agreement between men's and their wives' reports of the frequency with which the men ate various food items. The wives reported less frequent beer-drinking by the men. In a similar study of smoking, drinking and dietary habits in Hawaii, about 75% of the pairs agreed within acceptable limits: Kolonel L N, Hirohata H T, Nomura A M Y 1977 Adequacy of survey data collected from substitute respondents. American Journal of Epidemiology 106: 476.

For advice on interviews with *proxy respondents*, see Pickle L W, Brown L M, Blot W J 1983 Information available from surrogate respondents in case-control interview studies. American Journal of Epidemiology 118: 99. Walker A M, Velema J P, Robins J M 1988 Analysis of case-control data derived in part from proxy respondents. American Journal of Epidemiology 127: 905.

29. Harlow S D, Linet M S 1989 Agreement between questionnaire data and medical records: the evidence for accuracy of recall. American Journal of Epidemiology 129: 233.

30. Interview data about the remote past can sometimes be compared with old records. A study in Iowa found that the reported birth weights of adolescents were sufficiently similar to recorded weights to permit inferences about relationships with other factors: Burns T L, Moll P P, Rost C A, Lauer R M 1987 Mothers remember birthweights of adolescent children: the Muscatine Ponderosity Family Study. International Journal of Epidemiology 16: 550. Another study (which used old study records as criteria) showed that it is preferable to ask about past dietary practices, rather than assuming that the current diet is an indication of past diet: Byers T, Marshall J, Anthony E, Fiedler R, Zielezny M 1987 The reliability of dietary history from the distant past. American Journal of Epidemiology 125: 999. In Jerusalem, mothers were found to provide valid information (kappa = 80%) about the breastfeeding of army recruits (in their infancy); Kark J D, Troya G, Friedlander Y, Slater P E, Stein Y 1984 Validity of maternal reporting of breast feeding history and the association with blood lipids in 17 year olds in Jerusalem. Journal of Epidemiology and Community Health 38: 218. Records of a cohort study showed that 8% of 36-year-old men who said they had never smoked regularly had reported regular smoking when questioned at younger ages; Britten N 1988 Validity of claims to lifelong non-smoking at age 38 in a longitudinal study. International Journal of Epidemiology 17: 525.

31. Fowkes F G R 1988 The measurement of atherosclerotic peripheral arterial disease in epidemiological surveys. International Journal of Epidemiology 17: 248.

32. Blair S N, Haskell W L, Ho P et al 1985 Assessment of habitual physical activity by a 7-day recall in a community survey and controlled experiments. American Journal of Epidemiology 122: 794.

18. Constructing a questionnaire

Before a questionnaire is constructed the variables it is designed to measure should be listed. This done, suitable questions should be formulated, i.e. questions that have face validity (see p 152) as measures of these variables, and that also meet the other requirements listed below. To enhance validity, it may be decided to ask multiple questions on some topics, permitting the use of composite scales of measurement (see Ch. 13), both because it may not be possible to cover all facets of the variable in a single question, and because reliance on a single question may increase the chances of inaccuracy due to misunderstanding or other factors. In some cases, to enhance comparability with other studies, questions are borrowed from other sources rather than creating them anew.

'Something old, something new, something borrowed, something blue'—apart maybe from the last ingredient, this is the recipe for most questionnaires. The use of borrowed questions has the advantage that they have already been tested and found to be serviceable. But comparability is sometimes an illusion, since the same questions may differ in their validity in different kinds of population. The investigator should always consider the possible need to revalidate the questions in his own study population. The choice of questions to borrow is not always easy. According to a recent count, for example, a researcher wanting to measure social support can choose between at least 17 different questionnaires, varying in their conceptual framework, content, convenience, applicability, and validity.[1]

The sequence of the questions needs careful attention. The first questions should be easy to answer, of obvious relevance to the topic of the study and (if possible) interesting. 'Difficult' questions, which may occasion embarrassment or resentment, should be left until later—even questions about age, education, etc. are sometimes left to the end for this reason. The questions should follow an order that the respondent will see as natural, with smooth movement from item to item. On the other hand, if the questionnaire is long it may be wise to have breaks in the continuity by switching topics or altering the format of questions, since 'changes of scenery' may prevent boredom. Long successions of questions that are likely to elicit repeated identical responses (e.g. 'yes') should be avoided, as the respondent may fall into a rut (a 'response set') and continue to give the same response unthinkingly.

When arranged in order the questions should be gone through carefully to examine the implications of the sequence. The answer to an earlier question may commit the respondent to a specific answer to a later one (in which case the order should probably be reversed). A particular sequence may be awkward (such as 'Do you have children?' before 'Are you married?'). If the questionnaire includes both specific and general questions about attitudes, the general questions should come first, since specific questions tend to be answered in the same way, wherever they are placed. One study showed that the answer to a question about marital happiness was not influenced by a previous question about happiness in general, whereas the question on general happiness tended to be answered differently, depending on whether the marriage question was asked first.[2] Questions about general health and functional capacity should be put near the beginning, unless the investigator wants the appraisal to be influenced by questions about specific illnesses, symptoms and disabilities. With proper sequencing, irrelevant questions can be bypassed, so that (for example) subjects who say they take no alcohol are not asked for details of their consumption of alcoholic drinks.

If the questionnaire is a self-administered one, an introduction or explanatory note stating the purposes and sponsorship of the study will be necessary, and clear instructions and examples should be given. A statement about confidentiality should be included, but anonymity should not be guaranteed unless there is really no way of tracing which questionnaire belongs to whom. If the questionnaire is to be used by an interviewer, all the explanations and instructions may similarly be included in the form, or it may be preferred to prepare an accompanying guide or manual. The instructions to the interviewer should be full and explicit.

The format of the questionnaire should be one making for ease and accuracy in the recording and coding of responses (the planning of record forms will be discussed in Chapter 21).

When the questionnaire is reconsidered and discussed with colleagues, it is invariably found that it needs modification. Usually, more than one redraft is needed before a 'finished product' is ready—not ready for use, but ready for testing. A questionnaire should not be used until it has been tested in practice—'if you do not have the resources to pilot-test your questionnaire, don't do the study'.[3] It may be decided to try alternative versions of the same questions, in the same questionnaire or in questionnaires tested on different subjects. Pretests (see Ch. 23) are indispensable; they usually reveal a need for changes in the questions or their sequence or, very frequently, for shortening the questionnaire.[4]

OPEN OR CLOSED?

Questions may take two general forms: they may be 'open-ended' (or 'free response') questions, which the subject answers in his own words, or 'closed' (or 'fixed-alternative') questions, which are answered by choosing from a number of fixed alternative responses.

Open-ended questions often produce difficulties when it comes to interpreting the responses. Suppose, for example, we were interested in knowing how many people had given up smoking for reasons connected with health. The question 'Why did you stop smoking? State your main reason' might excite such responses as: 'I thought it was better not to smoke'; 'I'd been smoking for 30 years, and decided it was time to give it up'; 'Because my wife said I should'. There is obvious difficulty in categorizing these answers; in all three instances, it is impossible to tell whether the main reason was connected with health. In a self-administered questionnaire, even a question like 'What is your marital status?' may be answered 'Unsatisfactory' or 'Ask my wife'; a closed question ('Are you at present single, married, widowed or divorced?') is preferable. There is, of course, no difficulty in the use of open-ended questions in instances where the responses can be easily handled, e.g. 'How old were you at your last birthday?' or 'In what country were you born?'. Open-ended questions have an important role in exploratory surveys, where they indicate the range of likely replies and provide a guide to the formulation of alternative responses to closed questions. They may also be used to provide colourful case illustrations to brighten up an otherwise dull report. If followed by 'probe' questions, open-ended questions have certain advantages in the study of complicated or ill formed opinions or attitudes. Qualitative research (see p 134) uses open-ended rather than closed questions.

Closed questions make for greater uniformity and simplify the analysis, and are therefore preferred for most purposes, although they limit the variety and detail of responses. They may provide two responses (such as 'yes–no', 'agree–disagree') or more (such as 'never', 'seldom', 'occasionally', 'fairly frequently', and 'very often'). The range of responses is equivalent to the scale of measurement we have previously spoken of (Ch. 12); it should be comprehensive, and the categories should be mutually exclusive. An 'other (specify)...' category is sometimes included, as insurance against oversights in the choice of categories. Except in simple instances such as 'yes–no' choices, the alternative responses should be read to the subject, shown to him (e.g. on a card) or, in a self-administered questionnaire, printed after the question. To avoid the need to express all the alternative responses in words, use may be made of graphic rating scales. The subject is shown a line or ladder labelled at its ends with the two extreme responses, and asked to answer the question by indicating an appropriate point on the scale; some intermediate labels may also be printed on the scale. Points along the scale may be shown by numbers, or a score can be obtained by measuring the position of the point marked by the respondent.[5]

The formulation of response categories for a question like 'What was your main reason for giving up smoking?' often needs careful thought. A misguided selection of alternatives may, like a Procrustean bed, achieve conformity at a considerable price. It is sometimes advisable to use an open-ended question first (in a pretest), so that free responses can be collected and used as a basis for the design of 'closed' categories. Another approach is to follow the closed question with a suitable open-ended one on the same topic; in a pretest, this may demonstrate flaws in the closed question; in the study itself, the combination provides the advantages of both types of question.

REQUIREMENTS OF QUESTIONS

1. Must have face validity
2. Respondents can be expected to know the answer
3. Must be clear and unambiguous
4. Must not be offensive
5. Must be fair

The main requirement of a question is, of course, that it should have *face validity* as a measure of the variable it is wished to study. There are also other requirements.[6]

The questions should be ones to which the respondents can be *expected to know the answers*. There is little point in asking 'Did your grandmother have piles?', or in inviting opinions on a matter the respondent has never thought about, or asking the respondent to state attitudes or motivations of which he may not be aware. People who have not been told they have diabetes cannot report that they have the disease. There is little value in questions concerning events or experiences that had little impact and that many subjects will not recall, such as minor injuries or food eaten 3 days previously. Many mild illnesses not requiring medical care and not restricting activity fail to be reported after the lapse of 1 week, and many hospitalizations are not recalled after 1 year. Illnesses requiring a single consultation with a physician are reported more poorly than those requiring many consultations, and conditions requiring a long stay in hospital or involving surgery are reported more fully than other conditions.

It is often decided that since the respondents cannot be expected to supply the required information in a direct way, indirect questions will be asked, the desired information being inferred from the responses to questions on other matters. Instead of asking the subject if he is emotionally healthy, he may be asked about a series of symptoms from which his emotional health can be inferred.[7] Instead of asking a mother to state her attitudes concerning permissiveness towards children, she may be asked whether she carries or carried out specific actions, or what she would do in a specific situation, or how she thinks other mothers would feel or act, or how she thinks mothers *should* act. Instead of (or as well as) asking the respondent whether he is satisfied with his own medical care, he may be asked what he thinks of the medical care in his neighbourhood, or whether he agrees or disagrees with such statements as 'Most doctors take a real interest in their patients'.

The way in which questions are worded can 'make or break' a questionnaire. Questions must be *clear* and *unambiguous*. They must be phrased in language that it is believed the respondents will understand, and that all respondents will understand in the same way. This is more easily said than done—when a questionnaire is tested, unexpected double meanings are often found concealed in apparently crystal-clear questions. 'Single' may mean 'never married' to some people, and 'not married at present' to others; 'abortion' may mean different things to different people. 'Family' may be understood to mean the immediate family, or relatives in the same household, or the far-flung extended family, or forebears. The most everyday words may evoke different interpretations. In one methodological study it was found that when answering questions about 'usual' behaviour— where the intended meaning was 'in the ordinary course of events'—

20% of respondents gave it other interpretations (e.g. 'more often than not' or 'at regular (even if infrequent) intervals'), and 19% disregarded the term completely, and gave answers that were not constrained by it at all.[8]

Medical terms, even those commonly used in everyday speech, may occasion much difficulty. 'Anaemia' and 'heart disease' may have different connotations for the layman and the physician; to many laymen, 'palpitation' means a feeling of breathlessness or of fright, and 'flatulence' means an acid taste in the mouth.[9] If a difficult term must be used, a preliminary 'sieve' question should be asked, to screen out persons who do not know it; for example, before asking 'Do you think that people with a lot of cholesterol in their blood should give up smoking?', it might be wise to ask 'Do you happen to know what cholesterol is?'.

To ensure clarity, each question should contain only one idea; 'double-barrelled' questions like 'Do you take your child to a doctor when he has a cold or has diarrhoea?' are difficult to answer, and the answers are difficult to interpret.

If closed questions are used, all the alternative responses should be clearly expressed. The alternatives should be stated at the end, not the beginning, i.e. not 'Do you very often, frequently, seldom, hardly ever, or never do the Highland fling?', but 'How often do you do the Highland fling—very often, frequently, seldom, hardly ever or never?'

Where possible, it is wise to avoid questions that may *offend* the respondent, for example those that deal with intimate matters, those which may seem to expose the respondent's ignorance, and those requiring him to give a socially unacceptable answer, such as admitting to venereal disease or a shameful habit. If 'difficult' questions of this sort must be asked, special care must be taken (see below).

The questions should be *fair*. They should not be phrased (or voiced) in a way that suggests a specific answer, and should not be loaded. The question 'What are the main things that are wrong with the care you get from your doctor?' is an obviously unfair one. A format that 'begs the question' in this way should be used, if at all, only in studies of attitudes in which it is felt that the best way to get a respondent to voice his biases is to indicate that the interviewer shares them.

Short questions are generally regarded as preferable to long ones. But experiments have shown that length may sometimes be a virtue—longer questions may elicit fuller responses.[10] More symptoms or chronic disorders, for example, tend to be reported if longer questions are used. This may partly be because the additional material helps the respondent's recall. But a longer question may evoke a fuller response even if the added verbiage seems redundant. In one study, the question 'The next question is about medicines during the past 4 weeks. We want to ask you about this. What medicines, if any, did you take or use during the past 4 weeks?' yielded more information than the same question with the first two sentences removed. The reasons for this are not clear—maybe asking a longer question inclines the respondent to answer at equal length, or maybe the extra material simply gives the respondent more time to think. Short, terse questions appear to be preferable for the study of attitudes,[3] but longer questions may have advantages for symptoms, disorders, and practices. One recommendation that has ensued from these findings is that questions should be short when possible, but interviews should be conducted at a slow pace, so that respondents have time to think. Longer questions should be used with discrimination—'if we larded all questions with "filler" phrases, a questionnaire would soon be bloated with too few, too fat questions'.[11]

'SENSITIVE' QUESTIONS

It may not be possible to avoid asking 'sensitive' questions that may offend respondents, e.g. those that seem to expose the respondent's ignorance, or call for socially unacceptable answers. Embarrassment can often be mitigated by including a statement designed to show that the questioner's interest is non-judgemental: 'We know that all married couples sometimes quarrel with each other; how often does it happen that *you* quarrel with your husband?' Possible tactics, as amusingly described by Barton,[12] are:

1. *The everybody approach*: 'As you know, many people have been killing their wives these days. Do you happen to have killed yours?'
2. *The other people approach*: (a) 'Do you know any people who have murdered their wives?' (b) 'How about yourself?'
3. *The Kinsey technique*: Stare firmly into the respondent's eyes and ask in simple, clear-cut language such as that to which the respondent is accustomed, and with an air of assuming that everybody has done everything, 'Did you ever kill your wife?'

A study of reactions to questions concerning behaviour about which many people are reluctant to talk fully and honestly, in three large samples in the USA, showed that responses were little affected by the mode of administration (face-to-face, telephone, or self-administered) or the presence of a third party, but that the construction of the question made a great deal of difference.[13] In particular, there were two tactics that produced a two- to threefold increase in the amount of reporting of behaviour. The first was the use of a long introduction to the question, and the second was the use of an open-ended question. In this study the open-ended format was used only for questions about the amount or frequency of behaviour (how much liquor do you drink? how many times a week do you drink?), where the answers could be fairly easily coded. The findings suggested that long questions and an open-ended format should routinely be used when asking about the frequency of sensitive behaviour. The open-ended questions gave significantly higher frequencies for beer, wine and liquor drinking, petting, intercourse, and masturbation. A suggested reason is that the presence of low-frequency categories ('never, once a year or less, every few months, once a month, every few weeks...') made people less willing to admit to higher frequencies.

Another recommended approach, which increased the reported frequencies of socially undesirable behaviour by about 15%, is the use of words familiar to the respondent. A suggested method is to let the respondent decide what term should be used, and then to use this in subsequent questions. For example, 'Different people use different words for sexual intercourse [or marijuana, masturbation, etc.]. What word do you think we should use?' It may also be helpful to ask whether the respondent has engaged in the socially undesirable behaviour in the past ('Did you ever, even once...'), before asking about current behaviour.[3]

Another simple technique is putting the possible responses on cards, so that the respondent need only point to the answer, without letting the offending words sully his lips.

NOTES AND REFERENCES

1. Orth-Gomer K, Unden A L 1987 The measurement of social support in population surveys. Social Science and Medicine 24: 83.
2. Turner C F 1984 Why do surveys disagree? Some preliminary hypotheses and some disagreeable examples. In: Turner C F, Martin E (eds) Surveying subjective phenomena, vol 2. Russell Sage, New York.
3. Sudman S, Bradburn N M 1983 Asking questions. Jossey-Bass, San Francisco.

4. For more detailed guides to questionnaire construction, see Kornhauser A, Sheatsley P B 1976 Questionnaire construction and interview procedure. In: Selltiz, Wrightsman L S, Cook S W (eds) Research methods in social relations, 3rd edn. Holt Rinehart & Winston, New York, pp 541–573; Kahn R L, Cannell C F 1967 The dynamics of interviewing. Wiley, New York, pp 106–165; pp 541–573; Bennett A E, Ritchie K 1975 Questionnaires in medicine—a guide to their design and use. Oxford University Press, London.

5. For examples, see reports on the use of graphic scales to measure beliefs about diseases (Jenkins C D 1966 The semantic differential for health: a technique for measuring beliefs about diseases. Public Health Reports 81: 549); the coronary-prone behaviour pattern (Bortner R W, Rosenman R H 1967 The measurement of pattern A behaviour. Journal of Chronic Diseases 20: 525); and aspirations and fears (Cantril H 1965 The pattern of human conflicts. Rutgers University Press, New Brunswick N J, pp 22–26).

6. For far more detailed advice on the formulation of questions, see Payne S L 1965 The art of asking questions. Princeton University Press, Princeton, N J; Converse J M, Presser S 1986 Survey questions: handicrafting the standardized questionnaire. Sage Publications, Beverly Hills; Sudman & Bradburn (1983; see note 3).

7. For a review of the use of such questionnaires in psychiatric epidemiology, see Goldberg D P 1972 The detection of psychiatric illness by questionnaire. Oxford University Press, Oxford, pp 5–34.

8. Belson W A 1981 The design and understanding of survey questions. Gower, Aldershot, Hants.

9. Boyle C M 1970 Difference between patients' and doctors' interpretation of some common medical terms. British Medical Journal ii: 286.

10. Henson R, Cannell C F, Lawson S A 1979 In: Cannell C F, Oksenberg L, Converse J M (eds) Experiments in interviewing techniques. Institute for Social Research, Ann Arbor, Michigan; Laurent A 1972 Effects of question length on reporting behavior in the survey interview. Journal of the American Statistical Association 67: 298–305; Belson (1981; see note 8); Gower, Aldershot, Hants; Sudman & Bradburn (1983; see note 3).

11. Converse & Presser (1986; see note 6), p 12.

12. Barton A J 1958 Asking the embarrassing question. Public Opinion Quarterly 22: 67.

13. Bradburn N M, Sudman S et al 1981 Improving interview method and questionnaire design. Jossey-Bass, San Francisco.

19. Surveying the opinions of experts

There is sometimes interest in learning the opinions of people who are specially knowledgeable. The latter may be experts who have special skills and knowledge relevant to some field of health care, or they may be professionals or laymen who are especially well-informed about some situation, such as a specific community and its problems.

Surveys of experts' opinions may have two kinds of study objective:

1. To determine attitudes, concerns, appraisals of the relative importance of various factors or the desirability of various options, and the reasons for these judgements. When planning a health programme, for example, it may be helpful to know what knowledgeable people think are the chief problems and how they appraise the relative importance of these problems, or their opinions about the desirability, feasibility or pros and cons of various solutions. When a programme is to be evaluated, experts may be asked to choose criteria for the evaluation and to decide on the relative importance of these criteria, so that an appropriate weight can be allocated to each of them.[1]
2. If objective facts about a situation are difficult or impossible to obtain, experts may be asked what they judge the facts to be. These 'guesstimates' may in some circumstances provide a basis for programme planning, on the assumption that an informed guess is better than no information at all. This use of experts' opinions may be especially appropriate in developing countries in instances where 'hard' data cannot be gathered. In studies of cost-effectiveness, experts' estimates of the effectiveness of intervention procedures may be used as a substitute for objective measurements. In long-term planning, decisions may be based on experts' forecasts of the future situation.

Such surveys call for special methods. The main limitation of ordinary interview and questionnaire methods is that they permit no communication among the participants, and hence limit the exercise of expertise. One expert has no opportunity to influence others, or to reach a modified judgement after appraising the opinions of his peers. Group techniques that permit free communication—panel discussions, committee meetings and conference telephone calls—have other limitations. The group's decisions may be heavily influenced by the manner in which its members interact, and this may be determined by a chairperson's bossiness or ineffectiveness, dominance by verbose or forceful speakers, deference to authority, power, prestige or age, or friendships or antagonisms between participants. A group discussion designed to gather data on attitudes and perceptions requires a trained discussion leader who follows a prescribed set of rules, and a carefully prepared discussion guide.[2]

The problems of group techniques can be minimized by methods that avoid or restrict interaction between participants, but provide interim feedback of the opinions of the group as a whole, which each participant can take into account before stating his final judgement. This is then pooled with other contributions to yield a group decision.

The *nominal group technique* is a simple method that may be used if the experts can be brought together at a meeting. The *Delphi technique* needs more elaborate preparation and organization but does not require the experts to come together. With both techniques the findings depend, of course, on the selection of the participant experts.

NOMINAL GROUP TECHNIQUE

The nominal group technique (NGT) which was developed by Van de Ven and Delbecq,[3] is so called because although the participants sit together, discussion is permitted only during specified phases of the process. Hence during most phases they are a group 'in name only'.

The technique may be used in a variety of situations requiring group decision-making. The participants may be any knowledgeable or concerned individuals, professional or lay. The technique was originally developed as a method of involving disadvantaged citizens in community action agencies, and it has been recommended for use in exploratory studies of citizens' or professionals' perceptions of health care problems (see p 313).[3]

The procedure[4] is simple. Five to nine participants (preferably not more than seven) sit round a table, together with a leader. If there are more participants they are divided into small groups. A single session, which deals with a single question, usually takes at least 60–90 minutes (longer if the judgements of different groups are to be pooled).

For a typical meeting of a single small group, the following are the successive steps.

1. Silent generation of ideas in writing
2. 'Round-robin' feedback of ideas
3. Serial discussion of ideas
4. Preliminary vote
5. Discussion of preliminary vote
6. Final vote

1. *Silent generation of ideas in writing.* After making a welcoming statement, which stresses the importance of the task and of each member's contribution, the leader reads out the question that the participants are required to answer. This is usually an open-ended question that calls for a list of items, e.g. the elements of a specified problem or of a proposed programme for dealing with a problem. Each member is given a worksheet (at the top of which the question appears) and is asked to take 5 minutes to write his ideas in response to the question. The leader also does this. Discussion is not permitted.

2. *'Round-robin' feedback of ideas.* The leader goes round the table and asks each member in turn to contribute one of the ideas he has written, summarized in a few words. The leader also takes a turn in each round. Each idea is numbered and written on a large blackboard or on a flip pad, completed sheets of which are taped or pinned where they are visible to all members. Members are asked not to contribute ideas that they regard as complete duplicates. Members are encouraged to add ideas to their worksheets at any time; they may 'pass' in one round and contribute in a later one. The process goes on until no further ideas are forthcoming. Discussion is not permitted during this stage.

3. *Serial discussion of ideas.* Each of the ideas listed on the board or flip pad is discussed in turn. For each one, the group is asked whether there are questions, or whether anyone wishes to clarify the item, explain the logic behind it, or express a view about its relative importance. The object of the discussion is to obtain clarity and to air points of view, but not to resolve differences of opinion.

If there is much overlap between items it may be desirable to modify the list, after the serial discussion. One way of doing this is to rearrange the items so that variants of a single factor appear consecutively (retaining their original serial numbers) under a broad heading. Modest rewording may be undertaken if the group wishes to refine the list.

4. *Preliminary vote.* Each participant is asked to select a specified number (5–9) of 'most important' items from the total list, and copy them on to cards. If six are to be chosen, each participant is asked to write '6' (underlined or circled) on the 'most important' card, then '1' on the least important, then '5' on the most important of the remaining four, then '2', and so on. The leader also ranks the items. The cards are then collected and shuffled to maintain anonymity, and the votes are read out and recorded on a tally-chart that shows all the items and the rank numbers allocated to each.

5. *Discussion of preliminary vote.* Brief discussion of the voting pattern is now permitted. Members are told that the purpose of this discussion is additional clarification, and not to pressure them to change their votes.

6. *Final vote.* Step 4 is then repeated. The most important items may again be ranked, or they may be given ratings on a scale from 0 (unimportant) to 10 or 100 (very important). The rank numbers or ratings allotted to each item may be averaged by summing them and dividing by the total number of participants. Other rating methods may be used. For example, members may be asked to assign 100 points to the most important item and to give points to the other items in proportion to their relative importance, e.g. 50 points for an item half as important.[5]

If there are 10 or more participants they should be divided into small groups, and steps 1 to 4 are performed separately in each group. There is then a break, during which the group leaders meet to prepare a master list of items, including the top five to nine priorities identified by each group. Where necessary, items are reworded or combined. The master list shows the aggregated votes relating to each of the items included. All the participants then gather in a single large group, and discuss each item in the master list in turn, for clarification. The preliminary vote is then discussed. At any member's request, items not included in the master list can be added. A final vote is then conducted.

DELPHI TECHNIQUE

The Delphi technique (named after the oracle) is more elaborate. It was first used to forecast what atom bomb targets might be selected by a potential enemy of the USA and how many bombs would be needed. Since then its applications have broadened considerably. It has been defined as a 'method for structuring a group communication process so that the process is effective in allowing a group of individuals, as a whole, to deal with a complex problem'.[6]

The method has been extensively applied in the health field, for example to determine experts' opinions concerning ways of dealing with drug abuse[7] and sick absenteeism,[8] the likely effects on children's IQs of various nutrition intervention programmes in pregnancy and infancy,[9] the number of potential candidates for chronic haemodialysis,[10] expected changes in nurses' roles,[11] criteria for use in the evaluation of psychiatric care,[1] the extrapolation of the results of animal experiments to man,[12] and definitions of epidemiological terms.[13]

Face-to-face contact between the participants is not required, although the 'Delphi' label is sometimes attached to procedures that include group discussion.[1] A series of mailed questionnaires is usually used, each one sent out after the results of the previous one have been analysed. The process therefore usually takes weeks or months. The time taken may be cut down considerably by the use of modern telecommunications and a computer.

The elements that are usually included are an opportunity for individuals to contribute ideas of information, an assessment of the group judgement, clarification of reasons for differences, a chance for individuals to revise their views, and some degree of anonymity for the individual responses. Votes may be cast and results fed back repeatedly, until stability or consensus is reached.

The Delphi procedure is protean in its manifestations, and no simple prescription can be given.[14] A learned compendium on the technique states that 'if anything is true about Delphi today, it is that in its design and use Delphi is more of an art than a science'.[6]

NOTES AND REFERENCES

1. Clark A, Friedman M J 1982 The relative importance of treatment outcomes: a Delphi group weighting in mental health. Evaluation Review 6: 79. This describes a study in which a group of clinicians, administrators and researchers assigned weights to nine outcome measures, so that these measures could be combined to appraise the overall effectiveness of psychiatric care programmes.

Improvement in ability to support oneself was judged the most important outcome, with symptom reduction second (weights 0.19 and 0.17 respectively); frequency of drug abuse was judged the least important measure (weight: 0.03).

2. A *group discussion* technique, with a description of the role and training of the discussion leader, is described by Blum M I, Foos P W 1986 Data gathering: experimental methods plus. Harper & Row, New York, Chapter 14.

3. Van de Ven A H, Delbecq A L 1972 American Journal of Public Health 62: 337.

4. The *nominal group technique* is fully described by Delbecq A L, Van de Ven A H, Gustafson D H 1975 Techniques for program planning: a guide to nominal group and Delphi processes. Scott, Foreman, Glenview, Illinois. The procedure described in the text is based on detailed instructions given in Chapter 3 of that book.

The authors point out the importance of asking the right questions and the right people, likening the nominal group technique to a microscope and a vacuum cleaner: 'NGT is like a microscope. Properly focused by a good question, NGT can provide a great deal of conceptual detail about the matter of concern to you. Improperly focused by a poor or misleading question, it tells you a great deal about something in which you are not interested' (p 75). 'NGT is like a vacuum. It is a powerful means to draw out the insight and information possessed by group members. However, if there is nothing to "draw out" even a powerful vacuum is useless' (p 79).

5. If a fixed number of points are assigned to the referent item, it may be desirable to standardize the scores by expressing each one as a proportion or percentage of the sum of all the points allocated by the person. See Edwards W, Guttentag M, Snapper K 1975 A decision-theoretic approach to evaluation research. In: Struening E L, Guttentag M (eds) Handbook of evaluation research. Sage, Beverly Hills, California, p 155.

6. Linstone H A, Turoff M (eds) 1975 The Delphi method: techniques and applications. Addison-Wesley, Reading, Massachusetts, p 3.

7. Jillson I A 1975 The national drug-abuse policy Delphi: progress report and findings to date. In: Linstone & Turoff (1975; see note 6), p 124.

8. Williamson J W cited by Linstone & Turoff (1975; see note 6), p 79.

9. Longhurst R cited by Linstone & Turoff (1975; see note 6), p 80.

10. Hallan J B, Harris B S H 1970 Estimation of a potential hemodialysis population. Medical Care 8: 209.

11. Study by the School of Nursing of the University of Wisconsin, Madison; specimen questionnaires are reproduced by Delbecq et al (1975; see note 4), p 194.

12. Milholland A V, Wheeler M S, Heieck J J 1973 Medical assessment by a Delphi group technic. New England Journal of Medicine 288: 1272.

13. Last J M 1982 Towards a dictionary of epidemiological terms. International Journal of Epidemiology 11: 188.

14. Interested readers may refer to Linstone & Turoff (1975; see note 6) who give a number of detailed examples. Delbecq et al (1975; see note 4) provide simple guidelines for one form of Delphi procedure.

20. The use of documentary sources

The use of documentary sources is attractive because it is a relatively easy way of obtaining data; documents can provide ready-made information both about the study population as a whole, and about its individual members. Documents may also constitute the best or only means of studying past events. ('There are two ways of telling the age of a rhinoceros. The first is to examine its teeth. The second is to collect the evidence of those who remember the beast when it was young, and may even have kept some newspaper cutting recording its birth.')[1]

The documents may be written, printed, or recorded electronically (computer tapes or disks, tape recordings). They include clinical records, 'vital records' (certificates of birth, death, marriage, etc.), other personal records (such as health diaries specially maintained for the purpose of a study), and registers, databases and archives containing aggregations of data on individuals. Use may also be made of documents that provide ready-made statistics and other information on populations (demography, mortality, morbidity, hospitalization rates, etc.).

Documents are frequently the only or the most convenient source of information at the investigator's disposal. But it must be remembered they were generally produced for clinical, administrative or fiscal ends rather than for research purposes, and questions of validity may arise. There may be no uniform definitions (of diseases and demographic or other variables), methods of investigation may be unstandardized or used differentially, and the records may not have been maintained with the obsessive care that would be expected in a planned investigation. Even if uniform definitions and procedures were used, they may not be consistent with the investigator's concepts of the variables; for his purposes the data may hence be of low validity. Secondary data should always be used with circumspection.

CLINICAL RECORDS

Medical records may be very disappointing as a source of data, unless they have been planned and maintained as a basis for research. To quote Mainland, 'Most of the people responsible for hospital and clinic records are not trained investigators, and moreover the pressure of routine work is commonly heavy. From experience gained in the making of clinical records myself, from watching others making them, and in trying to use them, I have come to believe that the only records trustworthy for anything more than superficial impressions, or as hints for further research, are: (a) The records made meticulously by a physician regarding his own patients because he wishes to learn from them; (b) Records kept regarding a particular group of patients by a suitable and adequately instructed person, specially assigned to the task'.[2]

There are generally problems of reliability and validity. The information may have been collected by more than one person, using different definitions. Since the data are second-hand, it is possible that even if uniform definitions and procedures were used, these may not be consistent with the investigator's requirements. Moreover, recording may be patchy; occupations, body weights and blood pressures may be recorded in some instances, not in others. If the presence of a symptom, sign or specific disease is not recorded, this may mean that it was found to be absent, or that no attempt was made to establish its presence, or that its presence was established but not recorded, whether by oversight or because it was regarded as unimportant or irrelevant. Even in good hospital records,[3] the absence of information does not mean absence of the phenomenon. As an extreme illustration of this type of shortcoming, an analysis of the diagnoses recorded in an African hospital revealed that 2% of African and Indian outpatients were recorded as having avitaminoses or other deficiency states;[4] since field surveys had revealed that the majority of Africans and Indians in the region had clinical evidence of malnutrition, this finding threw light on the inadequacy of the records rather than on the prevalence of malnutrition.

Nevertheless, routine records that include reasonably well-recorded information of reasonable quality can be reasonably useful as a basis for investigations. Special care must be taken not to make errors when the information is extracted from the records. These are especially likely to occur if handwritings are difficult to read or if the required information has to be hunted for, e.g. if it is not recorded in a standard place or is buried in long works of prose. A study of reliability, based on replicate extractions by carefully trained personnel from a set of hospital records, showed a good deal of interextractor and intraextractor variation; for example, in 23% of instances there was disagreement between extractors on the presence of a history of hypertension, and in 21% there were discrepancies between two extractions (6 or more months apart) by the same person. In about half these cases the disagreement concerned the presence or absence of the history, and in half the conflict was between 'negative' and 'uncertain'. The main reasons for disagreements were failure to find information recorded in unexpected places, and errors (despite careful training) in the coding of data.[5]

However good the records and however carefully the data are extracted, it is important to remember that the information is unlikely to be complete. Use is being made of selected facts—those that clinicians determined and recorded—concerning selected people—those who came for care (see p 59). The possibility of bias is illustrated by a community survey in Mississippi, which showed that 42% of identified cases of Parkinson's disease had not previously been diagnosed as having this condition.[6]

Routine clinical records from services other than hospitals and certain clinics and health centres are generally of little value as a basis for research. This applies especially to general practice records, which usually give only a very rough guide to morbidity patterns and the utilization of services. Not only may the quality of the diagnostic information be unsatisfactory, for lack of suitable diagnostic facilities and other reasons, but the records are seldom full or maintained in a manner that lends itself to analysis. Records of home visits are usually especially incomplete; a study of the clinical records maintained in a medical care plan in New York indicated that half the home visits (as opposed to one-sixth of the office visits) were not recorded, and that respiratory diseases were consequently underrepresented in the diagnostic data.[7]

This is not to say that routine records from general practices or other primary-care services can never provide useful data. On the contrary, if pains are taken to collect and record information accurately, the records may be of immense value.[8] Not only do people who attend for primary medical care constitute a very much larger and more representative population group than patients treated in hospitals or specialty clinics, but the records of a primary-care service directed at a defined eligible population can sometimes provide data about all members of that population, including those who do not seek care. Moreover, primary-care records can yield data about mild illnesses as well as those that need specialized care, and in many instances can also provide information about incipient and potential illnesses and about factors that may endanger or promote health. They can provide a basis for research on the aetiology, natural history, prevention and care of common diseases and disabilities, processes of growth and development, and the effects of familial factors and social supports and pressures on health and health care. Networks of primary-care practices that engage in collaborative research have been set up in the UK, the USA and Canada, the Netherlands, Belgium and other countries.

The use of clinical records for epidemiological purposes is an essential element in community-oriented primary care (see Ch. 32).

A number of instruments (record cards, books, etc.) have been developed to enable physicians to conduct epidemiological, operational and other research based on their own work.[9] These include age–sex registers of the practice population, 'minimum data sets' that include a wider range of variables, and registers of patients with selected disorders or risk factors. Throughout the world, primary-care practitioners are experimenting with 'problem-based'[10] and other improved clinical records.

Recent years have seen an increasing interest in the computerization of primary-care records,[11] usually with an eye to the easy retrieval of clinical information at an individual level and the provision of reminders to practitioners, or as an accounting tool. The development of user-friendly software that permits statistical processing and analyses as well as supplying these needs is in its infancy.

MEDICAL AUDIT

In recent years much attention has been paid to the development of techniques of evaluating the quality of clinical care by measuring the performance of diagnostic, therapeutic and other procedures. These 'medical audit' and related techniques[12] are usually based upon an examination of clinical records. In order to enhance objectivity, use is generally made of explicit criteria. These may be *normative* standards, which express experts' opinions as to what procedures should be carried out in specific types of cases, or *empirical* standards, based upon studies of what is actually done in clinical facilities that are of an acceptable level. The review may cover all cases cared for, a representative sample, or defined categories, such as patients with selected 'indicator' conditions. It is often especially helpful to review the history of patients with poor outcomes, such as those with preventable disorders or complications. This may identify deficiencies not only in the care that was given, but also in compliance and in the availability and use of services.[13]

Audit techniques have their main application in evaluative reviews (as opposed to trials) of clinical services. The audit is based on the assumption that the performance of certain procedures is likely to benefit patients, and care is favourably evaluated if the audit shows that these activities have been satisfactorily performed. The assumptions themselves are not tested. This means, of course, that the evaluation is valid only in so far as the assumptions are valid. Sceptics point out that evidence of the efficacy of the procedures is usually lacking; that is, there is seldom convincing proof of a cause–effect relationship between the recommended procedures and the outcome.[14]

An important advantage of the audit method is the ease with which the evaluation results can be translated into practical recommendations. If the audit shows that X is *not* being done, then the recommendation is made that X *should* be done. It is also a useful educational tool—a new doctor or nurse in a clinic will rapidly learn that it is expected that X *will* be done.

In some audit systems, account is taken of outcomes. The outcomes that are measured include 'end-results' ('changes in the patient as a person or in the attributes of the disease or condition')[15] and intermediate outcomes, such as the establishment of correct diagnoses, or changes in the patient's health behaviour. The assumption is made that satisfactory end-results indicate that care was satisfactory. This is of course not necessarily true, but if patients do well, there is at least no cause for concern.

A basic problem of medical audit is that the records may not provide the required information unless they were planned for this purpose, and unless pains are taken to keep full clinical notes (computer recording does not necessarily solve these problems). Fuller notes may of course not mean better care. A comparison of the charts of patients treated for acute appendicitis, for example, revealed considerable disparity among three hospitals in the frequency of documentation of commonly sought symptoms and signs, yet at each hospital the disease was diagnosed with the same accuracy. Similarly, in cases with acute myocardial infarction the documentation of elements of the history, physical examination and special tests bore no relationship to the outcome of care, such as the length of time lost from work, or the occurrence of new angina pectoris, a repeated infarction, or death. 'Outstanding clinicians may keep

inadequate records, whereas others less competent may write pro-
fusely...The mere act of writing cannot improve a patient's
outcome.'[16]

HOSPITAL STATISTICS

Hospital records have come a long way since Florence Nightingale
wrote, 'In attempting to arrive at the truth, I have applied everywhere for information, but in scarcely an instance have I been able to
obtain hospital records fit for any purposes of comparison'.[17] In
most hospitals today, most diagnoses regarded as important are
recorded, and most recorded diagnoses are reasonably well substantiated. Despite their shortcomings, hospital statistics provide a
useful source of data on the morbidity pattern of a population.

Problems in the use of hospital statistics include the bias caused by
selective factors influencing hospitalization, including possible
Berksonian bias affecting associations between diseases and between
diseases and other factors (see p 59). Another problem is that diagnostic statistics based on hospital records are usually based on the
selection of a single one of the patient's diagnoses. There may be
little consistency in the way this diagnosis is chosen, even where
a standard criterion has been decided upon. A recommendation
made by WHO is that 'the condition to be selected for single-cause
analysis...is the main condition treated or investigated during the
relevant episode; if no diagnosis was made, the main symptom or
problem should be selected.'[18] A common procedure is to select the
condition that prompted the hospital admission (in terms of the final
diagnosis of this condition, not the tentative diagnosis recorded at the
time of admission). The choice may be made by a physician (often a
junior one) or a medical recorder. Diagnostic statistics based on
hospital records must be treated with a degree of reserve. In the USA
there was a substantial increase in reported hospitalizations for acute
myocardial infarction between 1981 and 1986, caused by a change in
the way diagnoses were selected.[19]

In some countries diagnosis-related groups (DRGs) are used for
determining rates of payment for hospital care. The classification is
based not only on the patient's main diagnosis, but on other factors
as well, such as age, the occurrence of complications and associated
disorders, and the form of treatment. Since the inclusion of additional data may increase the hospital's income, more information is
likely to be used than merely a diagnosis—there is a higher rate of
remuneration for 'complicated peptic ulcer' (such as a bleeding

ulcer), for example, than for an uncomplicated ulcer. But there may also be bias, since a choice is often available (depending on clinical judgement) between DRGs with very different rates of reimbursement; one author who warns of possible 'shift in a hospital's reported case mix in order to improve reimbursement' refers to this possibility as 'DRG creep—a new hospital acquired disease'.[20] A study of hospital diagnostic statistics in the USA before and after the introduction of payment by DRGs showed differences consistent with the hypothesis that 'within the range of accepted medical practice, diagnoses will be recorded which maximize hospital revenues'.[21] Nevertheless, say the authors of that study, 'while it is true that epidemiologists must operate in a world of imperfect information, they should not be paralyzed by this lack of knowledge; rather they must become as aware as possible of the nature and extent of these imperfections. As Major Greenwood said: "The scientific purist, who will wait for medical statistics until they are nosologically perfect, is no wiser than Horace's rustic waiting for the river to flow away."

DEATH CERTIFICATES AND MORTALITY STATISTICS

Mortality statistics are based on the causes of death reported in death certificates. As the following excerpt from the international form shows (Table 20.1), several causes may be entered. One of these is selected as the *underlying cause* of death; this is defined by WHO as '(a) the disease or injury which initiated the train of events leading directly to death, or (b) the circumstances of the accident or violence which produced the fatal injury'. If the certificate has been filled in correctly this is the last condition entered in part I of the certificate. This cause is not automatically selected—if it seems highly improbable that it was in fact the underlying cause of death, a different condition may be chosen, using a series of rules recommended by WHO. These rules are not simple.[22] The wording chosen for the diagnosis (e.g 'chronic ischaemic heart disease' or 'arteriosclerotic cardiovascular disease', or 'cancer of the uterus' or 'cancer of the cervix') may determine the coding category to which the cause is allotted.[23]

There are a number of obvious sources of inaccuracy. As any physician who fills in death certificates knows, it is not always easy to complete the form accurately. The certifier may not be sure of the true cause or causes of death, either because he has insufficient clinical information, or because the clinical picture is a complicated

Table 20.1   Part of the international form of the medical certificate of cause of death

	Cause of death
	I
Disease or condition directly leading to death*	(a) ....
	due to (or as a consequence of)
Antecedent causes: Morbid conditions, if any,	(b) ....
giving rise to the above cause, stating the	due to (or as a consequence of)
underlying condition last	(c) ....
	II
Other significant conditions	....
contributing to the death, but not related to	
the disease or condition causing it	....

* This does not mean the mode of dying, e.g. heart failure, asthenia, etc. It means the disease, injury or complication which caused death.

one—and may yet feel bound to specify a cause of death, so as to avoid forensic complications or for other reasons. It may not be easy to distinguish between direct, antecedent and contributory causes, or to determine a simple sequence of causes, as required by the certificate. The physician may in any case regard the certificate as 'red tape' rather than a scientific document, and not attempt to complete it conscientiously; even when an autopsy is performed, the certificate is often made out before the autopsy, and not modified in the light of the post-mortem findings. Add to this the known unreliability of clinical diagnoses, and the possibility that coders may vary in their selection of an underlying cause (largely because of disagreements as to whether what the physician has written can be taken at its face value),[24] and it is clear that death certificate data and mortality statistics must be treated with some reserve.[25]

In a study in England and Wales, where 9500 certificates completed by hospital physicians before autopsies were compared with certificates subsequently made out by pathologists (based upon both the autopsy and clinical findings), it was found that the underlying causes differed in 55% of cases. In half of these, the difference was one of wording or opinion; in the other half, there was a difference of 'fact'—either the clinician named an underlying cause that the pathologist did not mention in his certificate or notes, or the pathologist named one that the clinician did not mention even as a contributory cause or in the differential diagnosis that he was asked to append to his certificate. The proportion with differences of 'fact' was 16% in cases where the clinician had indicated that he was reasonably certain of his diagnosis (about two-thirds of all cases), 33% in cases where the clinician stated that his diagnosis was 'probable' (a quarter of all cases) and 50% where he stated that the diagnosis was 'uncertain' (one-tenth of all cases). For some disorders, the discrepancies tended to 'cancel each other out'; in other instances there was a definite bias, with a tendency for the clinician to 'underdiagnose' (e.g. chronic bronchitis, peptic ulcer and malignant neoplasms of the lung) or 'overdiagnose' (e.g. bronchopneumonia and cerebral haemorrhage).[26]

Although death certificate data and statistics based upon them must be treated with reserve, this certainly does not nullify their usefulness, since they undoubtedly contain a sufficient core of hard fact. Their lack of complete accuracy and possible biases must, however, be taken into consideration. One precaution to be taken is that mortality from broad groups of diseases, rather than specific diseases, should be considered. In the autopsy study cited above, for example, it was found that while for specific neoplasms there were differences between the statistics based on clinicians' and pathologists' diagnoses, there was fair agreement on the total number of malignant neoplasms. Similarly, when all categories relating to pneumonia and bronchitis were combined, this eliminated the inconsistencies shown by specific conditions.

It must of course be remembered that whatever the validity of death certificate data as a reflection of *causes* of death, they have less validity as a measure of the *presence* of diseases at death,[27] and still less as a measure of prevalence among the living.

NOTIFICATIONS

In most countries physicians are required by law to notify the public health authority of cases of certain (mainly communicable) diseases; doctors, laboratories and others may also be requested to make voluntary reports of certain other diseases to public health or other agencies.

The main problem besetting the use of disease notifications and statistics based on them is that reporting is often far from complete, even where notification is mandatory. One study showed that only 35% of cases of notifiable diseases treated in hospitals in Washington, DC were notified; the notification rates ranged from 11% for viral hepatitis to 63% for tuberculosis.[28] Reporting is likely to be fuller when the physician feels that notification will benefit the patient or the community and less complete when he feels that it will bring no benefit, or may embarrass the patient; a national survey in the USA indicated that only 11% of the cases of gonorrhoea and of infectious syphilis treated by private practitioners were reported to health departments.[29] Furthermore, reporting may be selective; cases of venereal disease treated in public clinics may be far more fully notified than those treated by private practitioners. Such selective factors may introduce biases, in social class or other characteristics, that must be taken into account when inferences are drawn from the data.

These shortcomings apply to all reporting systems, such as those set up for the surveillance of hospital infections, drug reactions, movements into or out of a neighbourhood, etc. The information collected tends to be far from complete, unless a great deal of trouble is taken to ensure full reporting. Despite these shortcomings, the number of notifications can be a useful rough guide to time trends, provided that notification practices have not altered greatly over the period studied.

REGISTERS

Health services and other agencies often maintain registers of people who have specific disorders or who require defined types of care. These registers[30] may list patients with cancer, tuberculosis, or other diseases, people who are blind, housebound, or otherwise handicapped, pregnant women, infants, the elderly, children or families who are at risk of disease, etc. The diagnostic index of a hospital may be used as a disease register. The registers may be simple lists, card indexes, or computerized. In many cases they fulfil important functions in the day-to-day provision of a service, e.g. by identifying patients who require care and by providing a check on the performance of procedures, apart from collecting data that can be analysed for epidemiological or evaluative purposes.

Registers, and the statistics based upon them, may provide valuable data. An investigator not connected with the responsible agency must remember, however, that the information is second-hand or, very often, third-hand—obtained by the agency from other sources—and he should acquaint himself with the definitions and procedures used, in order to decide on the suitability of the data for his purpose.

Registers should not contain more data than necessary: 'their failure . . . in many instances has been due to the collection of too much data . . . Some cancer registries have drowned under a weight of data suitable not for a register, but for a data bank'.[31]

Registers of patients with chronic or other selected conditions can be especially valuable in primary care settings, as a basis for the planning and conduct of organized programmes (see p 309). The maintenance of such registers is, however, not easy, unless clinical records are computerized, which can avoid the need to record the diagnosis twice, both in the clinical record and in a separate register. A register is likely to be complete only if the physician is convinced that it is helpful in his work or research. A check of computerized chronic disease registers in seven teaching general practices in Oxford showed that the registers included only 49–72% of all patients having care for diabetes, thyroid disease, asthma or epilepsy; in one practice, 97% of patients with diabetes were recorded; but in another, only 18%. Computers had been used in these practices for 4 or more years, but as an adjunct to, rather than as a substitute for, manual records; they were hardly ever used during consultations.[32]

HEALTH DIARIES AND CALENDARS

In some studies, people are asked to record symptoms, illnesses or other events, physician contacts, self-medication, food consumption, or other data in diaries or calendars. These documents can then be used as direct sources of data, or as memory aids in face-to-face or phone interviews. They generally lead to a considerable increase in the reporting of symptoms and illnesses, especially minor ones.

A drawback of these methods is that not everyone is able or willing to maintain such a record; non-response tends to be higher for poorly educated and elderly subjects. Even in uneducated populations, however, appropriate techniques may be devised; in a study in Bangladesh, for example, health calendars were prepared in which diarrhoea, scabies and conjunctivitis were indicated by appropriate drawings, and parents were asked to record episodes by putting the affected child's handprint in the appropriate space.[33]

Also, the value of the record tends to decline if it has to be maintained for more than a short period ('fatigue effect')—reported symptoms or illness rates tend to decline after a month, and sometimes during the first month. In a study in Detroit, subjects who were of a higher social status were more likely to persist with a diary for 6 weeks. There is also evidence of a 'sensitization effect'—maintaining a health diary may make respondents more aware of health problems and may spur them to take greater care of their health; in the Detroit study, the average number of days spent in bed because of illness increased during the 6-week period.[34]

OTHER DOCUMENTARY SOURCES

A large variety of other documents may be useful as sources of information on morbidity or other characteristics—medical certificates, sick-absence records, medical insurance records, certificates of birth and fetal death, social welfare records, police records, school records, census publications, etc. Parish records have successfully been used in a study of long-term trends in infant mortality.[35]

In each instance, the investigator should acquaint himself with the possible limitations of the information provided. It is important, however, not to expect too much. These documents were designed for someone else's purposes, and it is no more than a happy chance if they meet the investigator's needs (see Finagle's Third Law).[36]

RECORD LINKAGE

With the advent of computers there has been increased interest in the bringing together of records from different sources. Different records relating to the same person may be linked, such as records from various hospitals, or death certificates and hospital or census data. Alternatively, the linkage may be of records relating to different people, such as members of a family; this is a useful method in genetic research. Record linkage presents considerable practical problems, and may be beset by the ethical problem of possible breaches of confidentiality. When practicable, it has extensive applications in epidemiological and other health research.[37]

NOTES AND REFERENCES

1. Morton J B 1966 The best of Beachcomber. Penguin Books, Harmondsworth; p 102. ("Fancy that," said the man who handed a rhinoceros to the pigeon fancier.' ibid. p 219.)
2. Mainland D 1963 Elementary medical statistics, 2nd edn, p 147. W B Saunders, Philadelphia.
3. Kark S L, Gampel B, Slome C, Steuart G W, Abramson J H, Ward N T 1956 A Study of the King Edward VIII Hospital Out-patient Services. Department of Social, Preventive and Family Medicine, University of Natal.
4. A study at the Yale-New Haven Hospital showed that among post-menopausal women whose medical records provided no information on the presence or absence of certain phenomena, the proportion who reported the phenomenon at interview ranged from 72% (for hot flushes), through 39% (for benign breast disease) to 1% (for the taking of beta-blockers or reserpine). Horwitz R I 1986 Comparison of epidemiologic data from multiple sources. Journal of Chronic Diseases 39: 889.
5. Horwitz R I, Yu E C 1984 Assessing the reliability of epidemiologic data obtained from medical records. Journal of Chronic Diseases 37: 825.
6. Anderson D W, Schoenberg B S, Haerer A F 1988 Prevalence surveys of neurologic disorders: methodologic implications of the Copiah County Study. Journal of Clinical Epidemiology 41: 339.
7. Densen P M, Balamuth E, Deardorff N R 1960 Medical care plan as a source of morbidity data: the prevalence of illness and associated volume of service. Milbank Memorial Fund Quarterly 38: 48.
8. Wood M, Mayo F, Marsland D 1986 (Annual Reviews of Public Health 7: 357)

review the reasons for *using primary-care records in epidemiology*, discuss
methods and instruments, problems with diagnoses and their classification and
problems with numerators (what is an illness episode?) and denominators, and
give examples of collaborative and other research in primary-care settings.

9. Eimerl T S, Laidlay A J 1969 A handbook for research in general practice.
   Livingstone, Edinburgh.
10. See, for example, Sanderson G F B 1976 General practice. In: Acheson R M,
    Hall D J, Aird L (eds). Blackwell, Oxford, Seminars in community medicine,
    vol 2. Health information planning and monitoring pp 76–92; Spenser T 1978
    Principles of a problem-oriented record system. In: Medalie J H (ed) Family
    medicine—principles and applications. Williams & Wilkins, Baltimore,
    pp 337–342.
11. Barnett G O 1984 (The application of computer-based medical-record systems
    in ambulatory practices. New England Journal of Medicine 310: 1643) reviews
    the use of *computer-based medical recording* in ambulatory care. For a review of the
    use of a computer for morbidity recording in general practice, with emphasis on
    practical problems, see Dinwoodie H P 1970 Simple computer facilities in
    general practice: a study of the problems involved. Journal of the Royal College of
    General Practitioners 19: 269. Many physicians are at present reluctant to use a
    computer. 'Is the computer a devilish invention, to be avoided at all costs, or is it
    God's gift to general practice? Sheldon M G 1984 Computers in general practice:
    a personal view. Journal of the Royal College of General Practitioners 34: 647. Do
    doctors fear they may become redundant? In a test of one program in a general
    practice in Bombay, where symptoms were entered by a non-physician, the
    computer provided patients with prescriptions and instructions; in over
    two-thirds of cases these were similar to those given by the physician; the other
    patients were advised by the computer to see a doctor: Uplekar M W, Antia
    N H, Dhumale P S 1988 Sympmed I: computer program for primary health
    care. British Medical Journal 297: 841.—some patients feel the computer will
    Reported attitudes of patients vary—some patients feel the computer will
    remove the doctor's personal touch or impair confidentiality; but patients who
    have used a personal computer or previously encountered the use of a computer
    in a clinical setting tend to have more favourable responses. See Cruickshank P J
    1984 Computers in medicine: patients' attitudes. Journal of the Royal College of
    General Practitioners 34: 77; Pringle M, Robins S, Brown G 1984 Computers In
    the surgery. British Medical Journal 288: 289; Rethans J —J, Hoppener P,
    Wolfs G, Diederiks J 1988 Do personal computers make doctors less personal?
    British Medical Journal 296: 1446.
    Commercial systems for use in general practice are compared by Daniels A,
    Coulter A 1988 How to choose a general practice computing system: comparison
    of commercial packages. British Medical Journal 297: 838.
12. *Medical audit* and similar techniques for evaluating clinical care—'self-audit',
    'peer review' (by others), 'internal audit' (by colleagues in the same institution),
    'external audit', 'medical care evaluation studies', 'nursing audit', etc.—may be
    based upon routine records, upon specially modified or designed records, or upon
    special investigations, including direct observations of practitioners at work. A
    review by Sanazaro P J (1980 Quality assessment and quality assurance in
    medical care. Annual Reviews of Public Health 1: 37) stresses the need for the
    development of sound methods based on criteria whose validity has been tested.
    The use of medical audit in general practice is discussed by Acheson H W K
    1975 Medical audit and general practice. Lancet 1:511; most volumes of the
    Journal of the Royal College of General Practitioners contain one or more
    examples; for an example of the use of 'indicator conditions' in primary medical
    care, see Burdette J A, Babineau R A, Mayo F, Hulka B S, Cassel J C 1974
    Primary medical care evaluation: the AAFP-UNC collaborative study. Journal of
    the American Medical Association 230: 1668.

13. The value of investigating the reasons for poor outcomes is stressed by Blum H L 1974 Medical Care, 12: 999.
14. Brook R H 1973 Quality of care assessment: a comparison of five methods of peer review. DHEW Publication No. HRA-74-3100. US Department of Health, Education, and Welfare, Rockville.
15. Sanazaro P J, Williamson J W 1968 Medical Care 6: 123.
16. Fessel W J, van Brunt E E 1972 Assessing quality of care from the medical record. New England Journal of Medicine 286: 134.
17. Nightingale F 1873 Notes on a hospital.
18. World Health Organization 1977 Manual of the international statistical classification of diseases, injuries and causes of death, vol 1. WHO, Geneva, pp 697–741.
19. Statistics on hospitalizations for acute myocardial infarction in the USA were based on the 'first-listed' diagnosis until 1982, when it was decided that if this diagnosis was not the first one recorded, but occurred with other circulatory diagnoses, it would be moved to first place. As a result, the proportion of acute myocardial diagnoses that were regarded as the principal reason for hospitalization rose from 60% in 1981 to 87% in 1986. Vital and Health Statistics series 13, no. 96.
20. Simborg D W 1981 DRG creep: a new hospital-acquired disease. New England Journal of Medicine 304: 1602.
21. Cohen B B, Pokras S, Meads M S, Krushat W M 1987 How will diagnosis-related groups affect epidemiologic research? American Journal of Public Health 126: 1. The quotation is from Greenwood M 1948 Medical Statistics from Graunt to Farr. Cambridge University Press, Cambridge.
22. Illustrations of the *WHO rules for coding causes of death*: World Health Organization (1977 see note 18).

If the certificate reads:

I (a) Perforating duodenal ulcer
  (b) Hypertensive heart disease
  (c) —
II Anaemia

the death is assigned to perforating duodenal ulcer, since this, the reported direct cause of death, is very unlikely to have been caused by hypertensive heart disease. In the following case:

I (a) Dermatitis
  (b) Perforating duodenal ulcer
  (c) Hypertensive heart disease
II Anaemia

the death is again ascribed to the ulcer, since dermatitis is unlikely to cause death and is not reported as the cause of a more serious complication. If 'chronic pyelonephritis' is the last condition entered in part I and is acceptable as the underlying cause, but 'prostatic obstruction' is entered in part II, the death is assigned to prostatic obstruction.

23. Nelson M, Farebrother M 1978 (The effect of inaccuracies in death certification and coding practices in the European Economic Community (EEC) on international cancer mortality statistics. International Journal of Epidemiology 16: 411) show how differences in certification and coding practices may affect international comparisons of cancers of the cervix and body of the uterus. Sorlie P D, Gold E B 1987 (The effect of physician terminology preference on coronary heart disease mortality; an artifact uncovered by the 9th Revision ICD. American Journal of Public Health 77: 148) show how the change in the 9th revision of the ICD, whereby 'arteriosclerotic cardiovascular disease' is no longer

classified as 'ischemic heart disease', may account for part of the apparent decline in coronary heart disease mortality.

24. World Health Organization 1966 Studies on the accuracy and comparability of statistics on causes of death. Unpublished WHO document EURO-215.1/16. WHO, Geneva.

25. Sirken M G, Rosenberg H M, Chevarley F M, Curtin L R 1987 (The quality of cause-of-death statistics. American Journal of Public Health 77: 137) stress the need for periodic assessment of the quality of *cause-of-death statistics* in the USA. Grubb G S, Fortney J A, Saleh, S et al 1988 (A comparison of two cause-of-death classification systems for deaths among women of reproductive age in Menoufia, Egypt. International Journal of Epidemiology 17: 385) show how the findings of a detailed local survey can reveal biases in official cause-of-death statistics in a developing country.

26. Heasman L A, Lipworth L 1966 Accuracy of certification of cause of death. A report on a survey conducted in 1959 in hospitals of the National Health Service to obtain information on the extent of agreement between clinical and post-mortem diagnoses. General Register Office, Studies on Medical and Population Subjects no. 20 HMSO, London.

27. Beadenkopf W G, Abrams M, Daoud A, Marks R U 1963 An assessment of certain medical aspects of death certificate data for epidemiologic study of arteriosclerotic heart disease. Journal of Chronic Diseases 16: 249; Abramson J H, Sacks M I, Cahana B 1971 Death certificate data as an indication of the presence of certain common diseases at death. Journal of Chronic Diseases 24: 417.

28. Marier R 1977 The reporting of communicable diseases. American Journal of Epidemiology 105: 587.

29. Curtis A C 1963 National survey of venereal disease treatment. Journal of the American Medical Association 186: 46.

30. For a review of types and uses of *registers* and criteria for their evaluation (completeness and validity) see Goldberg J, Gelfand H M, Levy P S Registry evaluation methods: a review and case study. Epidemiologic Reviews 2: 210. Uses and problems are discussed by Thompson J R 1989 The role of registers in epidemiology: discussion paper. Journal of the Royal Society of Medicine 82: 151.

31. Brooke E M 1976 Problems of data collection in long-term health care. Medical Care 14: (suppl): 165.

32. Coulter A, Brown S, Daniels A 1989 Journal of Epidemiology and Community Health 43: 25.

33. Stanton B, Clemens J, Aziz K M A, Khatun K, Ahmed S, Khatun J 1987 Comparability of results obtained by 2-week home maintained diarrhoeal calendar with 2-week diarrhoeal recall. International Journal of Epidemiology 16: 595.

34. Verbrugge L M 1984 Health diaries—problems and solutions in study design. In: Cannell C F, Groves R M (eds) Health survey research methods. DHHS publication no. PHS 84–3346. National Center for Health Services Research, Rockville, MD, pp 171–192.

35. Armenian H K, Zurayk H C, Kazandjian V A 1986 The epidemiology of infant deaths in the Armenian parish records of Lebanon. International Journal of Epidemiology 15: 373.

36. Finagle's three laws on information state: '(1) The information you have is not what you want. (2) The information you want is not what you need. (3) The information you need is not what you can obtain'. Cited by Murnaghan J H 1974 Health indicators and information systems for the year 2000. New England Journal of Medicine 290: 603.

37. See Baldwin J A, Acheson E D, Graham W J 1987 Textbook of medical record linkage. Oxford University Press, New York.

21. Planning the records

Records cannot be properly planned until the study plan is almost complete. The planning of records requires prior decisions as to what variables will be studied, what scales of measurement will be used, and how the information will be collected and processed.

Apart from the forms used for recording the primary data collected in the study, a variety of other records may be required to ensure smooth working. These may include lists of people to be examined or interviewed, lists of potential controls from which some are to be chosen by matching or random selection, 'appointment book'-type records showing when examinations or re-examinations are scheduled, and so on. In a study in which various procedures are applied to the same subjects on different occasions or in different places (interview, physical examination, glucose tolerance test, chest X-ray, etc.), it is often helpful to maintain a 'record of procedures' for each individual, showing what has been performed (and if not, why not). Cards or a computer database program[1] can be used. In card registers, the cards of people awaiting different procedures can be kept in separate sections or marked with variously coloured tags. In a large study the organization of an efficient filing system may not be simple.

The most important forms are those used for recording the primary data of the study. These forms, or 'data sheets', may take the shape of questionnaires, examination schedules, forms for laboratory or other test results, extraction forms on to which data are copied from clinical or other records, etc., or they may be multi-purpose forms with different sections to meet these various purposes. It is usually advisable to use different forms for data (concerning a single individual) collected in different places, from different sources, by different observers or interviewers, or at different times. It may also be necessary to use different forms for different categories of subjects, e.g. when there are substantial differences in the questionnaires put to men and women, or to living patients and the surviving relatives of dead ones. If several types of forms are used, it may be helpful to use differently coloured paper.

These record forms should, if possible, meet the following four main requirements.

1. Only one individual per form

It is advisable to use a separate form for each individual studied. (As usual, 'individual' here means the individual unit of the study, even if this is a collective unit, such as a family or school.) This usually greatly facilitates the subsequent handling of the data. Lists showing many individuals, with columns for different pieces of information (the 'ledger', 'register', or 'exercise book' method), have limited value; if hand tallying (p 221) is used, errors are likely if more than two or three variables are recorded in the list. Swaroop tells a true story of a director of public health who analysed several thousand registers of cholera patients to determine how many had died, then repeated the process to obtain the same information for each sex, and when he found that he was unable to obtain the same total 'threw up his hands and exclaimed, "Now I *really* wish those people had not died" '.[2] Some of the records suggested by the Royal College of General Practitioners as an aid to research in general practice are of the 'ledger' type.[3] They contain little information about the patient, however, so that hand tallying is not impracticable; they also provide the physician with a diagnostic index to his individual clinical records, thus facilitating more detailed investigations.

As a corollary to the use of a separate form for each individual, it is necessary to identify the individual to whom the form refers. The identifying data are not necessarily used in the analysis. In addition to the person's name, use may be made of his or her sex, age, address, hospital number, personal identity number, etc. (In a long-term follow-up study, it is often helpful to add the name and address of a close friend or relative, to help in finding the person should he change his address.) Each record should also have space for a number that distinctively indicates the individual to whom it refers. This identifying number is usually a *serial number* or 'study number' arbitrarily allocated for the specific purpose of the study. The same identifying number should appear on all records pertaining to a single individual. In an investigation where anonymity is guaranteed, this number will be the only identification on the record.

In studies where computers are used, a 'check digit'[4] may be added to the serial number. This is a digit that is derived from the digits in the number, using a predetermined rule, and that is placed after it to make a new serial number that has a logical consistency. An error made in transcribing or computer entry is likely to produce an 'illogical' number, which the computer can detect. A simple method is to choose a digit that will provide zero or a multiple of 10 when alternate digits are added and subtracted. If the original number is 1568, the check digit is 6, since $(+1-5+6-8+6) = 0$, and the new serial number is 15686. If this is accidentally rendered as 16586, the error can be detected, since $(+1-6+5-8+6) = -2$.

2. All the required information should be specified

Physical examination schedules are frequently unsatisfactory, in that they do not specify all the variables about which the investigator wishes to obtain information. If we wish to know about swelling of the legs, for instance, there is little point in using a form which merely has a heading 'Lower extremities', with a blank space beneath it. If the space remains blank after the examination, or if some other abnormality is noted, we will not know whether the examiner looked for oedema; even if the researcher has carried out the examinations himself, he cannot be sure that he did not forget to carry out a specific test for oedema. At the least, then, the heading 'oedema of legs' should be printed.

Furthermore (and this applies to questionnaires as well as to examination schedules) all the alternative categories of measurement should appear on the form. If the heading 'oedema' has only a space beneath it, which the examiner leaves empty, we will still be uncertain that this sign was sought. The words 'present' and 'absent' should be printed, for the examiner to mark whichever is applicable; the findings are then clear and unequivocal. This item in the schedule might have the following format:

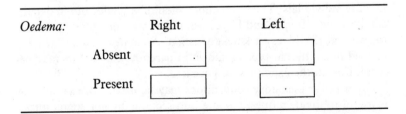

As an extra precaution, the examiner may be asked to write 'not examined' (and state the reason) if any part of the examination is omitted, or to enter a prearranged number, say 9, in the appropriate box.

The same principle applies to questionnaires, in which (except in the case of open-ended questions) all the possible responses to each question should be printed, including (if necessary) a category of 'other'—or, more usefully, 'other (specify)...' One exception to this rule is that some investigators prefer not to include a 'don't know' or 'unknown' category, in order to reduce the frequency of such answers, but leave such responses for the interviewer to write in. To avoid the possibility of ambiguous 'blank' responses when a question requests a numerical answer ('On how many days of a week do you eat meat?'), the instruction 'If not at all, write 0' should be stated.

3. The form should be easy to use

The easier the form is to use, the fewer errors there will be.

The items should follow the sequence in which the data are to be collected. This requirement may present especial difficulties in the planning of a schedule for a clinical examination, and flaws in the schedule may not be detected until the form is submitted to a pretest.

As far as possible, the need for writing should be avoided, both to simplify the task of the observer, interviewer or extractor, and to reduce the need to decipher unintelligible scrawls. Wherever possible, the relevant findings or responses should be marked with a tick or cross or by circling or underlining.

The form should, as far as possible, be self-explanatory. The main instructions should be clearly stated in the form itself, even if a more detailed manual has been prepared for examiners or interviewers. Although written instructions cannot replace oral explanations, they serve as a constant guide and reminder. Instructions are particularly important when, as often happens, certain items are applicable only to some individuals. The instructions should be spelled out in detail, e.g. by saying 'If male and 17 years or older, ask:' or 'If 'no', proceed to question 17. If 'yes', ask next question'. Such instructions are best printed in a different type or shown in parentheses. Arrows may be helpful, as in the examples on page 213.

Other self-explanatory conventions may be used. For example, it is useful to divide a questionnaire into sections by horizontal lines, and instruct the interviewers that whenever the response they receive is one that is marked by double underlining, they should go on to the next section (see the second example on p 213).

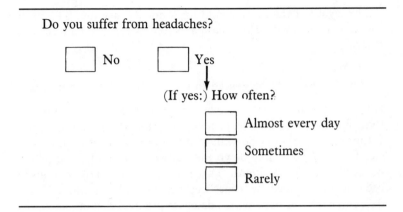

Do you suffer from headaches?

☐ No   ☐ Yes
                  ↓
       (If yes:) How often?

           ☐ Almost every day
           ☐ Sometimes
           ☐ Rarely

---

9. Do you suffer from headaches?

   0. No   1. Yes
   ‗   ↓
             10. How often?
                 0. Rarely   1. Sometimes   2. Almost
                 ‗   every
                                                  day
                                    │   ↓
                                    ↓
             11. Have you ever consulted a doctor about
                 them?
                 0. No   1. Yes
                 ‗   ‗

Clear and simple instructions are particularly important in self-administered questionnaires. The method of marking responses should be clearly explained. In a study to be carried out in Trinidad, for example, the introduction (after explaining who is performing the study and why, and inviting the respondent's co-operation) might state:

Most of the questions can be answered by putting an 'X' in the box next to the answer that fits you best. For example:

Do you live in Trinidad?   ☒ Yes   ☐ No

The layout of the form should make for its easy use. The items should not be crowded, and the spaces for answers should be clearly shown.

4. The form should be geared to the needs of data processing

If it is proposed to sort and count the records manually, the record form should, if possible, be printed on a card rather than on paper.

Computer entry may be facilitated by printing boxes for the codes (see Ch. 22), preferably down the right-hand side of the page opposite the respective items. This may avoid the need to transfer codes to an intermediate 'codesheet' before computer entry. Unless data entry is to be done with a database program that automatically puts data in the right place in the computer record (see p 237), it is advisable to mark each box with the number of the appropriate columns(s) in the computer record. (If such boxes are used in a self-administered questionnaire, they should be clearly labelled 'For office use only'.) If the data are to be entered into more than one computer record, e.g. in 'card image' format (see p 236), it is helpful to print each record's number (1, 2, 3, etc.) at its start.

In the example that follows, the intention is to code the number of rooms in the house and the number of persons in the household, and calculate the crowding index. A box for the crowding index is required if the crowding index is to be computed before entry, but not if the calculation will be done by the computer.

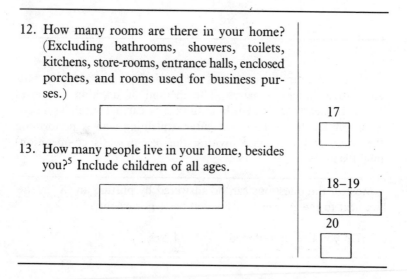

12. How many rooms are there in your home? (Excluding bathrooms, showers, toilets, kitchens, store-rooms, entrance halls, enclosed porches, and rooms used for business purses.)

    17

13. How many people live in your home, besides you?[5] Include children of all ages.

    18–19

    20

The use of a precoded form permits coding to be done at the time the data are collected. The code digits are printed on the form, and are either marked by circling or by checking an appropriately numbered box, or are written in a box provided for the purpose. A different approach is used in each of the pot-pourri of items on page 216. (In practice, the use of a medley of methods in a single form would be confusing.) The numbers on the right are the column numbers (not needed if a database program is used for data entry).

An alternative approach, preferred by some investigators, is to provide an interviewer with only a single questionnaire, on which the coded alternatives to each question are stated, and to have a separate 'answer sheet' filled in for each respondent. This sheet need contain only the subject's name, etc. and the numbers of the questions, with either a box or a row of the alternative code numbers (for ringing) next to each question number. This makes the form more compact, but there may be more errors when it is filled in.

Precoding is best avoided in self-administered questionnaires, since it may confuse the respondent. It may, however, be used if the code numbers are kept small and inconspicuous, as in the following example.

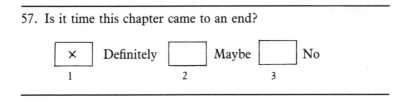

57. Is it time this chapter came to an end?

×	Definitely		Maybe		No
:-:		:-:		:-:	
1		2		3	

NOTES AND REFERENCES

1. There are many easy-to-use *PC database programs* (see note 3, p 34) that can be used for filing, updating, sorting, finding and printing individual records and for displaying or printing reports (lists and simple counts). Popular examples include *PC-File Plus* and *File Express*.
2. Swaroop S 1966 Statistical methods in malaria eradication. WHO, Geneva, p 20.
3. Eimerl T S, Laidlaw A J 1969 A handbook for research in general practice. Livingstone, Edinburgh, pp 39–82.
4. Acheson E D 1968 Record linkage in medicine. Livingstone, Edinburgh, pp 181–183.
5. The question is worded in this way to make things easier for the respondent. Before calculating the crowding index (persons per room), the number of persons stated is increased by one.

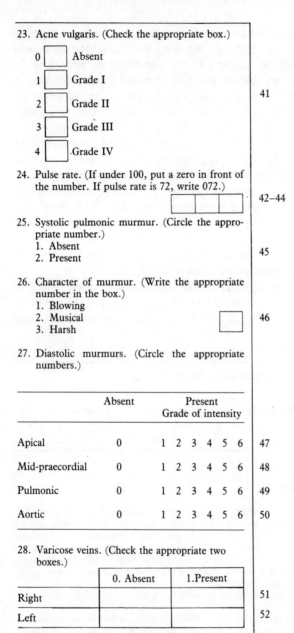

23. Acne vulgaris. (Check the appropriate box.)

0 ☐ Absent

1 ☐ Grade I

2 ☐ Grade II   41

3 ☐ Grade III

4 ☐ ·Grade IV

24. Pulse rate. (If under 100, put a zero in front of the number. If pulse rate is 72, write 072.)

☐☐☐ ·   42–44

25. Systolic pulmonic murmur. (Circle the appropriate number.)
   1. Absent
   2. Present   45

26. Character of murmur. (Write the appropriate number in the box.)
   1. Blowing
   2. Musical   ☐   46
   3. Harsh

27. Diastolic murmurs. (Circle the appropriate numbers.)

	Absent	Present Grade of intensity	
Apical	0	1 2 3 4 5 6	47
Mid-praecordial	0	1 2 3 4 5 6	48
Pulmonic	0	1 2 3 4 5 6	49
Aortic	0	1 2 3 4 5 6	50

28. Varicose veins. (Check the appropriate two boxes.)

	0. Absent	1.Present	
Right			51
Left			52

22. Planning the analysis

During the planning phase of a study, decisions must be made on the coding, processing and statistical analysis of data. These decisions are inter-related.

DECISIONS ABOUT CODING

To facilitate computer processing and analysis, codes must be assigned to the categories of variables that have nominal, ordinal or dichotomous scales. Numbers (0, 1, 2 etc.) are generally used for this purpose. The codes should be decided in advance, particularly if precoded records (see p 214) are wanted. Coding is not needed for simple numerical data or for verbal data that will not be analysed (e.g. subjects' names).

Coding requires the preparation of a *coding key* that shows the codes used for each variable, and their meanings. If coding is complicated, detailed *coding instructions* may be needed. These should be clear and unambiguous, in order to ensure coding reliability. Voluminous instructions may be needed if the responses to open-ended questions or statements made in relatively unstructured interviews have to be coded, particularly with respect to attitudes, motivation, etc. ('content analysis').

Standardized codes should be used wherever possible, so as to simplify both the coding process and the analysis. If there are 'yes–no' questions, for example, 1 might be allocated to all 'yes' answers and 0 to all 'no' answers. It is particularly important to use standard codes for 'unknown' and 'not applicable'—for example, 'unknown' might be entered as 9, 99, or 999, and 'not applicable' as 8, 88 etc. This is advisable for numerical as well as categorical data, to reduce errors during data entry or analysis.

A specimen portion of an imaginary coding key, incorporating coding instructions, is shown in Table 22.1. The position of each

217

variable in the computer record (column or variable numbers) may be added to the key.

Table 22.1   Code

Variable	Code	Coding instructions
Sex	1. Male 2. Female 9. Unknown	Precoded (question 1). If not shown, look at subject's name, and see whether questions 3–5 (for females only) have been asked. If sex is still uncertain, code 9
Marital status	1. Single 2. Married 3. Widowed 4. Divorced 9. Unknown	Precoded (question 2). If not shown, code 9
Social class	1. SC I 2. SC II 3. SC III 4. SC IV 5. SC V 8. Unclassifiable 9. No data on occupation	Code occupation stated in answer to question 6, using attached instructions. If occupation not stated, code 9
Height	999. Unknown	Centimetres (ignore fractions or decimals). If not measured, code 999
Relative weight	888. Unclassified 999. Unknown	Consult appended weight-for-height tables to find standard weight for a person of the subject's sex and height. Divide subject's weight by this standard weight, multiply by 100, round off to one decimal place, and enter. Code 999 if sex, height or weight is unknown. Code 888 if height falls outside range shown in tables

A more ambitious codebook may be prepared, including the operational definitions of the variables (see Table 9.1, p 98) as well as the coding key and instructions.

The computer may subsequently do manipulations that create *derived variables* from the variables that are entered. For example, a weight–height ratio may be calculated; data on the number of cigarettes smoked may be used to categorize subjects as non-smokers or light, moderate or heavy smokers; or diagnostic criteria may be brought together so as to categorize subjects in terms of the presence or absence of a disease. These derived variables should be documented, preferably in the same list or codebook as other variables. If their creation is planned in advance, they can be in the list from the outset; otherwise, they should be added later. A record should be kept of the computer instructions.

Coding is less important if the data are to be processed by hand. But even then, it may be convenient to make use of symbols or standard abbreviations such as + (present), − (absent), ? (unknown) M (male) and F (female).

Before record forms are printed it is necessary to decide whether coding will be done at the time data are collected (by having the examiner or interviewer do the coding). This is obviously cheaper and faster, and if the coding is simple this does not impose a burden. But it becomes impossible to detect and rectify coding errors, unless the full data are recorded as well as the codes. In one study in which subjects were interviewed twice, half the disagreements that were not caused by conflicting reports were attributable to coding errors by an interviewer.[1]

DECISIONS ABOUT DATA PROCESSING

The main decision to be made at this stage is whether the data will be processed by computer or manually (methods other than these[2] have been largely displaced by the computer), and whether a micro-computer (personal computer) or a large (mainframe) computer will be used (or both).

Computer processing has indisputable advantages,[3] and there is no need to sing its praises. But it is not an unmixed blessing, and some words of warning are not out of place. First, there is still a belief (especially among people with little experience of computers) that 'the computer is never wrong'. The computer is no mental giant, but a moron that slavishly does just what it is told to do. It cannot be accurate if the humans who operate it make errors, and to err is human. The data may be inaccurate or entered inaccurately ('garbage in, garbage out'), errors may be made in giving instructions, or the programs may have unknown bugs. 'Because of the faith that is placed in computers, the possibility of undetected human error may be greater when computers are used.'[4] Secondly, analysis by computer is so easy that there may be a temptation to examine trivial hypotheses, or hypotheses based on 'data snooping' (i.e. constructed only after examining the findings)—which may lead to unwarranted conclusions (see p 245). And thirdly, complex statistical procedures have become so readily available that they are often used even if they are inappropriate for the data or for answering the questions that the study asks. One statistician laments that 'in the past we have had misgivings about "cook book" statistics, and now what has evolved would have to be termed the "TV dinner"... Previously, we could believe that the user would at least have to read the recipe!'[5] Others observe that 'it is not hard to do a bad analysis... All that is needed is a canned computer program... and a lack of competence in bio-statistics. These resources are widely available'.[6] 'Output from commercial computer programs, with their beautifully formatted tables, graphs, and matrices, can make garbage look like roses.'[7]

Microcomputers are coming into wider use both for data entry (see p 236) and for data processing. Their use is likely to grow in popularity, as a result of the exponential increase in the speed, storage capacity and multitasking and networking potentials of these com-puters and in the availability of statistical software. Processing is slower than with a mainframe computer; but if the mainframe com-puter is busy (so that there is much queueing, or processing is spread over many time slices) there may be little difference in the total time taken to obtain results. Personal computer software is generally more user-friendly, providing on-screen explanations, warnings and instructions, and use of a personal computer facilitates an interactive functioning mode, whereby decisions about the analyses to do and how to do them are made and transmitted in an ongoing way rather than in advance. In the words of a microcomputer enthusiast: 'All of which must tend to make some people ponder the actual future of the mainframes themselves and wonder, specifically, whether they have one. Doubtless they have—but in the same way that main drains have a future. They will always be there. They will always deal with massive throughput. But, because of the subjective element involved in the user interface, there may come a time when the average human will never want to look at them again'.[8]

Manual data-processing methods (hand tallying and hand sorting), although tedious and appropriate for small-scale studies only, are favoured by some investigators on the grounds that they keep them 'close to their data'. 'The figures that we are analyzing represent the patients, animals, things or processes that we are studying, and the more familiar we become with them, the more likely we are to know about their interrelationships, oddities and defects; and the more likely we are to catch hints of explanations and clues for further research.'[9]

Hand tallying is the most primitive method. A tally sheet is prepared in the form of a skeleton table, and a tally mark is made in the requisite cell for each individual. The usual method is to make a vertical mark for each individual. Every fifth individual in a cell is indicated by a diagonal line drawn through the preceding four: ⨫

This facilitates subsequent counting. An alternative method[10] is to make dots (arranged in a square) for the first four, then to draw a line (joining two dots) for each of the next four, so that a square means 8 individuals. A diagonal is then drawn for each of the next two, so that a complete set of 10 looks like a little flag: ⊠

When a tabulation is done directly from lists (containing information on different individuals on the same page) or from unwieldy records (e.g. voluminous clinical files), hand tallying may be a convenient method. Its disadvantages are that it is laborious and time-consuming, and errors are prone to creep in, especially if a complicated cross-tabulation is being used. If an error is detected (e.g. if it is found that the total number shown in the table is one less than the actual number of individuals), this requires the repetition of the entire process, unless differently coloured inks have been used for different batches of records to help in the localization of errors.

Hand sorting is usually preferable to hand tallying. This requires a separate and easily handled record for each individual. The records are sorted and physically separated into piles conforming with the cells in the skeleton table, and the numbers in each pile are then counted, recounted, and entered. If an error is detected, it is usually necessary to repeat only part of the procedure. To prepare a cross-classification, the records are usually sorted 'hierarchically'; i.e., they are sorted into piles according to one variable, then each pile is sorted according to a second variable, and so on until the cross-classification is complete; each pile is then counted. The records used may be the forms or cards on which the data were initially recorded, or special forms or cards to which the data have been transferred for this purpose. If conveniently small cards are used, if information on each variable is written in a standard position on the card, and if heavy lines and writing in different colours are used to facilitate the visual identification of various items of data, sorting becomes relatively easy. Many investigators find that this is a satisfactory method, except in large or complicated studies. This form of card-playing has the advantage that it keeps the investigator 'closer to his data' than any other method of processing.

DECISIONS ABOUT STATISTICAL ANALYSIS

During the planning phase the investigator should decide, at least in broad outline, how the information he proposes to collect will be analysed. It is often helpful to draw up a number of specimen skeleton tables, showing the scales of classification of the variables they include, i.e. with column and row headings but containing no figures, and to consider how different kinds of result will be interpreted. This process of 'thinking forward' to the analysis often reveals gaps in the data (variables omitted, no information on the denominator population, etc.), defects in scales of measurement, or the superfluity of certain data. It provides a further opportunity for second thoughts as to whether the study, as planned, is likely to meet its objectives.

Consideration should be given not only to the format of tables, but to the statistical techniques to be used in the analysis. This often calls for the help of a statistician, although it is a consoling thought that the analysis of a well planned study often requires only the simplest of statistical techniques. It is foolhardy to decide to use complex procedures without adequate statistical knowledge or expert guidance.

If a statistician is to be consulted, this should be done during the planning phase, when he can still influence the design of the investigation, and not after the data have been collected, when he may find that they are unsuitable for analysis. In consulting a statistician it must be remembered that a silly question gets a silly answer. Unless the investigator can explain very precisely and specifically what he hopes to learn from his study, the advice he gets, however erudite and well meaning, may be inadequate and even misleading.

The general lines of the analysis should always be decided in advance. Sometimes a detailed plan can be prepared (this may be demanded if an application is made for research funds); but options should be left open—the findings, as they emerge, may call for new analyses.

NOTES AND REFERENCES

1. Horwitz R I, Yu E C 1985 Assessing the reliability of epidemiologic data obtained from medical records. International Journal of Epidemiology 14: 463.
2. *Peripheral punch cards* and *mechanical sorting*, and their coding requirements, are described in previous editions of this book.
3. Hunt A T, Morrison P R, Pagano M (1985 The effects of computer science advancements on public health research. Annual Reviews of Public Health 6: 325) review the effects of computers on public health research.

4. Blum M L, Foos P W 1986 Data gathering: experimental methods plus. Harper & Row, New York, p 80.
5. Schucany W R 1978 Comment. Journal of the American Statistical Association 73: 92.
6. Bross I D J 1981 Scientific strategies to save your life: a statistical approach to primary prevention. Marcel Dekker, New York, pp 42–43.
7. Tabachnick G B, Fidell L S 1989 try throughout their book (Using multivariate statistics, 2nd edn. Harper & Row, New York) 'to suggest clues for when the true message in the output more closely resembles the fertilizer than the flowers'.
8. Naylor C 1987 The PC compendium. Sigma Press, Wilmslow, p 23.
9. Mainland D 1964 Elementary medical statistics. Saunders, Philadelphia, p 168.
10. Tukey J W 1977 Exploratory data analysis. Addison-Wesley, Reading, Massachusetts, pp 16–17.

23. Pretests and other practical preparations

Before the collection of data can be started, it is usually necessary to test the methods and to make various practical preparations. If the planning phase was the gestation period, this is the stage of parturition. It may not be free of pain, and if there are practical problems that cannot be overcome the study may yet be stillborn.

PRETESTS

Pretests, or prior tests of methods, vary in their scope. A pretest may consist of a single visit to a clinic to see whether patients' weights or other items of information are routinely recorded on their cards, or may take the form of a large and well planned methodological study or a full-scale 'pilot study', a dress rehearsal of the main investigation. Pretests may be required in order to examine the practicability, reliability or validity of methods of study, and their planning varies according to their purposes. A pretest may be a well constructed study aimed at yielding definitive results, or it may be designed to provide only a 'feel' of the suitability of a method. Pretests of examination schedules and questionnaires are usually of the latter type.

In a typical small-scale pretest of a questionnaire, 10–30 subjects are interviewed.[1] These may be chosen haphazardly, but should not be members of the study population, since participation in the pretest interview may reduce willingness to be interviewed in the study proper, or may affect the responses given in the study proper. Subjects are usually chosen who are similar in their characteristics to the members of the study population. Sometimes, in order to highlight possible flaws in the questionnaire, 'difficult customers'—such as persons with an especially low or high educational level—are purposely chosen. The interviewer is asked to record not only the responses for which the questionnaire makes provision but also his observations of the respondent's reactions (boredom, irritation, impatience, antagonism—or even interest!), to make verbatim records of the respondent's comments, and to note his own criticisms and suggestions concerning the questions, their sequence, skip patterns ('If X, go to Question Y'), and the layout of the questionnaire form. He also records the time taken by the interview. The interviewer (or another interviewer, in a special call-back visit) may be requested to discuss the questions with the respondent after they have been answered, asking whether they seemed clear, what he meant by his answers, why he answered 'Don't know', etc. This may be done informally, or a formal procedure may be used: the interviewer explains that he wants to test some of the questions that were asked, and then reads out each of these with its response, and asks the respondent to explain exactly how he arrived at the answer; this is followed by preplanned questions designed to find out how particular terms were understood by the respondent.[2]

On the basis of all this information, it is often possible to identify 'difficult' questions—those that are offensive, hard to understand, or do not seem to elicit the information they are intended to get—and awkward sequences of items. If a question elicits many 'Don't know' answers, it is probably unsatisfactory; if it produces many qualifying comments, the response categories are probably not suitable. Inconsistencies between the answers to related questions, or uniform answers by all respondents ('all-or-none' responses) may also point to flaws. If questions were omitted or asked when they should not have been, the questionnaire's arrangement or provision of instructions is probably defective. The pretest usually points to a need for changes in the questionnaire and the interviewing instructions. These changes are made, and a new version is available for pretesting.

A useful distinction has been made between a 'participating' pretest of a questionnaire, in which respondents are previously told it is a practice run, and an 'undeclared' pretest, in which they are not.[1] A participating pretest—which may require hand-picked respondents ('investigators may find themselves relying on that familiar source of forced labor—colleagues, friends and family')[1]— permits detailed questioning about reactions to the questions. The best strategy is often to begin with a small-scale participating pretest.

ENLISTING CO-OPERATION

It is particularly important to enlist the good will of people who will be involved in the study (subjects who will be examined or interviewed, administrators and others who can provide access to records or various facilities and services, etc.), those who *think* they are involved in the study (such as physicians who feel that they own their patients), and those (such as some colleagues) who feel they *should* have been involved in the study. In a community study, co-operation can be enhanced by suitable public relations and preparatory educational work in the community.[3] The best results are provided by contacts with key individuals and organizations in the community, but use may also be made of mass media, such as radio talks, newspaper articles, pamphlets and posters. In such contacts, people should be told what they can expect to 'get out of' the study, but no false promises should be made; in medical surveys 'the two most generally effective motivations are the desire to contribute to the community effort to benefit health through science, and the subject's own interest in a free medical examination'.[4] Gimmicks are sometimes used, such as the offer of a prize to be raffled among participants; this is probably unlikely to help unless the prize is big (in a controlled trial in England, prizes of £50, £30 and £20 had no effect at all on response rates).[5]

In a household survey it may be decided to send out letters telling prospective respondents about the study and the impending visit by an interviewer (it is usually unwise to make the initial contact by telephone—this invites refusals). It may also be decided to prepare 'reminder' and 'thank you' letters. In studies in which access to confidential medical records is necessary, people may be required to give their approval in writing, and consent forms should be printed for this purpose.

OTHER PRACTICAL PREPARATIONS

There may be many other practical preparations before data can be collected. A budget may have to be prepared, and funds found (the expert in 'grantmanship' here comes into his own) and arrangements made for their administration. Approval may have to be obtained from an ethical committee. Accommodation, equipment and its maintenance, supplies, transportation, and access to laboratory, data processing, or other facilities may have to be arranged. Personnel may have to be found or trained. Record forms must be printed. Maps may have to be found or prepared, or a census of the study population may have to be performed. Sampling frames may have to be prepared, cases of a disease identified, and samples or controls selected. In a blind or double-blind experiment, complicated practical preparations may be needed to ensure secrecy (dummy medicinal preparations, containers identified by symbols, etc.). In a study involving a sequence of procedures performed by different examiners, logistic problems may require solution. An inspired researcher is not necessarily a good administrator (and vice versa, as the activities of many public health departments, hospitals and other medical services eloquently testify), and in a large investigation it is often wise to appoint a study co-ordinator or field-work director with a bent for practical matters.

If observational methods of data collection are to be used (by persons other than the investigator who has planned them), they should be carefully explained and demonstrated, and 'running in' exercises should be arranged. An 'examiner's manual' may be required, both for training purposes and for subsequent consultation. If necessary, reference standards should be made available, such as standard photographs of skin abnormalities or (for laboratory tests) solutions of known chemical composition.

If interviewers have to be found, they should be carefully selected, the main requirements being that they should be capable, personable, honest and interested.[6] If the interviewers are new to this job, they should be given a general training in interview methods.[7] All interviewers should receive an explanation of the objectives and methods of the study, and should be told, unhurriedly and in detail, what they are expected to do. An 'interviewer's manual' should be prepared if it is thought this will be helpful. 'Trial interviews' should be conducted and discussed before the interviewer starts to interview members of the study population.

If documentary sources are to be used, steps should be taken to ensure that there is access to them—confidentiality and poor systems of record storage and retrieval often pose problems—and that they contain the desired types of information. The persons who are to extract the data should receive detailed instructions.

Whatever methods are to be used, arrangements should now be made for 'quality control' during the stage of data collection. (This will be discussed in Ch 24.)

If the data are to be coded, practical preparations for coding should be made, although these may sometimes be delayed until a later stage. Coding keys and coding instructions should be prepared, coders trained, and arrangements made for the testing and control of coding reliability.

Finally, a word of advice from Cochran[8]—when the study plan is near completion, find a 'devil's advocate'—a colleague who is willing to examine the plan and find its methodological weaknesses (not recommended for sensitive souls.).

NOTES AND REFERENCES

1. Converse J M & Presser S 1986 (Survey questions: handcrafting the standardized questionnaire, 2nd edn. Sage Publications, Beverly Hills, California) who provide detailed advice on pretests of questionnaires, write: 'The Magic N for a pretest is of course as many as you can get. We see 25–75 as a valuable pretest range'.
2. Belson W A 1981 The design and understanding of survey questions. Gower, Aldershot, Hants.
3. Practical problems in the performance of epidemiological *surveys in developing countries*, with special reference to measures for ensuring the population's co-operation, are discussed by Bennett F J 1973 Fieldwork techniques. In: Barker D J P (ed) Practical epidemiology. Churchill Livingstone, Edinburgh, pp 92–101. For a simple guide to the collection of epidemiological data at a district level in developing countries, see Vaughan J P, Morrow R H (eds) 1989 Manual of epidemiology for district health management, WHO, Geneva.

    Practical preparations for the use of microcomputers in developing countries ('Buy enough supplies to last for at least 1 year . . . Train your own service personnel . . . make several backup copies of all software' etc.) are reviewed by Bertrand W E 1985 Microcomputer applications in health population surveys: experience and potential in developing countries. World Health Statistics Quarterly 3: 91. Also, see note 4, p 34.

    Rapid epidemiological assessment (REA)—i.e., the use of simple, undemanding and cheap methods as a basis for programme decisions in developing countries (or at a local level in developed countries)—is the topic of a number of papers in the International Journal of Epidemiology 1989 18: supp. 2. Methods include cluster sampling (see note 5, p 90), rapid ethnographic assessment (i.e., qualitative methods; see p 134), the use of portable computers, sentinel surveillance (e.g., reporting of infective diseases in sentinel practices or groups not necessarily representative of the total population), 'verbal autopsies' to clarify causes of death, simplification of examination methods, and evaluation by the use of case-control studies (see p 292). Allowance may be needed for poor accuracy and inbuilt biases.
4. Rose G A, Blackburn H 1968 Cardiovascular survey methods, WHO, Geneva, p 58.
5. Mortagy A K, Howell J B L, Waters W E 1985 A useless raffle. Journal of Epidemiology and Community Health 39: 183.
6. For a fuller list of criteria for evaluating and selecting interviewers, see National Opinion Research Center, University of Chicago 1967 Manual of procedures for hiring and training interviewers. University of Chicago, Chicago, Illinois, pp 14–18.
7. See, for example, National Opinion Research Center 1967 pp 19–33.
8. Cochran W G 1983 Planning and analysis of observational studies. Moses L E, Mosteller F (eds) Wiley, New York, p 71.

24. Collecting the data

After the intellectual stimulation of the planning phase, the investigator now comes to a rather dull period when data are collected in a routine and predetermined manner. The greater the forethought and effort that were put into the planning and preparation, the more uneventful this new phase is likely to be.

However, the best-laid plans of good and bad researchers gang aft agley.[1] All kinds of unexpected contingencies may arise, and the investigator must be prepared to make running repairs as they become necessary.

Apart from this kind of troubleshooting, the investigator should take positive steps to test whether the collection of the data is in fact proceeding as it should. This may be done by instituting 'spot checks' (in Carl Becker's words, 'we need, from time to time, to take a look at the things that go without saying to see if they are still going') or, preferably, by regular periodic or ongoing surveillance.

This surveillance has two aspects. First, an ongoing record should be maintained of the performance of procedures—how many persons have been examined? how many have refused to be interviewed? etc. Secondly, *quality control* measures, to test the quality of the information which is being collected, should be instituted.[2]

In a study where the investigator himself collects the data, all that may be required for quality control is that he should check each record form as he completes it, to make sure that it has been filled in properly. Coding may be done at the same time. In a study where the data are collected by others, each record form should, if possible, be similarly checked as it is handed in. Sometimes omissions and errors can be corrected on the spot by editing; at other times, it may be necessary to refer to the person who completed the form, or even, if the omission or error is an important one, to repeat part of the examination or interview. If it is not possible to check each form as it is handed in, a sample of forms should be scrutinized. Regular meetings with examiners or interviewers are advisable, to share problems and maintain interest, as well as reviewing completed forms.

Checks on reliability (see pp 142–144) form an important part of quality control. It is not often possible to conduct repeated examinations or interviews of the same persons, but sometimes the reliability of examinations is tested by having the same subjects examined simultaneously by two examiners. Sometimes, limited analyses of the findings are performed, to permit comparisons of the data obtained (for different individuals) by different examiners or interviewers, or at different times by the same examiners or interviewers. If, for example, one examiner finds a far higher rate of varicose veins than others, it is worth exploring the possibility that this is due not to a difference in the subjects, but to his method of diagnosing varicose veins. Similarly, if the hypertension rate springs up in a specific month, this may be due to a defect in the instrument used. All measuring equipment should be checked periodically. If laboratory procedures are used, reliability should be checked by periodic comparisons with standards and by the examination of replicate specimens. In addition, systematic differences between laboratories, or in the same laboratory at different times, may sometimes be detected by comparing the results of determinations (of different batches), in terms of their average values or the proportions of determinations falling above or below predetermined cutting points.

Throughout this stage, detailed records should be kept of people who are omitted from the study—subjects who are replaced, nonrespondents, persons who drop out or are excluded because of side-effects, etc.—so as to permit possible sample bias to be taken into account in the analysis (see p 247). A record should be kept of their demographic characteristics and any other relevant information that can be easily obtained. Sometimes it is feasible to concentrate resources upon an attempt to obtain full information about a sample of non-respondents.

Identifying the subjects, finding them and persuading them to co-operate may require hard work, patience and ingenuity. In a case-control study, the identification of cases may involve tedious searches through clinical records, disease registers, diagnostic indexes of hospitals, or other sources. The selection of controls too may be far from easy, especially if they are matched. If the subjects were identified from old or incorrect records, it may be difficult to locate them. Names change—especially those of nubile females—and are often wrongly spelt. Recorded addresses may be incomplete, incorrect, or out-of-date. People who have moved may be difficult to trace, especially those who were living alone or as lodgers and the divorced and widowed.[3] With luck, the present residents at the previous address may know where the subjects went, or a letter may be forwarded by the post office. In other cases, intensive detective work may be needed, including contacts with ex-neighbours, known relatives and friends, local shopkeepers, the postman, the local doctor or public health nurse and so on.

Even in a simple household survey, it may not be easy to make contact, especially if the family is childless or all its members go out to work. The only solution, of course, is to try, try, try again, sometimes in the morning, sometimes in the late afternoon or evening, sometimes at weekends. Once contact has been made, obtaining co-operation usually presents little difficulty in an interview survey. More non-response is to be expected if medical examinations or blood samples are needed. The examination process should be made as painless as possible—flexible schedules, no waiting around, and above all a pleasant atmosphere—but broken appointments and frank refusals can be expected, however convenient the arrangements. Here too, perseverance is needed. Response rates can be boosted by establishing rapport, by repeated contacts and patient persuasion, by a judicious unreadiness to take 'no' for an answer (at least the first or second time it is said)—and, often, by a readiness to call for the help of a more irresistible member of the study team.

The longer these efforts go on, the more subjects will be traced and the more non-respondents will turn into respondents. But a line has to be drawn, and it is important to know where to draw it. A time comes when the added benefits fall far short of keeping pace with the added investment of effort, and the investigator should not hesitate to cry halt. This law of diminishing returns has been rephrased as the Ninety-Ninety Rule—'The first 90 per cent of the task takes 90 per cent of the time, and the last 10 per cent takes the other 90 per cent'.[4]

NOTES AND REFERENCES

1. So do the stylistic efforts of writers of books about survey methods—some readers have complained that this phrase is Greek to them. It is not, it is Scottish—'gang aft agley' means 'often go wrong'. ('The best-laid schemes o'mice an' men gang aft agley'—Robert Burns. Cohen J M, Cohen M J 1960 The Penguin dictionary of quotations. Harmondsworth: Penguin Books, p 84.

2. For a detailed account of the quality control measures used in a large-scale health examination survey, see National Center for Health Statistics 1972 Quality control in a national health examination survey, Vital and Health Statistics, series 2, no 44. Public Health Service, Washington, DC.
3. For descriptions of methods used to trace hard-to-find subjects, see Skeels H M, Skodak M 1965 Techniques of a high-yield follow-up study in the field. Public Health Reports 80: 249; Modan B 1966 Some methodological aspects of a retrospective follow-up study. American Journal of Epidemiology 82: 297; Bright M 1967 A follow-up study of the Commission on Chronic Illness Morbidity survey in Baltimore: I. Tracing a large population sample over time. Journal of Chronic Diseases 20: 707; 1969 A follow-up study of the Commission on Chronic Illness Morbidity survey in Baltimore: III. Residential mobility and prospective studies. Journal of Chronic Diseases 21: 749.
4. Wallechinsky D, Wallace I, Wallace A 1977 The book of lists. Cassell, London, p 300.

25. Processing the data

The analysis of findings has two components—data processing (which includes statistical analysis) and interpretation of the results. Processing is dealt with in this chapter, and interpretation in the next. These aspects are interdependent, and should be seen as activities that go hand in hand rather than as separate stages. Except in the simplest of investigations, the investigator produces or obtains a set of analytic results, then carefully considers them, seeing what inferences may be drawn from them and what further questions these open up, decides what further facts are needed in order to test the inferences or answer the questions, produces or obtains the new tabulations or calculations that are required, thinks about the new facts, and so on. Both processing and interpretation are carried out step-wise. This should apply even if a computer is used. . . . If 'the investigator tries to ask at one time for everything which he might possibly want (far more than he ever uses and often lacking what later turns out to be of critical importance) . . . we question that this is really efficient use of expensive equipment . . . it is a horrible waste of time of talented investigators'.[1]

Except in small studies, data processing is today usually done by a computer (see p 219). Many investigators have the expert knowledge of computer operation and specific programs that this requires; others can themselves handle the statistical analysis, but leave the creation, maintenance and management of data files to professionals. An investigator who does not have the necessary expertise or is not a 'do-it-yourself' enthusiast should give a very detailed explanation of his objectives and study plan to an expert, so that he can receive the best possible aid and advice with regard not only to data processing, but to the planning of forms and record systems.

Ready-made statistical programs for mainframe computers, microcomputers and pocket calculators are now widely available.[2] Even if the investigator does not run these himself, he should try to read the documentation, so that he knows what they do and what options are available, and can understand the printout; if he can make sense of the instructions given to the computer, he can satisfy himself that what he has got is what he wanted.

CODING AND DATA ENTRY

If a computer is to be used, the data must first be coded and entered.

Accurate coding may not be easy to achieve, even if there are detailed written instructions (see p 217). Careful training and monitoring may be needed; as a check on coding reliability, double coding (by the same or different coders) may be done for all records, a sample of records, or selected hard-to-code variables. The codes may be written or marked on the original data sheets, or may be copied to codesheets. Unnecessary transcription should be avoided, to minimize errors; if the codes are copied, this process too may need checking.

The process is simplified if coding is done at the time the data are collected, by the person who collects the data. But later checks and corrections are then possible only if the original data were recorded as well as the codes.

Data are generally entered manually, using a keyboard. Exceptionally, results of chemical, electrocardiographic and other examinations by instruments may go straight to the electronic record. The use of devices that can read written material is likely to increase.

Each variable is entered into a separate *field*, which can accommodate one or more characters (numbers, letters or other symbols). Before entering data, a plan is needed: what variables will be entered, in what order, how large will each field be, and so on. The data for each individual go into one or more *records*, which are often 'card-images' that are limited to 80 'columns', i.e. that can accommodate up to 80 characters (the old IBM punch card had 80 columns, and most computer screens display lines of 80 characters). All the records of all individuals make up a data *file*, which may be stored on disk, tape, or other medium.

Data should be entered in a format appropriate for the statistical programs to be used. If necessary, expert help or advice should be sought. Some data entry programs provide numerous options. A *fixed format* is generally used—each variable is recorded in the same place on the same record for all cases in the file. Sometimes a *freefield format* is used—the variables are recorded in the same order for each case, but not necessarily in the same locations; they may be separated by blank spaces, commas, carriage returns, or other delimiters.

Microcomputers are coming into wider use for data entry, even if the data will be analysed by a mainframe computer. Database programs are generally used, although word-processing programs can also be used (which requires simple typing of strings of digits or other characters, with or without delimiters, in the correct format). Database programs ask for information about each variable, e.g. its name, the width of the field, whether the entry will be treated as a number or as a string of text ('alphanumerical'), and how many decimal places. It is usually easy to get the program to provide a screen image of the record form, so that during data entry the items appear on the screen in the same order and with the same spatial arrangement as on the record form. A program written or adapted by an experienced programmer can also audit the data as they are entered, and identify errors, i.e. entries that do not fall into the variable's legitimate range or that are not logically consistent with entries for previous variables. Sophisticated programs can also incorporate 'skip patterns' that bypass irrelevant variables (a drawback of these patterns is discussed on p 168). Many database programs can create *derived variables* (see p 218) during the data entry process.

One trial of methods of data entry showed that use of a word processor, which required minimal computer experience, was more than adequate for short record forms. For longer records, a simple program using a screen image of the form was fastest and most liked. A more sophisticated program, with inbuilt logical checks and skip patterns, did not realize its theoretical advantages; it was slower, and identified only 10% of errors. Most errors caused by incorrect key-punching (about 1% of all digits entered can be expected to be wrong)[3] are not detected by these checks. The recommended method was the simple one using a screen image of the record form, with verification by repeated keying.[4]

The data entry procedure can be greatly simplified by the use of a program that asks for no information about the variables, but 'reads' a questionnaire or schedule of items that has been produced on a word processor in ordinary text format and shows it on the screen, so that each individual's values can be typed in and are automatically stored in the database.[5]

DATA PROCESSING

The data should always be checked before they are analysed. The minimal check—one that should never be forgotten—is a simple count. Data forms have a nasty habit of going astray.

If a computer is used, a 'machine edit' based on a set of checks should always be performed before the data are analysed. The values of each variable are examined, to see whether any fall outside the acceptable range. In addition, acceptable or unacceptable combinations of values (of different variables) may be defined ('logical checks'). It is then possible to pick up such obvious errors as a person aged 342 years, a woman who was married before she was born, or a man who is still menstruating. The errors, which may arise from inaccuracies in the original data or in coding or data entry, are corrected if this is possible. Otherwise the unacceptable values may be changed to 'unknown', and the individuals concerned may be excluded from specific analyses, or from the analysis as a whole. Erroneous and missing values are also sometimes changed to 'imputed'[6] ones.

For each analysis, the investigator must decide not only on the statistical procedure and indices wanted, but also who should be included (all? a subgroup? a separate analysis for each subgroup?), and how missing values are to be handled.

Adequate documentation of the analysis should be kept, whether processing is done by computer or manually. Tables and other results should be fully labelled, even if they are only for one's own use; it is amazing how much one can forget as time goes on. There should be a record of the categories of individuals who were included or excluded and how 'missing values' were handled, and the variables and their categories should be explicitly spelt out. All this information may come ready-printed in computer outputs; but the investigator should make sure he can decode it.

If there are many tables they should be numbered, and an index may be a good idea. This makes it easy to record the source of findings used when drafting the report, and may obviate a tedious search if confirmation or additional facts are needed.

Figures should be checked and cross-checked whenever possible, even if they come from a computer. Totals and marginal totals[7] can usually be compared with numbers known from previous tables. Sometimes errors are shown by the fact that the figures just 'don't make sense' (the interocular traumatic test[8]).

STATISTICAL ANALYSIS

The detailed analysis plan must obviously depend on the objectives of the study. We will deal with general strategy, not detailed tactics. No attempt will be made to explain statistical techniques, but some commonly used indices and methods will be briefly described in footnotes.

The investigator should start with a clear conception of the main kinds of result he wants. We have previously discussed the use of skeleton tables as an aid in planning the analysis (p 222). At this stage, such tables not only help to crystallize ideas about the analysis, they also provide frameworks (work sheets) for the manual entry of results, or a basis for instructions to be given to the computer.

No hard and fast rules can be laid down for the sequence of the analysis, but the inexperienced investigator is advised to keep to the following order:

1. Examine each variable separately
2. Examine pairs of variables
3. Examine sets of three or more variables

Multivariate methods of analysis, which permit the simultaneous examination of relationships involving a number of variables, are today easily available, and it is tempting to start with them. Most experts consider this unwise:

> We regard this approach as unsound, and instead recommend a more orderly application of analytic methods, beginning with simple descriptive statistical displays and summaries. Gaps, patterns and inconsistencies in the data can be discovered and further analyses suggested by this examination. Next, relationships between variables can be explored by means of simple cross-tabulations, scatter plans, and measures of association ... Once again, patterns and inconsistencies are sought and, when found, lead to additional tabulations. Finally, multivariate methods may be applied to the data after a full exploration has been conducted using simpler techniques.[9]

A textbook on multivariate statistics stresses that detailed prior screening of the data — 'cleaning up your act' — is fundamental to an honest multivariate analysis.[10]

It is usually advisable to start the analysis by *examining the frequency distributions* of all variables. That is, a separate table is prepared for each variable, showing how many individuals fall into each category or at each value of the variable. It is best to use detailed scales of measurement at this stage, i.e. narrow categories, with little or no 'collapsing' — so that the distributions can provide a basis for decisions about the categories to be used in subsequent stages.

The frequency distribution may influence decisions about subsequent steps in the analysis. Plans for detailed studies of relationships between social class and illnesses, for example, may have to be abandoned if the study population turns out to be very homogeneous in social class. ('Make sure your variables vary.'[11]) If there are only three cases of gout, there is little point in planning complicated tables on the epidemiology of this disease.If there are an excessive number of individuals in an 'unknown' category, it may be decided that the variable cannot be studied. Moreover, peculiarities in a distribution may throw doubt on the accuracy of the data (low face validity). *Outliers* may be found—specific values that differ very markedly from the others. These isolated values can have an unduly large effect on statistics, and may need special handling;[12] even if there is no reason to doubt the correctness of the extreme values, their presence may make it difficult to draw conclusions that can be applied more generally than to the particular sample studied.

Simple indices that summarize frequency distributions,[13] such as means, percentages and rates, may be calculated at this time or later. They may of course come ready-made from a computer together with the frequency distributions.

A major part of the analysis usually involves pairs or sets of variables— a dependent variable and one or more independent variables—rather than single variables. Even in the simplest descriptive survey the investigator will probably want to look separately at the findings in the two sexes and in various age groups; in a simple programme review he may want to see whether the performance of care procedures varied for different categories of patients or at different times of the year. In epidemiological studies aimed at testing causal hypotheses and in clinical and programme trials, the examination of *associations between variables*—putative causes and putative effects— is the main focus of the analysis.

In seeking evidence of associations, emphasis is given to those the study was designed to investigate—that is, the associations that are specified or implied in the stated objectives of the study—and to other possibly important relationships with the dependent variables. In most community medicine studies it is helpful if associations between the dependent variables and age, sex, and other selected 'universal' variables (see p 95) are explored early in the analysis. The process of examining a body of data in order to determine which variables are associated with one another may be referred to as 'screening for associations'.

Simple methods may suffice to reveal associations between pairs of variables. A relationship between pregnancy and anaemia, for example, may be revealed by a *contingency table* (cross-tabulation) in which each woman is simultaneously classified according to her pregnancy status and the presence or absence of anaemia. For an example of such a table, see p 252; but note that a different format[14] is called for if *paired data* are used — that is, if pairs of individually matched cases and controls were studied, or if 'before' and 'after' measurements were made of the same subjects. An association may be revealed by simple scrutiny of the figures in the table, or by elementary summarizing statistics[13], e.g. means or percentages, based upon these figures. Any measure of the strength of an association (see p 252) may be used to determine whether an association is present. A number of these measures are based upon data obtained from contingency tables, and there is much to be said for the prior use of contingency table analysis even if the use of more elaborate techniques is contemplated.

Associations may also be revealed by simple diagrams, such as a scattergram or a graph showing a frequency distribution.[15] A graph showing time trends is often used to demonstrate the effect of a new health programme.

Once identified, the associations can be studied more intensively, in terms of their strength, statistical significance, and other characteristics (see Ch. 27).

The next step is to consider a number of variables at the same time. The simplest way of doing this is by *stratification (subclassification)*, i.e. the construction of multiple contingency tables that allow for simultaneous cross-classification by three or more variables; for an example, see Table 27.2 on p 255. Multiple linear regression analysis, multiple logistic regression analysis, and other techniques of multivariate analysis may also be used. These analyses permit an examination of *modifying effects* (does one variable modify the relationship of another with the dependent variable?) and of *confounding* (see p 256).

Age, sex and other 'universal' variables are among those most frequently introduced into the analysis. In addition, consideration is usually given to other variables known or suspected to be associated with the dependent variable. No set rules can be laid down. Decisions depend on the aims of the study, on feasibility, and above all on the imaginativeness and ingenuity of the investigator.

It is of course not essential to follow the above sequence. Instead, other variables may be built into the analysis from the outset. This applies especially to 'universal' variables; tables are often broken down by age and sex[16] from a very early stage of the analysis. When there are two or more study populations, e.g. cases and controls, they are often analysed separately from the outset.

Complex methods are available which permit the simultaneous examination of relationships involving a number of variables. These techniques of *multivariate analysis* require considerable statistical expertise. It is often helpful to do an analysis by stratification techniques first, so as to identify important variables and get some understanding of their inter-relationships.

NOTES AND REFERENCES

1. Hammond E C, Irwin J, Garfinkel L 1967 Data-processing and analysis in epidemiological research. American Journal of Public Health 57: 1979.
2. Well-known *statistical packages for computers* include *SPSS*[x], *SAS*, *BMDP* and *SYSTAT*, which have versions for microcomputers as well as for mainframe computers.

   About 50 commercial packages for microcomputers are reviewed in PC Magazine 1989 8: 94, as well as 15 mathematical toolboxes and 10 scientific graphing programs. Quotable quotes: 'When you get right down to it, the phrase "easy-to-use statistics", like "military intelligence", is an oxymoron'. 'Bugs are as common in the PC stat package landscape as they are on a June day in Maine.'

   There are also many public-domain and user-supported programs for microcomputers (see note 3, p 34), some in packages (e.g. *Abstat, Epistat, Kwikstat, MyStat, SPPC, Stat-Sak, Superstat* and *Stat 5.3*) and some for single procedures. *Epi Info* (see note 5, below) does simple analyses.

   Some microcomputer programs require a great deal of disk space. Some can analyse stored data, others require input from the keyboard. Complicated and reiterative procedures may be slow unless the microcomputer has a fast processor (e.g. 80286 or 80386) or a coprocessor.

   Programs for *pocket calculators* are provided by Rothman K J, Boice J D Jr 1982 Epidemiologic analysis with a programmable calculator, 2nd edn. Epidemiological Resources, Chestnut Hill, Maryland; Abramson J H, Peritz E 1983 Calculator programs for the health sciences. Oxford University Press, New York.

   New epidemiological programs for computers and calculators are described in the American Journal of Epidemiology from time to time.
3. Martin J N T, Morton J, Ottley P 1977 Experiments on copying digit strings. Ergonomics 20: 409.
4. Crombie I K, Irving J M 1986 An investigation of data entry methods with a personal computer. Computers and Biomedical Research 19: 543.
5. *Epi Info* (available from the Epidemiology Program Office, Centers for Disease Control, Atlanta, Georgia) is a public-domain program that streamlines data entry. The user types a questionnaire or data entry form in the ordinary way (but using certain conventions for numeric, Yes/No and other fields), and this is subsequently shown on the screen so that each subject's data can be entered and automatically stored. The program allocates variable names, field lengths, etc. using information derived from the form. To cite the manual, the program 'might be called "an automatic, questionnaire-driven, full-screen, multipage, data entry program. Only those who have spent hours defining "fields" and weeks waiting for programmers and keypunching operations will fully appreciate what this means'. Questionnaires typed with this program can be used in computer-assisted interviews (p 168). Data entry constraints (the range of

acceptable responses, etc.' can be built in. The program can also perform very simple analyses and draw simple graphs. A valuable feature is that it can convert the data to formats suitable for use with various statistical packages (e.g. *SPSS*, *SAS*, *EpiStat*) and other database programs.

Also worthy of mention is *PC-Edit* (Department of Technical Cooperation for Development, United Nations, New York) a simple data-entry program that cannot read questionnaires, but has skip patterns and checks for errors (including inconsistencies between variables), can compute derived variables, and permits verification by the re-entry of data; for data-entry screens in questionnaire format, use version 3.

6. Erroneous and missing values are sometimes replaced by *imputed* ones, especially if exclusion of the subjects from the analysis is likely to cause bias. Use may be made of the mean or usual value of the variable in the total study population or in people similar to the subject who has a wrong or missing value. Other methods are listed by Kelsey J L, Thompson W D, Evans A S 1986 Methods in observational epidemiology. Oxford University Press, New York, pp 269–271. Whatever method is used, it is often wise to do the analysis without as well as with the 'guessed' values, so that the effect of their inclusion can be observed and (if necessary) taken into account.

7. In a table showing a cross-classification, the totals of the figures in each column and row are referred to as 'marginal totals'. These are the totals in each category of the variables shown, i.e. simple frequency distributions. When one inspects the frequency distributions of variables (see p 239) one can puzzle the uninitiated by saying that one is looking at the marginals.

8. It hits you between the eyes.

9. Stolley P D, Schlesselman J J 1982 Planning and conducting a study. In: Schlesselman J J (ed) Case-control studies: design, conduct, analysis. Oxford University Press, New York, pp 69–104.

10. Tabachnick B G, Fidell L S 1989 Using multivariate statistics, 2nd edn. Harper and Row, New York. This book is a methodical guide to the use of BMDP, MYSTAT, SAS and SPSS for multivariate analyses.

11. Davis J A 1971 Elementary survey analysis. Prentice Hall, Englewood Cliffs, N J, p 23. 'If the heart of research is to compare cases which fall in different categories, the research worker must have plenty of cases which differ in their classification. It is hard to argue with such a truism, but it is easy to forget it.'

12. There is no simple solution to the problem of *outliers*. The least that should be done is to be aware of their presence, and it is generally worth seeing how their exclusion affects the findings. It may be decided to modify the scale of measurement (e.g. by collapsing categories) so that they are grouped together with less extreme values, or to exclude them, or to change them to less extreme values. See Tabachnick & Fidell (1989, see note 10), pp 66–70.

13. Indices that may be used to describe frequency distributions include measures of central tendency, measures of dispersion, and proportions.

The commonest *measures of central tendency* are the arithmetic *mean* (used for interval or ratio scales) and the *median* or *50th percentile*, which is the value of the middle observation when all the observations are arranged in ascending order (for ordinal, interval or ratio scales). Using a mean, the average human being has one testis.

The commonest *measures of dispersion* around the mean are the *standard deviation* (not to be confused with the standard error of the mean) and the *coefficient of variation* which is derived from it. *Quartiles* (the values below which fall one-quarter, one-half, and three-quarters, respectively, of all values) or the *interquartile range* between the upper and lower quartiles may be used to measure dispersion around a median. Use is frequently made of percentiles (the values below which fall 3%, 10% etc. of the observations), especially to summarize anthropometric data.

The number of individuals in a category may be expressed as a *relative frequency*, i.e. as a *proportion* (e.g. a *percentage*) of the total. The data may be combined to show what proportions of individuals have values that lie above (or below) successive levels (*cumulative frequencies*).

Rates are briefly discussed in note 1 on p 99.

14. *Paired data*, such as those derived from pairs of individually matched cases and controls (in a retrospective survey) or matched pairs of persons exposed and not exposed to a putative causative factor (prospective survey or experiment), or from pairs of observations made on the same persons before and after exposure to some factor, need special attention. Pairs and not individuals should be classified, using a contingency table of the following kind:

	Cases	
	Factor absent	Factor present
Controls		
Factor absent	a	b
Factor present	c	d

A disparity in size between b and c provides evidence of an association. A measure of the strength of the association is described in note 4 on p 264.

For methods to be used when each case has multiple individually matched controls, see Fleiss J L 1981 Statistical methods for rates and proportions, 2nd edn. Wiley, New York, pp 123–126.

15. In *histograms, bar diagrams* and *line diagrams* showing frequency distributions, the variable (e.g. haemoglobin value) is usually placed on the X (horizontal) axis and the frequency (e.g. the number or percentage of women in each haemoglobin category) on the Y axis. A *scattergram* or *scatter diagram* may be used if both variables are measured by ordinal, interval or ratio scales. It is a practicable method if the number of observations is not very large. Each observation is plotted as a point on a graph in which one variable (usually the independent one) is placed on the X axis and the other on the Y axis. The number of cigarettes smoked per day during pregnancy, for example, might be plotted against the baby's birth weight. If an association is present the points will tend to follow a sloping or curved path.

16. Hopefully, unlike the investigator.

26. Interpreting the findings

At the outset of his study the investigator formulated his objectives, specifying the questions he wished it to answer. At the present stage, his first and main task is to use the information he has since collected, in order to answer those questions. Careful consideration should be given to the ways in which the methods used, and their imperfections, may have influenced the results. The investigator should initially concentrate on 'understanding' his findings, on 'making sense' of what he has found in the study population he has investigated. In doing this, he may sometimes extend his interest to finding answers to questions that were not originally posed; but this must be done with reservations—as the study was not designed to answer these other questions, the answers may be inadequate or misleading. The testing of hypotheses that the study was not designed to test, but that are suggested by the data, has been referred to as 'data dredging'.[1] Any body of data will show some associations which have occurred only by chance; and if too much attention is paid to these, ignoring the fact that they are rare events among a large number of associations that might have arisen, misleading conclusions may be reached. An association brought to the surface by data dredging is best treated not as evidence that the relationship exists, but as a clue suggesting that it may exist. Other studies can then be designed to test this hypothesis.

To derive full value from the study, it is not enough to 'make sense,' of the findings, and the investigator should also give thought to their broader 'significance'—the extent to which they may be generalized beyond his study population, their wider scientific implications, the research questions they raise or leave unanswered, their practical implications in terms of the provision of medical care or other aspects of public health action, and so on.

The interpretation of findings may be child's play,[2] or may present formidable difficulties. Usually the task is a more exacting one than it seems on the surface. In one investigator's words of warning:

An eminent British biostatistician, Major Greenwood, remarked that once the proper questions are asked and the relevant facts collected, any sensible person can reach the correct conclusions. There are two limitations. The facts are never quite complete nor completely accurate, and, as Voltaire pointed out in his *Dictionnaire Philosophique*, 'Common sense is not so common'.[3]

The specific problems of interpretation will depend on the nature of the investigation and on its detailed findings, and cannot be fully discussed here. We will content ourselves with considering three aspects. First we will briefly review the ways in which the findings and their interpretation may be affected by bias, and then (in the next two chapters) we will deal with the interpretation of associations between variables and with problems of generalization.

BIAS

Bias is defined as 'any effect at any stage of investigation or inference tending to produce results that depart systematically [i.e. one-sidedly] from the true values'.[4] The term is here not used as a synonym for 'prejudice'. Of course the investigator's prejudices—his preconceived opinions and preferences—are among the factors that may lead to bias, both in the findings and in their interpretation.

Bias may affect both the *internal validity* of the study—i.e. its capacity to yield sound conclusions with respect to the study population—and its *external validity*—the ability to make valid generalizations to a broader reference population.

At this stage of the study, the investigator should systematically review his findings and consider the possibility that they may be biased, as a result of short-comings either in the study plan or (by the ineluctable operation of Murphy's Law[5]) in its execution. It may not be too hard, if he does not yet know his study's imperfections, to find a colleague who will gladly point them out.

We will here consider two kinds of bias of the findings—*selection bias* and *information bias*. (*Confounding*, which may also be regarded as a kind of bias, will be discussed on p 256).

First, the individuals for whom data are available may not be representative of the study population or populations. This *selection bias* may impair the *validity* of the findings as a measure of whatever it is that the investigator wants to know about the target population—the prevalence of a disease, the strength of an association with a disease, and so on.

Selection bias may be due to failure to choose a representative sample (*sample bias*), or to short-comings in the way that cases, experimental subjects or controls were chosen (see Chs 6 to 8). It may also be due to incomplete coverage—failure to obtain information about all members of a sample or population (*non-response bias*), refusal to participate in a trial (*non-participant bias*), or the loss of members of the study population during an experiment or longitudinal survey (*drop-out bias*).

Another kind of selection bias may be present—the whole study population may be a 'special' or 'different' one (see pp 59, 271). This may result from selective admission to the population, as in a study of hospital patients (Berksonian bias, see p 51) or of bus drivers, vegetarians, or other groups characterized by their occupations or behaviour (*membership bias*). It may also result from *selective migration* into or out of a population, or from *selective survival*.

The 'special' nature of a study population of course does not lead to bias if the investigator is interested only in the population he has studied or sampled. But generalizations that go beyond this population may not be valid. The prevalence of a disease or of breast feeding in one neighbourhood is not necessarily the same as that in the nation as a whole, and an association detected between diseases in a hospital population does not necessarily exist in the population at large.

Selection bias may occur in any type of study, and its presence should always be explored. To do this, the way in which the sample or samples were chosen should be critically reviewed. Special attention should be paid to substitutions (see p 85), non-respondents, non-participants, patients who were removed from a clinical trial because of side-effects, and drop-outs. How numerous were these, and what were the reasons? Bias is particularly likely if the selective factors were illness, death, or other reasons that might be connected with the variables under study. Unless the rates of substitutions, non-response and dropouts were negligible, the individuals included in the study should be compared with those who were omitted, using whatever demographic and other information may be available. Even at this stage, it may not be too late to collect further data for this purpose. Any differences that are found, such as an under-representation of working mothers among the respondents, may be helpful in the interpretation of the findings. An absence of such differences increases the likelihood that there is no important selection bias, but unfortunately it can never guarantee this, especially if non-response or drop-out rates are high. Occasionally it is possible to control selection bias by statistical procedures during the analysis (see p 271).

The second kind of bias, *information bias* ('non-sample bias') is caused by shortcomings in the collecting, recording, coding or analysis of data. This bias may have its source in the people who collected information (*observer bias, interviewer bias*), in the use of defective questionnaires or other instruments, or in one-sided responses by the people studied (*recall bias, response bias*). It may have arisen because 'blind' procedures were not used (see p 146), or because of deviations in compliance with experimental or other study procedures or because of misclassification errors (see p 159). Or (among other possibilities) the data for the various groups under comparison may not have been collected in a standard way. There may have been different observers or interviewers in various groups, or different operational definitions and criteria may have been used, or different instruments or techniques, or different follow-up periods. Evidence of exposure to a suspected cause may have been sought more energetically when the outcome was known to be present (*exposure suspicion bias*), or vice versa (*diagnostic suspicion bias*). If *measures* are of low validity, or if their validity varies in different parts of the study population, the *study* may be of low validity.

When possible bias is suspected, evidence of its presence should be sought. In a case-control study of the association between cataract and previous episodes of severe diarrhoea, for example, exposure suspicion bias was a possibility although the interviewers were not told whether they were interviewing a case or a control, since the cataract and its effects were often obvious. A comparison showed, however, that histories of diarrhoea were elicited as frequently from patients with obvious blindness as from patients with mild cataracts; this enhanced confidence in the findings.[6] In another study, the presence of interviewer bias caused by awareness that respondents had cancer was tested by examining data for patients whose cancer diagnoses were subsequently disproved.[7]

When possible the direction and magnitude of the bias should be appraised, so that allowances can be made when inferences are drawn. The effects of the bias can sometimes be controlled or corrected. If, for example, there is a constant bias in laboratory results, due to a mistake in the preparation of a standard solution, it may be rectified by applying a correction factor to the results. Special analyses may be required, as in a case-control study of a form of cancer, where there was a suspicion that the differences observed between patients and controls might be partly due to the fact that proxy informants had been far more often used for patients (many of whom had died) than for controls. Special analyses were therefore conducted, restricted to data with a high face validity. When parity was investigated, attention was confined to data obtained from the women themselves. When the subjects' home circumstances in their childhood were investigated, use was made of information provided by the subjects or their parents or siblings, not by other informants.[8] Computations may be used to allow for the effects of misclassification, if quantitative information about the bias is available.[9]

The above comments refer to bias of the findings. There is little that can be usefully said about the other form of bias, namely one-sidedness in the interpretation of findings. Biased interpretation is especially likely if the investigator has strong preconceptions, and it is usually due to unconscious processes. By a selective blindness to awkward facts, a failure to look for contrary evidence, and a too-easy acceptance of incomplete proof, he may readily find what he expected to find. This is part of the 'Self-fulfilling Prophecy' syndrome.[10] The investigator should seek insight into his motivations—how important is it to him to prove his case or to come up with a 'discovery'? He should interpret his findings as objectively and fairly as he can, and should take every opportunity to discuss his interpretation with colleagues, and then not only hear but listen to what they have to say.

NOTES AND REFERENCES

1. Selvin H C, Stuart A 1966 Data-dredging procedures in data analysis. American Statistician 20 (3): 20. Finding something by data dredging and then using the same data to test the finding may lead to unwarranted conclusions; this has been termed 'post hoc bias'; Feinleib M, Detels R 1985 Cohort studies. In: Holland W W, Detels R, Knox G (eds) Oxford Textbook of Public Health, vol 3: Investigative methods in public health. Oxford University Press, Oxford, pp 101–112.
2. See Abramson J H 1988 Making sense of data: a self-instruction manual on the interpretation of epidemiological data. Oxford University Press, New York.
3. Mann G V 1977 Diet-heart: end of an era. New England Journal of Medicine 297: 644.
4. Definition of bias from Last J M (ed) 1983 A dictionary of epidemiology. Oxford University Press, New York. An annotated catalogue of biases is provided by Sackett D L 1979 (Bias in analytic research. Journal of Chronic Disease 32: 51), quod vide for explanations of 'hot stuff bias', 'looking for the pony bias', 'rumination bias', 'tidying-up bias' etc. For a detailed discussion of bias, with special reference to the study of associations between two dichotomous variables, see Kleinbaum D G, Kupper L L, Morgenstern H 1982 Epidemiologic research, part II. LifeTime Learning Publications, Belmont, California. Sources of bias in case-control studies are reviewed by Schlesselman J J, Stolley P D 1982

Sources of bias. In: Schlesselman J J (ed) 'Case-control studies: design, conduct analysis. Oxford University Press, New York, Chapter 5.

5. Murphy's Law states: 'If anything can go wrong, it will'. O'Toole's commentary on this law: 'Murphy was an optimist'. Cited by Wallechinsky D, Wallace I, Wallace A 1977 The book of lists. Cassell, London, p 299.

6. Minassian D C, Mehra V, Jones B R 1984 Dehydrational crises from severe diarrhoea or heatstroke and risk of cataract. Lancet 1: 751.

7. Lilienfeld A M, Lilienfeld D E 1980 Foundations of epidemiology, 2nd edn. Oxford University Press, New York, pp 208–209.

8. Abramson J H, Pridan H, Sacks M I, Avitzour M, Peritz E 1978 A case-control study of Hodgkin's disease. Journal of the National Cancer Institute 61: 307.

9. The statistical control of misclassification errors is explained by Fleiss J L 1981 Statistical methods for rates and proportions, 2nd edn. John Wiley and Sons, New York. Chapter 12; and Kleinbaum et al (1982; see note 4) Chapter 12.

10. 'This is the bias a researcher is inclined to project into his methodology and treatment that subtly shapes the data in the direction of his foregone conclusions.' Isaac S, Michael W B 1977 Handbook in research and evaluation for education and the behavioral sciences. EdITS, San Diego, p 58. Maier's Law is relevant here: 'If the facts do not conform to the theory, they must be disposed of'; listed by Wallechinsky et al (1977; see note 5) p 300. If the investigator's prejudice is a reflection of a conventional or fashionable belief, his findings may tend to confirm this belief. This is the 'Self-perpetuating Myth' syndrome; see Fleiss (1981; see note 9) p 208.

27. Making sense of associations

The exploration of associations[1,2] between variables is usually the most challenging and rewarding part of the analysis. This is especially true in analytic epidemiological studies in which causal hypotheses are tested, and in clinical and programme trials, which aim at testing hypotheses about the effects of health care.

Simple methods of detecting associations are listed on page 240. Whenever an association is found, there are six basic questions that may be asked.

QUESTIONS ABOUT AN ASSOCIATION

1. Actual or artifactual? (Influence of bias?)
2. How strong?
3. Non-fortuitous?
4. Consistent? (Influence of modifying factors?)
5. Influence of confounding factors?
6. Causal?

Questions 1, 2 and 4 should usually be asked, in any kind of study, and 3, 5 and 6 are important if the investigator wants to explain his findings and not only describe them.

As will be pointed out, some of these questions may also be asked about the *absence* of an association.

ARTIFACTS

The first question, always worth asking, is whether the finding actually exists, or whether it may be an artifact—i.e. ask *whether* before asking *why* there is an association.

Artifactual ('spurious'[3]) associations may be produced by flaws in the design or execution of the study, that result in bias (see Ch. 26).

The prevalence of anaemia may appear to be higher in one town or one group of patients than in another because of selection bias or the use of different sources of data, different definitions of anaemia, different methods of measuring haemoglobin, etc. Artifactual associations may be caused by errors, often remediable ones, in the handling of data. Not uncommonly they result from mistakes in arithmetic.

Flawed methods may of course not only produce an artifactual association, they may also weaken, obscure, strengthen, or change the direction of an actual association.

If marked bias is strongly suspected and there is no way of correcting or controlling its effects, further examination of the association is usually pointless.

STRENGTH

The strength of an association is a measure of its importance. If anaemia is found among 30% of pregnant women and 2% of non-pregnant women (see Table 27.1), this marked disparity (a difference of 28%, or a ratio of 15) indicates a strong and important relationship between anaemia and pregnancy.

Table 27.1 Contingency table showing relationship between pregnancy and anaemia among 10 000 women (imaginary data)

	No anaemia	Anaemia	Total
Pregnant	a: 1400 (70%)	b: 600 (30%)	2000 (100%)
Not pregnant	c: 7840 (98%)	d: 160 (2%)	8000 (100%)

How strong an association must be if it is to be regarded as important is a matter of judgement. A difference of 2% in anaemia rates would probably be considered trivial, but a similar difference in infant mortality rates—i.e. 20 extra infant deaths per 1000 live births—would be more likely to be regarded as important.

As will be seen below, conclusions about the strength of an association may sometimes be modified when additional variables are incorporated into the analysis. An association should therefore not be prematurely discarded as unimportant. This, it must be said, is not easy advice to follow; it is very tempting to restrict further analysis to associations that 'come through loud and clear' from the beginning.

Measures of the strength of an association[2] include the *difference between rates or proportions* and the *rate ratio* (both used in the above example), the *odds ratio*,[4] the *difference between means* (e.g. of haemoglobin values), and *correlation and regression coefficients*.[5] Ratios (rate ratios or odds ratios) are generally appropriate in studies of causal processes or the influence of interventions, and absolute differences between rates are suitable if there is interest in the magnitude of a public health problem. *Attributable (aetiological), prevented and preventable fractions* (which are based on differences between rates) measure the *impact* of a harmful or protective factor on the health of people exposed to it, or on the total community; the *population attributable risk percentage*, for example, is the percentage of the disease in the population that can be attributed to a given cause.

Whatever measure is used, a confidence interval may be informative. This is the range within which we can assume the true value (in the population from which the study sample was drawn) to lie, with a specified degree of confidence.[6]

NON-FORTUITOUSNESS

Anything[7] may happen by chance. However strong the association that is observed between two variables, it may be fortuitous, unlikely though this may be. 'The "one chance in a million" will undoubtedly occur, with no less and no more than its appropriate frequency, however surprised we may be that it should occur to *us*.'[8] The absence of an association may also be a fortuitous occurrence.

The question is not whether the association observed in the study may have occurred by chance—the answer to which is almost always 'yes'—but whether we are prepared to regard it as non-fortuitous. Occasionally—e.g. if there is a big difference between the rates observed in two groups, and the groups are large—just looking at the results may enable us to decide whether to regard the association as non-fortuitous. When this 'eye test'[9] is not enough, a test of statistical significance[10] may be used to enable us to make this decision.

Significance tests should not be done when they are not needed. In some studies, especially in simple descriptive surveys and programme reviews in which probability sampling was not used, the issue of fortuitousness may have little importance. For practical purposes it may be enough to know that housebound patients are concentrated in certain neighbourhoods of a city or that the proportion of women given postnatal guidance on family planning is lower in one clinic than in others, without worrying about deciding whether these associations may be regarded as non-fortuitous. There is little point in doing a significance test on an association that is likely to be an artifact, or one that is so weak that it would be of no consequence even if it were regarded as non-fortuitous.

An association is adjudged to be statistically significant if the test yields a P value[10] that is less than an arbitrarily chosen *significance level (alpha)*. Critical levels often selected are 5% (0.05) and 1% (0.01). Whatever level is chosen, it must be remembered that significance tests have 'built-in errors'. Using a significance level of 5%, purely random processes will produce a verdict of 'statistically significant' in about five of every hundred significance tests performed, even if no real associations exist ('making a fool of yourself five times out of every 100,[11]). This is an important consideration if many tests are performed. The chance of such errors may be reduced by lowering the critical level, but can never be eliminated. Statistical significance can also be appraised by the use of confidence intervals.[10]

If the association is statistically significant we may regard it as non-fortuitous, without forgetting that, because of the 'built-in errors', we have not proved beyond doubt that the difference is not due to chance. A 'statistically significant' result does not mean that the relationship is necessarily strong, and it tells us nothing about the importance of the relationship. If the prevalence of anaemia is 30% in one group of pregnant women and 32% in another, this difference would be considered negligible even if it were statistically significant, which it would be if each group contained 5000 women.

If the result is 'not statistically significant' we can of course not conclude that an observed association is non-fortuitous. On the other hand, this negative result does not necessarily mean that the association is fortuitous (any more than a negative sputum test for the tubercle bacillus necessarily means that a patient does not have tuberculosis). The verdict is 'not proven'. If the samples are large such a result may, however, be taken to mean that there is unlikely to be a non-fortuitous association of any great strength.

CONSISTENCY OF THE ASSOCIATION

An association may vary in different parts of the population or in different circumstances. The simplest way of detecting this is to stratify the data in accordance with the categories of another variable, and then inspect the findings in each stratum separately. In Table 27.1, for example, we saw an association between pregnancy and anaemia. In Table 27.2 the same data are additionally subclassified according to educational level, so that education can be 'held constant' in the analysis. (This could of course be done better by using more than two educational categories, so as to ensure greater homogeneity in the educational strata.) This table shows a much stronger association between pregnancy and anaemia among the poorly educated (relative risk = 50% ÷ 2%, i.e. 25) than among the better educated (relative risk = 5).

Table 27.2   Multiple contingency table showing relationship between pregnancy and anaemia among 10 000 women, by educational level (imaginary data)

	No anaemia	Anaemia	Total
High educational level			
Pregnant	900 (90%)	100 (10%)	1000 (100%)
Not pregnant	3920 (98%)	80 (2%)	4000 (100%)
Low educational level			
Pregnant	500 (50%)	500 (50%)	1000 (100%)
Not pregnant	3920 (98%)	80 (2%)	4000 (100%)

In such analyses the additional variable (education) may be called a *modifier variable*,[12] since it 'modifies' the relationship between pregnancy and anaemia. In statistical parlance, there is *statistical interaction*[12] between education and pregnancy. This means that the association between anaemia (the dependent variable) and pregnancy differs when educational level varies, and also (check this in the table) that the association between anaemia and poor education differs among pregnant women (relative risk = 50 per cent ÷ 10 per cent, i.e. 5) and non-pregnant women (relative risk = 1).

The different findings in different strata are often of interest in their own right. They may have important practical implications. It may be possible, for example, to identify vulnerable 'high-risk' population groups—in our instance, poorly educated pregnant women—who may require special health care. In an evaluative study, a care procedure or programme may be found to be more effective among some categories of patients or population groups than among others.

The detection of inconsistent relationships is also a fruitful source of clues for the investigator who wishes not only to describe associations but to explain them. It often suggests what directions the subsequent analysis should take.

Consistency may sometimes be worth investigating even when no association has been found, since an association that occurs only in a relatively small stratum can be drowned by the findings in other strata, so that no association is observed in the data as a whole. An association may also (less commonly) be concealed if there are positive and negative associations in different strata, so that they cancel each other out.

Consistency may depend on what measure of association is employed. When the relative risk is used, the data in Table 27.2 show a stronger association between pregnancy and anaemia among the poorly educated. The same disparity is shown when rate differences are used; the difference is 50 minus 2, i.e. 48% among the poorly educated, and it is only 8% among the better educated. The results could, however, differ. If the rates were 40 and 20% in one stratum, and 4 and 2% in another, the rate ratio would be 2 in each stratum, but the differences would be 20 and 2% respectively. Effect modification always refers to a specific measure of association.

CONFOUNDING EFFECTS

It sometimes happens that an association between two variables can be explained by the influence of another variable and has little meaning in itself. This possibility is of obvious concern to an investigator who wants to understand his findings.

As an example, a survey in Massachussetts revealed that the children of fathers who smoked tended to have lower birth weights than those of fathers who did not smoke. This apparently occurred because smokers tended to have wives who smoked, and women who smoked during pregnancy tended to have light babies.[13] As another curious illustration:

> consider the association between storks and babies (which, depending on time and place, is almost always small but positive). Few people believe that storks bring babies, and the small positive relation is undoubtedly due to rural areas having both a large number of storks and a higher birth rate than urban areas.[14]

People who give up cigarettes have a high death rate in the next year or two. This occurs not because smoking is good for you, but because decisions to give up smoking are commonly due to the onset of diseases that carry a high fatality. Statistics show that the larger the number of fire engines that come to deal with a fire, the greater the fire damage. But does this necessarily mean that it is the fire engines that cause the damage?

In each of these instances the association that was originally observed was a *secondary* one, resulting from the fact that both variables were related to a third, *confounding* variable.[15] This may be portrayed as A—C—B, where A and B, the independent and dependent variables respectively, are both linked with C, the confounding factor. Variable A is a *passenger variable*[16] that C has carried into its association with B. It follows that the variables that should be investigated as possible confounders are those with known or suspected associations with both the dependent and independent variables.

As a numerical illustration, we can use our fictional data on 2000 pregnant women, among whom there was an association (relative risk = 5) between anaemia and poor education (Table 27.2). In Table 27.3 these data are subclassified according to an additional variable, the presence of hookworm infestation. When separate attention is paid to women with hookworm and those without, no association between anaemia and poor education is found in either stratum, although in the total sample of pregnant women the relative risk was 5. The association observed in the total sample is a distortion of the true situation, caused by the strong relationships between hookworm and anaemia (shown in the table) and between hookworm and poor education (750 of the 1000 poorly educated women in our sample suffered from hookworm, as compared with 100 of the 1000 well educated).

Table 27.3 Multiple contingency table showing relationship between education level and anaemia among 2000 pregnant women, by presence of hookworm infestation (imaginary data)

	No anaemia	Anaemia	Total
Hookworm infestation			
High educational level	36 (36%)	64 (64%)	100 (100%)
Low educational level	260 (35%)	490 (65%)	750 (100%)
No hookworm infestation			
High educational level	864 (96%)	36 (4%)	900 (100%)
Low educational level	240 (96%)	10 (4%)	250 (100%)
Total			
High educational level	900 (90%)	100 (10%)	1000 (100%)
Low educational level	500 (50%)	500 (50%)	1000 (100%)

It must be stressed that if an association disappears or is altered when another variable is controlled, this does not necessarily mean that there is a confounding effect. This could also happen if the pattern of associations was A→C→B, i.e. if A produces or affects C, and C produces or affects B. In this pattern, C is an *intermediate* or *intervening cause*; A is an *indirect cause* of B. In the present instance, the possibility must be considered that poor education, or some closely related factor for which poor education serves as a proxy, is a cause of hookworm infestation and hence, indirectly, of anaemia. To the extent that this is true, the relationship between education and anaemia may be causal. Even the association between fathers' smoking habits and their babies' birth weights may to an extent be causal, if men's smoking habits affect their wives'. To confound an association between A and B, variable C must cause or influence B, and it must also be related to A, but not simply because it is caused or influenced by A.

The way that a confounding variable distorts an association depends on the strength and direction of its relationships with the other variables. Controlling a confounding variable may make an association disappear (as in the above example); it may weaken it, strengthen it, or change its direction (from positive to negative or vice versa); and it may reveal an association not previously apparent.

There are three main approaches to the detection or control of confounding effects at this stage of the study:

1. The variable suspected of being a confounding factor can be held constant by *stratification*. The study population is divided into strata in accordance with the categories of the suspected confounder, and the association between the dependent and independent variables is measured separately in each stratum and compared with the association found in the data as a whole. If, as in the above example, this comparison reveals a difference large enough to be considered meaningful by the investigator (there are no statistical tests for this), and if the suspected confounder is not an intermediate cause, the difference is evidence of a confounding effect. The stratum-specific data provide estimates of the strength of the 'true' association when the confounding variable is controlled. As pointed out on page 254, stratification also permits the inspection of modifier effects.

2. The confounder can be *neutralized*. The strength of the association is measured by a statistical technique, such as standardization, multivariate analysis, etc., that nullifies the effect of the suspected confounder or confounders.[2] The difference between this *adjusted* measure of strength and the corresponding *crude* measure (not controlling for confounding) is an indication of the degree of confounding. It should be remembered that 'overadjustment' may have the same effects as overmatching (see p 72): the association that the investigation was designed to study may be masked, and unnecessary adjustment (for variables that are not confounding) may impair the precision with which this association can be measured.[17]

3. Confounding factors can occasionally be *reasoned away*; that is, it may be possible to deduce that an observed association between A and B is unlikely to be a secondary one caused by their common association with C. The reasoning is based on known and assumed facts about the relationships between C and the other two variables. An appreciable confounding effect can be produced only if these relationships are very strong—'the spurious effect is only a relatively weak echo'. Also, the direction of these relationships (positive or negative) influences the direction of the confounding effect.[18]

These methods of handling confounding effects can be used only if there was sufficient forethought in the planning stage of the study to ensure that possible confounders were selected as study variables (see p 94), and hence measured. It should be remembered that it is possible to cope with confounding effects when planning the study design, by *restricting* the study to a homogeneous group (see p 58) or by using *matching* (Ch. 7) or *randomization* (Ch. 30). During the analysis it is wise, if the latter methods were used, to check the similarity of the groups that are to be compared.

CAUSALITY

Finally, we come to the question of causality. How can we know whether the association between A and B (i.e. A—B) is a cause–effect one? Does A, or a factor of which A is a proxy measure, produce or affect B (i.e. A → B)? (Or, of course, vice versa: A ← B.)

Let us pause to consider what we mean by 'causality'. For our purposes, a causal association is best defined pragmatically, as 'an association between categories or events or characteristics in which an alteration in the frequency or quality of one category is followed by a change in the other'.[19] Basically, we wish to obtain information that can be put to practical use, now or in the long run. We want to identify factors that, if altered, would lead to a reduction in something we consider undesirable—premature deaths, disease, etc.—or to an improvement in something we regard as desirable, such as health care. For us, these factors are causes, even if their manipulation is unfeasible or unacceptable. In a clinical or programme trial, we want to know what effects, desirable and undesirable, can be attributed to intervention.

Not only do we want to know whether A causes B, we also want to know what the mechanism is—by what process is this influence exerted? In the chain of causation A→X→Y→Z→B, we are interested not only in A, but also in the intervening causes X, Y and Z. Having learned about X, Y and Z, we may endeavour to modify them as well as or instead of A, so as to modify B. In an evaluative study we may be interested not only in the achievement of changes in health and other desirable outcomes, but also in the chain of activities and intermediate outcomes that led to these end-results. What we actually want (but can probably never attain) is a complete picture not only of all the links in the chain of causation, but also of the other variables that influence A, X, Y, Z and B or the processes by which they affect each other (Fig. 27.1).

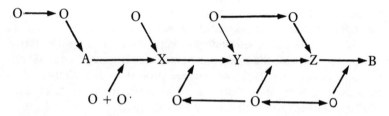

Fig 27.1   The web of causation.

In fact, we want to know the total nexus, the 'web of causation'.[19] From our immediate pragmatic viewpoint, all these variables, A, X, Y, Z, and the various Os shown in the above diagram, can be regarded as causes of B. Various micro-organisms, dirty feeding bottles, early weaning, malnutrition, respiratory infections, treatment by traditional practitioners, a lack of clinics or hospitals—all these, and more, are causes of deaths from gastroenteritis. Causes are always multiple.[20]

The best evidence for a causal relationship comes from a randomized experiment (especially if the findings are replicated in other experiments). The value of evidence from a non-experimental study depends on how well the study was designed and conducted—how close was it to a good experiment, with respect to the avoidance or control of selection and information bias and confounding? This is not easy to achieve, and it is not unusual for non-experimental studies to yield conflicting findings about causal relationships—a recently published list includes 56 topics with contradictory results—or findings that differ from those of experiments; an observational study may show a clear relationship between formula supplementation in early infancy and a low breast-feeding rate 2 months later, whereas a trial may show no relationship at all.[21]

Whatever kind of study the evidence comes from, three conditions must be met before we can seriously entertain the possibility that A may be the cause of B. First, we must be sure that A preceded B, or at least that A *may* have come before B. This is essential, although a time sequence cannot by itself prove causation; 'if winter comes, can spring be far behind?'—but does winter cause spring? Secondly, we must satisfy ourselves that there is little likelihood that the association is an artifact (see p 251) caused by shortcomings in the study methods. And thirdly, we must decide that the association is probably not wholly attributable to confounding (see p 256). We can of course never be quite sure that there are no confounding factors that were not taken into account in the design or analysis of the study, and that we may not even suspect. We can never really 'prove' a causal relationship. What we want, however, is 'reasonable proof', strong enough to be used as a basis for decision and action. To this end, we should review the way that possible confounders were handled in the study. Can we think of any important factors that were not measured, in themselves or by proxy, or that were measured unsatisfactorily? How well were possible confounding influences explored and controlled in the analysis? Do the size of the sample and the nature and complexity of the findings permit a thoroughgoing analysis of these influences? If not, to what extent can confounding influences be 'reasoned away' (see p 259)?

If these conditions are met, we can consider other evidence.[22] Basically, we see how well the facts fit in with what we might expect to find if the association were causal. This is not quite the same thing as 'proving' a causal association, but it is the best we can do. For this purpose, use may be made of the following additional criteria, which (taken together) may strengthen or weaken the case for causality, although none of them is essential or conclusive. These are:

1. *Statistical significance* supports the case for a causal association; its absence weakens the case, but only if the test is powerful[10] (i.e. if the sample is large).
2. *Strength* of the association—the stronger it is, the more likely that it is causal, and not produced by bias or confounding; but a weak association may also be (weakly) causal.
3. *Dose-response relationship*—the case for causality is supported if there is a correlation between the amount, intensity or duration of exposure to the 'cause' and the amount or severity of the 'effect'. But there may also be a correlation with the dose of a placebo.[23] Also, there may be an 'all-or-none' response that appears only

when the causative factor reaches a threshold level, or a relationship between cause and effect that is U- or J-shaped (or inverted U- or J-shaped) rather than linear.

4. *Time-response relationship*—if the incidence of the 'effect' (e.g. the rate of new cases of a disease) rises to a peak some time after a brief exposure to the 'cause' and then decreases, this supports the case.

5. *Specificity*—in particular, the finding that the 'effect' is related to only one 'cause' or constellation of causes—may be regarded as supporting the case.

6. *Consistency*—the evidence for causality is much strengthened if the association occurs in different groups and under different conditions, and has been found in other studies (of other populations, in different circumstances, by other investigators and by various methods of study). If results are inconsistent, and the variation cannot be attributed to modifying factors or differences in study methods, this weakens the case.

7. *Coherence* with current theory and knowledge—in particular, the availability of a satisfactory explanation of the *mechanism* by which A may affect B—supports the case; but the investigator who cannot think up *some* plausible explanation for his findings must indeed be a rare bird.[24] Incompatibility with known *facts* weakens the case.

The 'rules of evidence'[22] are not clear-cut, and the appraisal of causality is a matter of judgement. Experts often differ in their conclusions.

There is usually interest in knowing not only *whether* A is a cause of B, but also *how* it inter-relates with other causes in producing B. We have seen how even simple techniques of analysis can point to the role of an intervening cause (p 257) and demonstrate the occurrence of statistical interaction between independent variables (p 254). The temporal relationship of causes may be of interest: a distinction may be made between a *predisposing cause* or *precondition*, a *precipitating cause* or *initiator*, and a *promotor* (a later-acting cause in carcinogenesis); *concomitant causes* act simultaneously.

Multivariate analysis can streamline the production of information about the inter-relationships among a series of factors. It does not, unfortunately, provide a short-cut solution to the problem of causal interpretation.

Before leaving the subject of causality, it must be stressed that things may be more complicated than they seem, since not only may one cause have many effects and one effect many causes, but variables may simultaneously have more than one kind of association with each other. For example, there may be a reciprocal causal relationship, where A affects B, and B affects A (A ⟷ B). Poverty may be a cause of chronic illness, for example, and chronic illness may lead to poverty. At the same time there may be a secondary association between poverty and chronic illness, due to a common association with an identifiable factor such as ethnic group (A←C→B), or with unknown, possibly remote, common causes (A←?←?→?→B). The association between A and B may thus be partly causal and partly non-causal. A third variable may be both a confounding factor and an intervening cause; or it may have both confounding and modifying effects, and so on. 'O, what a tangled web we perceive.' Even Sir Isaac Newton observed that 'to myself I seem to have been only like a boy playing on the sea-shore, and diverting myself in now and then finding a smoother pebble, or a prettier shell than ordinary, whilst the great ocean of truth lay all undiscovered before me'.[25] But let us take heart—we don't have to find *all* the answers (not all at once, anyway), only *some* useful answers, and this we can do.

NOTES AND REFERENCES

1. The variables that are associated are usually designated as *dependent* and *independent* (see p 93). In community medicine, the dependent variable is usually a measure of health status, health behaviour or health care. The terms *criterion variable* and *response variable* refer to a dependent variable, and independent variables may be called *predictor, explanatory, stimulus* or *exposure* variables.

   Associations may be referred to non-specifically as *relationships* or *concomitant variation* or by a variety of other terms. *Statistical dependence* is a non-specific statistical term synonymous with 'association'.

   An association is *positive* if the two variables tend to 'go along' with one another. It is *negative*, or *inverse*, if the variables tend to go in opposite directions, e.g. if the presence of one characteristic is associated with the absence of another, or if high values of one variable are associated with low values of another.

2. The *appraisal of associations* and the indices used are discussed in all epidemiology textbooks. For exercises, see Abramson J H 1988 Making sense of data: a self–instruction manual on the interpretation of epidemiological data. Oxford University Press, New York. For detailed mathematical treatments, see Kleinbaum D G, Kupper L L, Morgenstern H 1982 Epidemiologic research: principles and quantitative methods. Lifetime Learning Publications, Belmont, California; Anderson S, Auquier A, Hauck W W, Oakes D, Vandaele W, Weisberg H I 1980 Statistical methods for comparative studies: techniques for bias reduction. Wiley, New York.

   To keep up with the latest analytic methods, watch the American Journal of Epidemiology, the Journal of Clinical Epidemiology, etc.; but don't expect to learn much more from your data than you would with simpler but less state-of-the-art techniques.

   The *logical basis for epidemiological inferences*, especially concerning causality, is discussed by Susser M 1973 Causal thinking in the health sciences: concepts

and strategies in epidemiology. Oxford University Press, New York; Susser M
1987 Epidemiology, health and society: selected papers. Oxford University Press,
New York, and in two recent symposia: Greenland S (ed) 1987 Evolution of
epidemiologic ideas: annotated readings on concepts and methods. Epidemiology
Resources, Chestnut Hill, Massachusetts; and Rothman K J (ed) 1988 Causal
inference. Epidemiology Resources, Chestnut Hill, Massachusetts.

3. Authors writing about associations between variables vary in their terminology
   and often use the same terms with different connotations. 'Spurious' for example,
   is variously used to refer to artifactual associations, fortuitous ones, secondary
   ones, and non-causal associations as a whole. The terms used in the text of this
   chapter were chosen because they are relatively clear and unambiguous.
   Alternative terms are mentioned in footnotes.

4. Using the symbols shown in Table 27.1, the simplest formula for the *odds ratio*
   (also called the *cross-ratio* or *cross-product ratio*) is $ad \div bc$. For the data in the
   table this gives a value of 21.0. A slightly more elaborate formula, which carries
   certain advantages, is $\dfrac{(a + 0.5)(d + 0.5)}{(a + 0.5)(c + 0.5)}$. This gives a value of 20.9. The
   numerators and denominators in these formulae may be transposed, giving a
   value of 0.048 (i.e. one twenty-first instead of 21). These findings may be
   interpreted as meaning that in this sample the odds in favour of having anaemia
   are 21 times higher among pregnant than among non-pregnant women, or
   alternatively that the odds in favour of being pregnant are 21 times higher among
   anaemic than among non-anaemic women.
   For *paired data* the estimated relative risk is $(b \div d)$ or $(d \div b)$, using the
   symbols shown in note 14, page 244.
   See note 2, above.

5. A *correlation coefficient* measures how closely the points plotted on a scattergram
   (see note 15, p 244) follow a single slanting straight-line path. It measures
   whether a linear relationship is present, but does not measure the slope of the
   path; that is, it does not indicate how much each variable changes when the other
   one changes; this requires regression analysis.

6. See note 1 on p 273, and note 10 below. The 95% confidence interval for the
   difference between rates (28%) shown in Table 27.1 is from 26 to 30%.

7. Well, almost anything.

8. Fisher R A 1966 The design of experiments, 8th edn. Oliver & Boyd, Edinburgh,
   p 13.

9. Mainland D 1963 Elementary medical statistics, 2nd edn. Saunders,
   Philadelphia, p. 73.

10. *Significance tests* are usually concerned with random sampling variation
    (see p 269). At the risk of oversimplification, most tests can be said to measure the
    probability (P) that an association that is as strong as or stronger than that actually
    observed will occur in a random sample drawn from a wider population in which
    this association does not exist (i.e. in which the null hypothesis holds true). That
    is, if a large number of random samples were drawn from this population, all of
    the same size as the sample actually studied, in what proportion of them could
    such an association be expected?
    When these tests are used in non-random samples or total populations they are
    generally based on the notion that the study sample or population is drawn from
    'a hypothetical population which would be generated if an indefinitely large
    number of observations, showing the same sort of random variation as those at
    our disposal, could be made.' Armitage P 1971 Statistical methods in medical
    research. Blackwell, Oxford, p 100. Many statisticians reject this use of what
    Feinstein (1977 Clinical Biostatistics. C V Mosby, St Louis, p 311) has called
    'a great imaginary parent population out there somewhere in the sky', and they
    limit the use of the tests to situations where there is random sampling variation or

another 'chance' process, such as random intrapersonal variation, random measurement error, and random permutation of the observations.

Two-tailed or two-sided significance tests test the null hypothesis (e.g. that there is no difference between the rates of anaemia in two groups) against the alternative that there is a difference, no matter in what direction. For a one-tailed (one-sided) test the alternative is that there is a difference in a prespecified direction (e.g. that there is a higher rate in group 1), and the null hypothesis is that there is not a difference in this direction. It is easier to obtain significance with a one-tailed test. Such a test should be used if, and only if, the null hypothesis and its alternative, stated before the analysis, are such as to warrant its use.

The P value is the probability of rejecting the null hypothesis when in fact it is true, i.e. of concluding that there is a real association when actually there is none. This is a type I error. A type II error is the erroneous missing of a true association; the power of a test is its capacity to avoid type II errors.

A more informative way of taking account of random or sampling variation is to calculate the confidence interval. If the value 0 is included in the 95% confidence interval for a difference between two rates, or if 1 is included in the confidence interval for the relative risk, the rates are significantly different (by most two-tailed tests) at the 5% level.

The relative merits of significance tests and statistical estimation (i.e. confidence intervals) are debated, inter alia, by Walker and Fleiss. See Walker A M 1986 Reporting the results of epidemiologic studies. American Journal of Public Health 76: 556; Fleiss J L 1986 Significance tests have a role in epidemiologic research: reactions to A M Walker. American Journal of Public Health 76: 559; Walker A M 1986 Significance tests represent consensus and standard practice. American Journal of Public Health 76: 1033; and Fleiss J L 1986 Dr Fleiss responds. American Journal of Public Health 76: 1033. Also, see Thompson W D 1987 Statistical criteria in the interpretation of epidemiologic data. American Journal of Public Health 77: 191; Poole C 1987 Beyond the confidence interval. American Journal of Public Health 77: 195; Poole C 1987 On the comparison of effects. American Journal of Public Health 77: 491; Gardner M J, Altman D G 1986 Confidence intervals rather than P values: estimation rather than hypothesis testing. British Medical Journal 292: 746; and Goodman S N, Royall R 1988 Evidence and scientific research. American Journal of Public Health 78: 1568.

11. Hamilton M 1974 Lectures on the methodology of clinical research. Churchill Livingstone, Edinburgh, p 43.

12. A modifier variable may also be termed an effect-modifier or a moderator or qualifier variable. It may also be called a specifier or conditional variable, terms which do not imply that the association is in fact inconsistent—the variable specifies the conditions in which the association will be examined. The form of analysis shown in Table 27.2 (subclassification or stratification) may also be termed specification.

The associations observed in the separate strata of analysis are called conditional relationships. If these differ in their strength or direction, there is statistical interaction between the independent and modifier variables.

Effect modification may be detected and appraised by multivariate analysis procedures.

See note 2, above.

13. MacMahon B, Alpert M, Salbert E J 1966 Infant weight and parental smoking habits. American Journal of Epidemiology 82: 247.

14. Labovitz S, Hagedorn S 1971 Introduction to social research. McGraw-Hill, New York, pp 80–81.

15. A confounding variable may also be referred to as a disturbing or nuisance variable. The term 'intervening variable' is best avoided, as it may be misinterpreted as meaning an intervening cause (see note 20, below). A secondary association may

also be called an *indirect association*—which may be misconstrued as an indirect causal association (see note 20, below)—or a spurious association, a term which has several other connotations (see note 3). The effect of a confounding effect may vary, depending on what measure of association is used. See note 2, above.

16. A happy term suggested by Susser (1973; see note 2).
17. *Overadjustment*: see Day N E, Byar D P, Green S B 1980 Overadjustment in case-control studies. American Journal of Epidemiology 112: 696, and subsequent correspondence in American Journal of Epidemiology 1982 115: 797 and 799.
18. Rules for deciding whether C's relationships with A and B are strong enough to account for the association observed between A and B are provided by Bross I D J 1966 Spurious effects from an extraneous variable. Journal of Chronic Diseases 19: 637 and 1967 Pertinency of an extraneous variable. Journal of Chronic Diseases 20: 487. For the 'direction rule', see Abramson (1988; see note 2), pp 208, 211–212.
19. MacMahon B, Pugh T F 1970 Epidemiology: principles and methods. Little, Brown, Boston, Massachusetts, pp 17–27.
20. Causes are always multiple. We can never speak of A as *the* cause of B. A always has its own determinants, and these are also causes of B. Moreover, as we learn more about the mechanism by which A affects B we can usually interpose *intervening (mediating) causes*, thereby changing A from a *direct* cause (A → B) to an *indirect* one (A → X → Y → Z → B). A cause is seldom *sufficient* to produce an effect without the participation of other causes—the outcome of exposure to pathogenic germs, for example, depends upon the susceptibility of the persons exposed. Sometimes A can be defined as a *necessary* cause of B, without which B cannot occur. But this need not mean that there are no other causes of importance; only a small fraction of people infected with the tubercle bacillus become ill with tuberculosis, indicating that factors other than the bacillus (the necessary cause) play a crucial role.
21. For papers on the *use of experimental principles is non-experimental studies*, see Esdaile J M, Horwitz R I 1986 Observational studies of cause–effect relationships: an analysis of methodologic problems as illustrated by the conflicting data for the role of oral contraceptives in the etiology of rheumatoid arthritis. Journal of Chronic Diseases 39: 841 and note 42, p 298. Contradictory results from case-control studies are listed by Mayes L C, Horwitz R O, Feinstein A R 1988 A collection of 56 topics with contradictory results in case-control research. International Journal of Epidemiology 17: 680.

    In a prospective survey in which precautions were taken to control bias and confounding, Gray-Donald K & Kramer M S (1988 Causality inference in observational vs. experimental studies: an empirical comparison. American Journal of Epidemiology 127: 885) found a clear association between formula supplementation of newborn babies in hospital, and a low breast-feeding rate at 9 weeks; but a controlled trial conducted in the same hospital demonstrated no association at all. This discrepancy was probably mainly attributable to confounders that were controlled in the trial but not measured (and therefore not controllable) in the survey (mothers' motivation to breast-feed and the occurrence of sore nipples or other indications for formula feeding).
22. *Criteria for the appraisal of causality* are discussed in more detail by Susser (1973; see note 2) and Susser M 1986 The logic of Sir Karl Popper and the practice of epidemiology. American Journal of Epidemiology 124: 711, and Lilienfeld A M, Lilienfeld D E 1980 Foundations of epidemiology, 2nd edn. Oxford University Press, New York, Chapter 12 (see p 317 for *Evans's criteria*, a set of rules for use in deciding whether a factor is a cause of a disease). For an illustration of the way in which judgements (using the same criteria) may differ, see a debate published in Journal of Chronic Diseases: Burch P R J. The Surgeon General's 'epidemiologic criteria for causality'. A critique: 36: 821; Lilienfeld A M The Surgeon General's 'epidemiologic criteria for causality': a criticism of Burch's critique: 36: 837; and

Burch P R J. The Surgeon General's epidemiologic criteria for causality'. Reply to Lilienfeld: 37: 148. See note 2.
23. Coronary Drug Project Research Group 1980 Influence of adherence to treatment and response of cholesterol to mortality in the Coronary Drug Project. New England Journal of Medicine 303: 1038.
24. The story (possibly true) is told of a trial comparing two treatments. When the statistician announced that one drug was superior, the researchers explained why this result could have been predicted, on the basis of prior knowledge about absorption, metabolism, tolerance, etc. When the statistician announced that he had confused the drugs, and it was the other that was superior, there was a short silence, and then a discussion that explained why the new result was consistent with expectations. Park C B 1981 Attributable risk for recurrent events: an extension of Levin's measure. American Journal of Epidemiology 113: 491.
25. Brewster D 1885 Memoirs of the life of Sir Isaac Newton, vol 2, Chapter 27.

28. Generalizing from the findings

We will often want to generalize from our findings. We may in fact have chosen the population we studied or sampled because we believed it was typical of a broader 'reference population' or 'external population' to which we wished to generalize the findings. Even if the study population was not chosen on these grounds, every population may be regarded as a part of a wider population, and we are often tempted to make generalizations. Having studied varicose veins in a single study neighbourhood, we may want to draw conclusions about their prevalence in the population at large, or to arrive at generalities, going beyond the population that was studied, about the strength of the association of varicose veins with fatness or leanness, the importance of occupation or tight garments as causal factors, the pros and cons of various forms of treatment, and so on.

The need to generalize is often thrust upon us even if our interest is limited to the specific population we studied. Unless data were obtained for all members of this population, i.e. with no sampling and 100% coverage, we will need to 'generalize' from the results in the sample we studied, by using these results as a basis for inferences about the study population as a whole.

In this chapter we will consider random sampling variation and the effects of selection bias on inferences concerning the study population, and will discuss distinctive features of the study population that may affect the 'generalizability', 'representativeness', or 'external validity' of the study with respect to generalizations that go beyond this population.

RANDOM SAMPLING VARIATION

Even when the whole of a satisfactory representative sample has been investigated, we must be cautious in applying the findings to the population from which it was chosen, since chance differences may be expected between different samples drawn randomly from the same population. Chance differences may similarly arise in a trial in which subjects are randomly allocated to experimental and control groups.

One of the advantages of random sampling and random assignment, however, is that it is easy to estimate the probable findings in the sampled population. By using formulae or tables, or a computer program, we can estimate, with a specified degree of certainty (usually 95 or 99%— this is the *confidence level*), within what range (*confidence interval*) the value in the sampled population lies.[1] The narrower this range, the greater the *precision* of the estimate. If a prevalence rate of 10% is detected in a simple random sample containing 200 individuals, there is a 95% probability that the rate in the parent population is between 6.4% (the *lower confidence limit*) and 15.2% (the *upper confidence limit*). If the sample had contained only 30 individuals, the 95% confidence interval would have been considerably wider, from 2.6 to 27.7%. Confidence limits can also be calculated for means and other measures of a distribution.

They can also be calculated for rate ratios, odds ratios, and other measures of the strength of an association. In comparing random samples drawn from different populations or allocated to different treatments, it is generally more useful to know the range in which the true value probably lies, than merely to know whether the difference is statistically significant. This has been illustrated by a review of 71 randomized controlled clinical trials that yielded 'negative' results—i.e. there was no statistically significant difference between the outcomes in the experimental and control groups.[2] When 90% confidence limits were calculated, it was found that in half the studies the interval included a 50% reduction in mortality or whatever other endpoint was used in the study. Hence an appreciable positive effect of the therapy could not be ruled out.

Confidence limits are sometimes calculated when it is wished to generalize from a study population to a broader 'reference population' that it is believed to represent (e.g. 'patients with peptic ulcer' or 'white men in the USA'), even if the study population is not a random sample of this broader sample. We are then estimating what findings might be expected in a hypothetical large population, if the study population were a random sample of this larger population.[3] This use of confidence limits is open to criticism.

SELECTION BIAS

If selection bias (see p 246) is present or suspected, it is not possible to make unqualified generalizations from a sample to the study population, let alone to a broader reference population.

It is sometimes possible to use statistical procedures to compensate for selection bias. If there was a low response rate in some age groups, for example, the findings can be weighted in accordance with the age composition of the total study population, to obtain an estimate that compensates for this selective response.[4] This method of adjustment becomes complicated if many variables (age, sex, social class, etc.) are taken into account, and is especially unwieldy if stratified sampling was used, so that different weights are needed in each stratum. A disadvantage of this method is that it is based upon the assumption that, within each defined category of the population, respondents and non-respondents are similar. This is not necessarily true. Weighting may actually increase bias, if a greater weight happens to be given to a stratum where the respondents are especially unrepresentative.

Adjustments may also be based upon assumed dissimilarities between the individuals for whom data are and are not available. In a study of causes of death, for example, the data were adjusted to compensate for the fact that (in different years) between 4 and 16% of deaths were not medically certified. Two alternative assumptions were made: (1) that the proportion of deaths from each cause (in a given age–sex stratum and in a given year) was twice as high among the uncertified as among the certified cases; and (2) that it was half as high. The two sets of alternative estimates yielded similar conclusions concerning trends of mortality from specific causes.[5] Extreme assumptions are sometimes made—e.g. that all or no non-respondents smoke—so as to obtain maximal and minimal estimates.

Probably the best way of handling non-response bias, although seldom a practicable one, is to invest concentrated efforts in an attempt to obtain full information about a sufficiently large and representative sample of non-respondents. These can then be compared with respondents in respect of the characteristics the investigator wishes to study.

DISTINCTIVE FEATURES OF THE STUDY POPULATION

Every study population has its own distinctive features, and generalizations cannot be undertaken lightly. Some study populations are representative of nothing but themselves. Populations vary in their characteristics, and associations detected in one population may not exist in another. Not only may the prevalence of anaemia differ in a slum and a well-off neighbourhood, but different causes may operate in the two populations. The risk associated with a particular cause, e.g. dietary iron deficiency, may differ,[6] and so may the effectiveness of the routine administration of iron or other supplements to pregnant women.

We have previously discussed the specific features of various types of study population (see p 59) and the artifactual associations that may result from the conditions that determine entry to special populations (see p 247). All this may seem obvious, yet how often do we read a statement like 'Conflicting findings are reported in the literature; A and B found something or other, C and D found something quite different, and E found something else again, which was not confirmed by F et al', without any designation or description of the populations studied by these investigators.

Although wide use has been made of the results of the Framingham Heart Study concerning risk factors for heart disease, for many years there was uncertainty about the generalizability of the results; the study started with a set of volunteers, who were then supplemented by a random sample of the town's population—with a response rate of 69%. Only in 1987, almost 40 years after the inception of the study, was it possible to compare the findings with those of a cohort study of a national probability sample and confirm that the Framingham risk model predicted coronary deaths in the national sample 'remarkably well'.[7]

Two questions that may not be obvious but are often worth asking are:

1. *Why was this study population chosen?* The reasons for the choice may be reflected in the findings—was the population chosen because of a high prevalence of a disease or drug addiction or broken homes, or because of its ethnic heterogeneity or residential stability, or a local community's special interest in a health problem, etc.? In an evaluative study, reasons with a possible bearing on health care are of particular importance. The study population may have been 'chosen' simply because the investigator was responsible for its health care, or because the staff of a particular clinic or health centre were motivated to perform or join in a study. Might this interest in research be a symptom of a high general standard of care? Was there special enthusiasm about the

treatment or programme that was evaluated? And may this have influenced effectiveness? Was the study population chosen because there were especially good clinical records, or because special facilities were available? Was it chosen because a high level of co-operation or compliance was expected? Or was a captive population selected, whose diet or medical treatment could be manipulated with ease? If the population was selected because it was exposed to a novel health programme, *why* was this programme provided in this particular setting?

2. *May the study itself have produced an effect?* One distinctive feature of every study population is that a study was performed in it. Sometimes the performance of the study may in itself affect the results. Interviews and examinations, and especially the 'feedback' of examination findings to subjects, may lead to changes in health practices and health care. This possibility should be considered in longitudinal studies, particularly if investigations were repeated frequently; weekly weighing of infants, or weekly interviews about their diet, may modify the growth pattern. The effect of the study itself is especially important in evaluative studies, where the subjects may be affected by their awareness that they are participating in an experiment, as well as by the experimental situation as a whole (see p 74).

NOTES AND REFERENCES

1. More strictly, the 95% confidence interval for a value is the interval calculated from a random sample by a procedure which, if applied to an infinite number of random samples of the same size, would, in 95% of instances, contain the true value in the population. See a statistics textbook. Calculation methods for commonly used confidence intervals are given in a series of papers in the British Medical Journal: Gardner M J, Altman D G 1986 Confidence intervals rather than P values: estimation rather than hypothesis testing. 292: 746; Campbell M J, Gardner M J 1988 Calculating confidence intervals for some non-parametric analyses. 296: 1454; Altman D G, Gardner M J 1988 Calculating confidence intervals for regression and correlation. 296: 1238; Machin D, Gardner M J 1988 Calculating confidence intervals for survival time analyses. 292: 1369.

2. Freiman J A, Chalmers T C, Smith H J Jr, Kuebler R R 1978 The importance of beta, the type II error and sample size in the design and interpretation of the randomized control trial: survey of 71 'negative' trials. New England Journal of Medicine 299: 690.

3. See citation from Armitage in note 10, p 264.

4. For a numerical example of this method of adjusting for non-response bias, see Moser C A, Kalton G 1972 Survey methods in social investigation, 2nd edn. Heinemann, London, pp 181–184. This book also describes the Politz-Simmons technique for dealing with the 'not-at-home' problem in household interview surveys (pp 178–181). The results are weighted in accordance with the proportion of days the respondent is ordinarily at home at the time he or she was interviewed.

Most weight is given to respondents who are seldom at home, who represent a group with a high non-response rate.

5. Gofin R, Abramson J H 1977 The causes of death of Moslems, Druze and Christians in Israel. Brookdale Institute of Gerontology and Adult Human Development in Israel, Jerusalem.
6. Rothman K J (1976) presents a conceptual framework for *causes*, in which he points out that most causes of disease are not in themselves sufficient to produce the disease, but are components of *constellations of causes* that together (acting in concert) suffice to cause disease. The risk associated with a particular cause therefore varies in different populations, depending on the prevalence of the other component causes that participate in these constellations. What is a strong risk factor (carrying a high relative risk) in one population may be a weak one in another. Modern Epidemiology. Little Brown, Boston, p 11.
7. Leaverton, P E, Sorlie P D, Kleinman J C et al 1987 Representativeness of the Framingham risk model for coronary heart disease mortality: a comparison with a national cohort study. Journal of Chronic Diseases 40: 775.

29. Writing a report

'"Ouch! Have a heart, Doc!" spluttered shapely Dolores X, the last of my hundred age and sex-matched controls, as I struggled to find her vein. "Do you really *have* to have my blood to find out whether people with malignant lymphogranuloma have a lot of antibody to some silly old virus?"' may be overdoing it somewhat as an introductory paragraph in a scientific report. But it serves to draw attention to the need for readability—a report should be written so as to attract, or at all events not repel, potential readers. To do this, it need not be written as a farce, a whodunit, or a lyric poem, but it should fulfil the following criteria:

1. The title should clearly explain what the report is about; if necessary, a subtitle can be added for extra clarity. A prospective reader usually looks first at the contents page of a journal, to see which titles 'tickle his fancy'. A journal is 'an open market where each salesman must cry his goods if he wishes to get an audience at his stall'.[1]
2. The abstract should be informative. A reader who has been attracted by the title will usually look at the abstract next, to decide whether the report is worth reading. 'The summary is your advertisement',[2] and should provide a picture in miniature of the whole report. It should include the objectives, specify the study population, and summarize the findings and discussion. Salient numerical details may—even should—be included.
3. The report should be easily intelligible.[3] This requires clarity of language (this is preferable to elegance of style), a logical presentation of facts and inferences, the use of easily understood tables and charts, and an orderly arrangement of the report as a whole. The report may be Greek to the layman, but it should be easily understood by the readers for whom it is written.
4. The report should be no longer than is necessary. Unnecessary

275

verbiage should be removed, and the report pruned to the minimum required for clearly communicating what has to be communicated. This process of pruning and condensing is not an easy one (who was it who apologized for sending a long letter by saying that he had not had the time to write a short one?).

Writing a good report may take much time and effort. The most difficult task is usually the preparation of the first draft, since this requires a crystallization of the investigator's ideas on how best to express his facts and inferences; subsequent revisions are usually easier. Comments from colleagues are often useful. Many writers find it helpful to tuck a draft in a drawer—or let it rest in peace on a computer disk—and bring it out for a fresh look after a few weeks.

No investigation is complete until a report has been written. Even if the results are of interest only to the investigator, they should be placed on record, albeit in a short and even handwritten form. If they are of wider interest, they should be made available to a wider audience. Whether they should be published in print is a question for the investigator (and later, of course, an editor or publisher) to decide. Particularly in academic fields, there is a tendency to publish whenever possible.

Colleges and universities are normally administered by busy people . . . called upon to make decisions concerning the hiring and firing, promotion and tenure of their faculty personnel. What criteria should they use in these decisions? They cannot be expected to read what their professors write, having no time for such activities and, expecially in the more technical disciplines, lacking the necessary qualifications to judge the material . . . The . . . option most common today is to fall back on the criterion of productivity as used in the business world . . . the number of books or articles that publishers or editors of professional publications are willing to accept from the man in question.[4]

This 'Publish or perish!'[5] motivation apart, publication may often be seen as an obligation. The investigator may feel a duty to communicate his results, 'positive' or 'negative', to others who may be able to replicate his findings, build their own research efforts upon them, or apply them in action. An editorial in the *British Medical Journal* relates that Kocher's method of reducing dislocations of the shoulder was regarded as an innovation when it was described in a German medical journal in 1870. His method had been portrayed 3000 years earlier, however, in a wall painting in a tomb in the Nile Valley. 'The moral of this episode,' says the editorialist, 'is clear.

Recognition of original work can be ensured only by publication in a reputable journal.[6]

Succinct advice on the writing of a paper is to be found in a document describing 'uniform requirements for manuscripts submitted to biomedical journals (the Vancouver style)', prepared by a committee of editors.[7] Over 300 journals have sanctioned these guidelines. Some journals, however, have their own requirements, particularly for the format of references; consult the journal's 'advice to contributors'.

To be useful, a report should not only give the results of the study and the inferences that have been drawn from them, but also enough information about the methods to enable a critical reader to appraise the validity of the findings and conclusions or (ideally) to check the findings by replicating the study. The report should include a description of the study population and its characteristics and information (if relevant) about methods and criteria used for choosing subjects or groups, sampling and randomization procedures, response rates, representativeness of samples, comparability of groups, reasons for non-participation and withdrawals, etc. Operational definitions (including diagnostic criteria) should be specified. Ideally, the description of the methods should be a detailed one. Unfortunately (or fortunately?) this is usually practicable only in books or dissertations required for university degrees, and only the highlights can be described. The rest has to be taken on trust.

To help the reader to make his judgement, the investigator should himself offer an honest and critical appraisal of the study, and point out and discuss the main sources of possible error. Possible biases should be stated and not left for others to reveal.

Where possible, facts should be presented in a form that may be useful to other investigators who prefer to use different categories or indices when measuring variables, e.g. by presenting full frequency distributions rather than 'collapsed' scales and combinations of categories.

Tables and figures should be well enough titled and captioned and (if necessary) have enough footnotes to be reasonably intelligible without reference to the text.

The tables should be well constructed,[8] and without anomalies such as totals that do not tally, percentages that do not add up to about 100% (say between 99.8 and 100.2%, and the use of too many decimal places. If percentages are used, no doubt should be left as to what the denominator is (it is often helpful to add '100%' in the requisite place).

Diagrams should clarify and not complicate, and care should be taken that they do not mislead[8]. They should serve to explain tables and should not replace them, unless the investigator is sure the reader will not require numerical data. If curves have been 'smoothed', the method used should be stated. There are many computer programs that can draw diagrams.[9]

The results of statistical procedures should be given in numbers and not just words (and preferably not only in pictures). Until lately, many writers and some editors felt that a sprinkling of P values lent a report an aura of scientific respectability. But the pendulum has now swung away from significance tests towards confidence intervals.[10] The advice in the 'Vancouver style' guidelines is:

> When possible quantify findings and present them with appropriate indicators of measurement error or uncertainty (such as confidence intervals). Avoid sole reliance on statistical hypothesis testing, such as the use of P values, which fails to convey important quantitative information.[7]

References should be carefully checked. A few small errors are probably inevitable; but an examination of a random sample of references in three public health journals found that in 15% the cited reference 'failed to substantiate, was unrelated to, or even contradicted the author's assertation', and 3% had major citation errors ('reference not locatable'). Minor citation errors were rife.[11]

NOTES AND REFERENCES

1. Asher R 1958 Why are medical journals so dull? British Medical Journal ii: 502.
2. Dart R A, Galloway A 1934 Memorandum on writing a scientific paper. Department of Anatomy, University of the Witwatersrand (Roneo), Johannesburg.
3. The need for intelligibility was realized by Geoffrey Chaucer in the 14th century when he departed from tradition and wrote a scientific treatise in simple English rather than in Latin, in order to explain the astrolabe to his son: 'This tretis, divided in fyve parties, wole I shewe thee under ful lighte rewles and naked wordes in English; for Latin ne canstow yit but small, my lyte sone. But natheles, suffyse to thee thise trewe conclusiouns in English, as wel as suffyseth to thise noble clerkes Grekes thise same conclusiouns in Greek, and to Arabiens in Arabik, and to Jewes in Ebrew, and to the Latin folk in Latin'. Chaucer G A Treatise on the astrolabe. Cited by Gordon I S, Sorkin S 1959 The Armchair Science Reader. Simon & Schuster, New York, p 294.
4. Berger P L 1969 Invitation to sociology: a humanistic perspective. Penguin Books, Harmondsworth, pp 20–21.
5. The pressure to publish is so strong that some investigators are led to falsify data or to pirate papers. For examples of *scientific fraud*, see Broad W J 1981 Fraud and the structure of science. Science 212: 137, 264; Broad W J, Wade N 1982 Betrayers of the truth. Simon & Schuster, New York; Stewart W W, Feder N

1987 The integrity of the scientific literature. Nature 325: 207. One researcher who submitted reports containing repeated falsifications received nearly $1 million in cancer research funds.

6. Editorial 1968 Where to publish? British Medical Journal 4: 344.

7. The *Vancouver style* guidelines (3rd edn) are published by the International Committee of Medical Journal Editors in British Medical Journal 1988 296: 401 and Annals of Internal Medicine 1988 108: 258. The paragraphs on the reporting of statistical aspects are amplified by Bailar J C III, Mosteller F 1988 Annals of Internal Medicine 108: 266. For guides to the writing of informative 'structured' abstracts, see Ad Hoc Working Group for Critical Appraisal of the Literature 1987 A proposal for more informative abstracts of clinical articles. Annals of Internal Medicine 106: 598 and Mulrow C D, Thacker S B, Pugh J A 1988 A proposal for more informative abstracts of review articles. Annals of Internal Medicine 108: 613.

8. See Hill A B 1977 A short textbook for medical statistics. Hodder & Stoughton, London; pp 48–51 deal with tables, and pp 51–59 with graphs, frequency polygons, histograms, bar charts, and scatter diagrams. The main types of diagram are described in Abramson J H 1988 Making sense of data. Oxford University Press, New York, pp 17–21. For misuses of diagrams, see Huff D 1973 How to lie with statistics. Penguin Books, Harmondsworth.

9. '*Graphics*. This is the one area where PCs outshine most mainframes' (Schordt P A 1987 Microcomputer methods for social scientists, 2nd edn. Sage Publications, Newbury Park, California). Many public-domain programs for microcomputers can draw charts, especially simple bar and line diagrams and pie charts. But commercial programs are generally preferred for preparing charts for publication. 'Good graphics can be produced on even the least expensive home computer, but excellent graphics require . . . expensive hardware and sophisticated software.' (Schrodt, 1987, as above). The best graphics programs are versatile. They offer many kinds of chart, including three-dimensional ones, permit changes in the positioning and scaling of the axes, offer a variety of lettering and symbols for data points, and provide for the printing of titles, subtitles, keys and arrows. Consult a computer magazine. PC Magazine, for example, reviewed graphics programs in two issues in 1988 (vol 7, nos 7 and 16), and 'scientific graphing software' (for logarithmic scales, error bars, etc.) in 1989 (vol 8, no. 5).

10. See note 10, pp 264–265 for references on the 'P values or confidence intervals?' debate.

11. Eichorn P, Yankauer A 1987 Do authors check their references? A survey of accuracy in three public health journals. American Journal of Public Health 77: 1011.

30. Clinical trials

Clinical trials are experiments or quasi-experiments that test hypotheses concerning the effects (favourable or unfavourable) of intervention techniques applied to individuals. These techniques may be therapeutic agents, devices, regimens or procedures (*therapeutic trials*), preventive ones (*prophylactic trials*), or rehabilitative, educational, etc.; (trials of screening and diagnostic tests were discussed on pp 160–162). The main objectives are usually to measure the efficacy and safety of the procedure, and their variation among patients with different characteristics. Attention may also be focused on efficiency, e.g. by comparing the costs of different ways of achieving a similar benefit. Other questions (concerning compliance, satisfaction, etc. — see p 48) may also be asked, but are usually seen as subsidiary, serving only to explain why the outcome is or is not satisfactory; they may, however, be dominant features if the study centres on the feasibility or acceptability of a procedure.

A distinction has been made between *explanatory* clinical trials, whose purpose is mainly to provide biological information (e.g. about the way drugs act and the way the body reacts to them) and *pragmatic* ones, which aim to test procedures under the conditions in which they would be applied in practice. Trials conducted in community medicine are generally of the latter sort.[1]

In community medicine, clinical trials may be set up not only to appraise the effects of individual-focused procedures, but (in some instances) to evaluate programmes. The latter use of clinical trials will be discussed in the next chapter.

Trials are prospective studies; i.e. they have a forward-looking directionality (see p 15). The use of retrospective (case-control) studies to appraise the effects of treatments and other procedures is discussed on page 292.

Here are six examples of trials. In the first four the subjects were randomly allocated to the groups that were compared. (For the findings, refer to the footnotes: no prizes.) The study objectives were:

1. To compare case fatality rates in patients with suspected myocardial infarction who were treated at home or sent to hospital.[2]
2. To compare the prevalence of symptoms of adenoidal hypertrophy, before and after operation, in children who had only their tonsils removed or who had their adenoids out too.[3]
3. To compare the proportions of people with common colds who were cured or improved 2 days after starting treatment with antihistaminic tablets or indistinguishable dummy placebo tablets.[4]
4. To compare the relief of symptoms in patients with angina pectoris after ligation of the internal mammary arteries (an operation designed to increase blood flow to the heart) or a sham operation (in which only a skin incision was made).[5]
5. To compare the occurrence of complications in soldiers whose wounds were treated with boiling oil or with a mixture of egg yolks, oil of roses and turpentine.[6]
6. To compare the countenances of four children fed on legumes and water for 10 days (Daniel, Shadrach, Meshach and Abednego) with those of children fed on King Nebuchadnezzar's meat and wine.[7]

STUDY DESIGNS

The following are the basic study designs.[8] If the intervention is not under the investigator's control—i.e. if decisions on who gets what, and when, are not made by the investigator—the study is a quasi-experiment. (As noted on p 10, some writers refer to any un-randomized trial as a quasi-experiment; the terminology used is less important than an awareness that careful consideration must be given to the possible biases in all experiments, whether 'true' or 'quasi'.)

1. *Parallel studies*, in which two or more independent groups are studied prospectively and compared.
2. *Externally controlled studies*, in which a single experimental group is studied and the findings are compared with data obtained from other sources.
3. *'Self-controlled'* studies, in which the subjects are their own

controls. These may be based on observations before and after a single treatment (*before–after studies*), or *crossover studies*, in which two or more treatments are applied in sequence to the same subjects.

These designs may be combined. Other designs (e.g. factorial, Latin squares) may also be used.[9] An example of a simple factorial design is the Physicians' Health Study, which examined the effect of aspirin on cardiovascular mortality and the effect of beta-carotene on cancer incidence; participants were randomly divided into four groups, who were respectively given aspirin and a placebo, beta-carotene and a placebo, aspirin and beta-carotene, or two placebos.[10]

Types of clinical trials

1. Parallel (concurrent controls)
2. Externally controlled
3. 'Self-controlled'

Parallel studies, or trials with *concurrent controls*, compare groups exposed to different interventions. A treated group may be compared with a control group that receives no treatment (or a placebo), or two or more groups who are having different treatments may be compared with each other or with an untreated group. If the allocation of subjects to the groups is random, the study is a *randomized controlled trial* (*RCT*). A well done RCT provides more convincing evidence and more precise estimates of the effect of an intervention than any other study method, and is generally regarded as the standard with which other methods should be compared.

Parallel comparisons require information about the subjects before as well as after the intervention (i.e. they should be 'premeasure-postmeasure' or 'pretest–post-test' studies). This not only permits a check on the comparability of the groups before the intervention, it also makes it possible to take proper account of possible confounders and modifiers in the analysis. Many studies are based on a comparison of the changes observed in different groups; the measurement of change, e.g. in blood pressure or other characteristics, requires baseline data. Trials with no information about prior status ('postmeasure only' trials) have unknown and possibly serious biases; Daniel's biblical trial (see p 282) is an example.

In *externally controlled studies* the findings in the experimental group are compared with control data obtained from other sources. In a therapeutic trial of this sort the latter data usually come from experience with cases treated in the past (*historical controls*). This approach may sometimes be of unquestioned validity, for example if the disease being treated is one that, according to previous experience, never disappears or is always fatal. Ethical constraints may compel the use of historical controls; a physician who is convinced of the merit of a new treatment and therefore cannot ethically use randomization may decide to perform a pilot trial using historical controls, in the hope of convincing sceptical colleagues that a randomized trial should be done. There may, however, be serious bias in externally controlled studies; the results of treatment may differ because the controls differed from the experimental subjects, or were treated by other clinicians, or at another time (when circumstances affecting the prognosis, such as other components of patient management, were different), or were appraised differently, etc. Even patients treated in the same centre and in the same way, but at different times, may have very different outcomes.[11] Trials with historical controls may provide the first clues to real breakthroughs in medical science; on the other hand, results may be misleading, and yet make a subsequent RCT ethically unacceptable. Historical controls are sometimes used as a check on the results of a trial using concurrent controls; if the randomized controls fared worse than previous experience would lead one to expect, this needs explaining.

In *self-controlled studies*, use of the subjects as their own controls prevents confounding by many characteristics that may influence the outcome. But there are possible biases in a simple 'before–after' study—those connected with extraneous events or changes that occur with time, non-specific effects caused by the performance of the experiment itself, changes in methods of measurement, and regression to the mean (see p 74); in a parallel study, comparison is made with a control group that is subject to the same effects. However, such studies may be appropriate in some circumstances (e.g. testing a treatment in patients with refractory disease, appraising the value of supplementary feeding for children in refugee camps[12]).

In a *crossover study* each subject is given the different treatments (or treatment and placebo) under comparison, one after another. Each subject is his own control. The sequence of assignment is generally randomized, so that this is a kind of RCT. A 'washing-out period' may be required between treatments, to permit the effects of the previous treatment to disappear, and the method is not feasible if a treatment has protracted 'carry-over' effects. The *'N of 1' clinical trial* or 'single-case experiment' is a special kind of crossover study aimed at determining the efficacy of a treatment (or the relative value of alternative treatments) for a specific patient. The patient is repeatedly given a treatment and placebo, or different treatments, in successive time periods.[13]

RANDOMIZATION

Randomization is a procedure whereby the assignment of treatments is left to chance. The allocation is decided by tossing a coin or some other strictly random method. Randomization does not guarantee that the groups will be identical, but it makes misleading results less likely, by ensuring that the only differences between the groups are those that occur by chance. This applies both to known risk and protective factors and to unsuspected ones. Unless the groups are very small, marked differences become unlikely.

Table 30.1   A typical randomized controlled trial

1. Eligible? ————→ If not, exclude
2. Consent? ————→ If not, exclude
3. Randomize to Groups A and B
4. Treat (subjects may be blinded to treatment)
5. Follow up all members of Groups A and B
6. Compare outcomes or changes in Groups A and B

The procedure of random assignment should be applied to *all* the subjects included in the study—to all the volunteers entering a prophylactic trial, or to all the patients whose diagnosis, clinical condition and other features make them eligible for inclusion in a therapeutic trial, and who have agreed to participate in it (Table 30.1). Exclusion criteria (too old, too ill, etc.) should be laid down in advance and, if possible, applied before the subjects are assigned to groups. If there is an objection to putting a subject in any one of the groups, he should be excluded from the trial before he is allocated. Such exclusions do not bias the results of the comparison (internal validity), although they may limit the applicability of the results (external validity). The results of a well conducted RCT can validly be applied to the kind of person who entered the trial ('no bias is caused by exclusion, even if for silly reasons'[14])—but not to anyone else.

Sometimes, as a convenient and theoretically adequate alternative to randomization, a systematic method of assignment is used, such as the allocation of alternate patients to treatment and control groups. Such methods have been criticized on the grounds that they are too easily manipulated by well-meaning clinicians. In a controlled trial of anticoagulant therapy for myocardial infarction, in which the patient's treatment was determined by whether he was admitted on an odd- or even-numbered day of the month, it was found that the physicians (convinced of the value of the treatment) saw to it that more patients were admitted on odd-numbered days.[15]

Whether random or systematic allocation was used, before drawing conclusions it is wise to compare the groups to check whether they were similar before the trial started. A large-scale trial of the effect of extra milk on the height and weight of schoolchildren was invalidated by biased allocation. The 10 000 subjects and 10 000 controls were allocated 'by ballot' or by using an alphabetical system, but the teachers were permitted to 'improve' the selections if they thought they were unbalanced. As a result, the children allocated to the experimental group were shorter and lighter than the control children.[16]

Randomization may be achieved by tossing a coin or throwing a die, using tables of random numbers[17] or random permutations,[18] or letting a computer[19] do the work. Use may be made of *balanced randomization*, which imposes a constraint on the randomization process so as to prevent the allocation ratio from diverging (by chance) from the intended ratio of, say, 1:1 or 2:1. Various methods are available for this purpose.[20]

Blocked (or *stratified*) *randomization* is sometimes used—the subjects are divided into 'blocks', and randomization (usually balanced) is carried out separately in each block. (This word comes from agricultural experiments in which a field was divided into blocks, in each of which a number of treatments was tried.)

The purpose of blocking (also called *prestratification*) is generally to control for the effects of important prognostic factors that may be confounded with the effects of the treatment—the blocks are pairs or sets of matched subjects. The candidates are stratified according to characteristics that may affect the outcome, such as age, severity of the disease, or month (if seasonal factors are deemed important), and balanced randomization (or systematic assignment) is then performed separately in each stratum. Blocking is often used in studies where the accrual of patients continues over a long period (with separate randomization of each pair or set of successively enrolled subjects) and in multicentre trials (with separate randomization at each centre).

Matching and prestratification may be useful in small studies, but statisticians disagree about their value in large studies (the collective noun for statisticians is 'a variance of statisticians'). The grounds for opposition are that these procedures complicate the trial unnecessarily, and the effects of important prognostic factors can just as well be taken into account during the analysis, e.g. by *post-stratification* ('retrospective stratification')—i.e. stratifying the subjects according to characteristics that are found to be related to the outcome.[21]

MAKING THE TRIAL EASIER

Randomized controlled trials are often unfeasible, and are always difficult. The constraints include ethical problems, insufficiency of resources or subjects, and the rapid evolution and obsolescence of treatments in some fields. 'It is hard to argue with the concept that every medical therapy should be evaluated in an RCT', says one expert, who also points out that the method 'is slow, ponderous, expensive, and often stifling of scientific imagination and creative changes in treatment protocols', and declares that it 'is a last resort for the evaluation of medical interventions'.[22]

There are a number of designs that try to lessen logistic or ethical difficulties, while still endeavouring to limit potential bias. For example:

1. Assign fewer patients to the less favourable therapy. In a trial that compares treatments whose success can be adjudged rapidly, each patient's treatment may be determined by the previous patient's result ('Play the winner'). Or two treatments may be tried in a half or third of the patients, and the more successful of the two can then be used in the remaining subjects.[23]
2. Reduce the number of randomized concurrent controls, but compensate for this by also using historical controls who were treated at the same institution with the same eligibility criteria and methods of appraisal, and use both sets of controls in the analysis.[24]
3. Stop accepting new subjects as soon as there is a definitive answer. A *sequential design* of this sort is practicable if subjects enter the trial serially and results are available soon. It requires the prior establishment of 'stopping rules', and ongoing analysis.[25]
4. In a trial comparing a new treatment with the best current standard therapy, randomize the subjects before obtaining their consent (this is Zelen's *prerandomized design*).[26] Give Group A the standard

Table 30.2　Prerandomized controlled trial

1. Eligible? ─────→ If not, exclude
2. Randomize to Groups A and B
3. Consent? (requested in one or both groups)
If refused, give treatment preferred by subject
4. Treat (subjects cannot be blinded to treatment)
5. Follow up all members of Groups A and B
6. Compare outcomes or changes in Groups A and B

therapy, and ask the members of Group B for their consent to the new treatment. If they consent, give them the new treatment; if not, give them the standard treatment. (Alternatively, ask the members of Group B to choose between the two treatments.) Then compare the outcomes in Group A (all of whom received the standard treatment) and Group B (some of whom received the new treatment). This is a valid comparison of randomized groups, although the design 'dilutes' the difference between the treatments (but this may be offset by the higher participation rate that may be expected in such studies). The only ethical problem is that members of Group A are not offered the experimental treatment. This is overcome in the *double prerandomized design*, where members of Group A are asked for their consent to the standard therapy (otherwise, they are given the new therapy); if they tend to consent, the comparison of Groups A and B remains useful. Disadvantages of prerandomized trials are that the subjects cannot be kept unaware of their treatment, and that it becomes difficult to examine the modifying effects of factors that are associated with the patient's decisions; the latter difficulty can be partly overcome by using 'blocking' for selected factors when randomizing. These designs and their analysis are vigorously debated by statisticians (See Table 30.2).

5. Let the patient select his own form of treatment, and then control for the confounding effects of differences between the groups by using appropriate analytic methods. The potential biases of this kind of quasi-experiment are the same as those of non-experimental studies, and the results cannot be expected to be as convincing —or necessarily the same—as those of randomized trials. This approach is advocated by opponents of randomization ('One is uncomfortable with a randomized protocol that lets chance dictate the medical care a human being receives'), who also plead for data banks for the accumulation of clinical experience, to provide material for evaluative studies ('One randomized trial with 100 patients can dramatically change physician behavior, whereas the experience of 100 000 patients might be neglected')[27].

PLANNING AND RUNNING A CLINICAL TRIAL

For a clinical trial to yield convincing conclusions it must be designed and conducted with meticulous attention to detail.[21] Unless the effects of the intervention are very marked and specific, they can be convincingly attributed to the intervention (and not to extraneous factors) only if special precautions are taken, such as the use of controls (Ch. 7), 'blind' methods (p 146), randomization, and appropriate methods of analysis; matching (p 72) and prestratification may also be used.

Study objectives should be formulated precisely, in the form of clear and specific hypotheses (see Chs 4 and 5). The study population should be defined explicitly (Ch. 6) and eligibility and exclusion rules formulated (as in case-control studies—see p 64). Attention must be given to intervention allocation methods, the size of the groups (p 86), the selection and precise definition of variables (Chs 9–11), including the outcome variables, the use of reliable and valid methods of data collection (Chs 14–16), quality control (p 231), surveillance of compliance, and data monitoring.

A written study protocol[28] is generally desirable, and essential in multicentre trials.[29] The protocol of a therapeutic trial should include a detailed description of the treatment and its permissible modifications.

The selection of a study population for a trial is determined by the reference population the investigator has in mind—i.e. to whom does he want to apply the results? This is the basis for decisions on the source of subjects and the method of enrolling them, and the formulation of eligibility and exclusion criteria. The results of a trial of the treatment of middle-aged adults with moderate hypertension may not be applicable to patients with mild hypertension, or to the elderly.

The generalizability of results depends on who is studied. The results of a trial conducted on volunteers, such as a trial of immunization performed by comparing outcomes in randomly allocated groups of volunteers, may not be directly applicable to the population at large. In all trials there are selective factors—the subject's wishes, the views of his treating physician, family, etc.—that the investigator cannot control. It is therefore important to try to appraise the importance and nature of selection bias by determining what proportion of eligible people enter the trial and how those who enter differ from those who do not. The rules and actual reasons for exclusions should of course be recorded, so that it is clear to what kinds of subject the results of the trial do not apply.

In a typical RCT the sequence of steps is: determine eligibility; request informed consent; assign randomly; treat; and follow up. In a prerandomized study, consent and randomization are reversed. In some studies, e.g. where compliance with the taking of medications is regarded as an essential condition for participation, it may be necessary to have a 'run-in' period before eligibility can be finally determined; this period may precede or follow randomization. In others, where treatment cannot be delayed until all diagnostic test results are available, eligibility may not be certain before treatment is started. In principle, randomization should be done as late as possible—i.e. when eligibility is certain and, in a trial where the initial treatment is the same for all patients, only after the initial treatment phase.[21]

In randomized trials, clinicians may be asked to consult a list showing how successive subjects should be treated, or to open a sealed envelope specifying the next patient's treatment, or to contact a co-ordinator and be told what treatment to give. It may not be easy to avoid divergence from the random allocation, even if sealed envelopes are used.[30] Drugs should look the same and their containers should not have distinctive labels, if the clinician is to be kept unaware of the treatment.

Rules for withdrawals from the randomized treatment should be laid down in advance. 'Escape hatches' must always be provided, to enable patients to be withdrawn whenever this is in their best interests—if, for example, they develop worrisome side-effects, illnesses or complications, or whenever (in a double-blind study) it becomes necessary for the clinician to know what treatment is being administered. Subjects may also be withdrawn because they turn out to be ineligible.

Follow-up should be as complete as possible. Subjects who are withdrawn from the study and those who drop out may be highly selected groups, and if they are numerous their exclusion from the analysis may cause serious bias. Wherever possible, the reasons for drop-outs should be ascertained. In a trial with defined end-points, such as death, the occurrence of a disease or complication, recovery, etc., the aim should be to follow up every member of every study group until the occurrence of an end-point, the lapse of a predetermined study period, or the conclusion of the study. Patients who turn out to be misdiagnosed or ineligible for other reasons are exceptions to this rule; they can usually be withdrawn without causing bias. In some clinical trials it may also be helpful to follow up members of the study population who were eligible for inclusion in the study but did not agree to participate; the findings in the randomized study groups can then be supplemented by information on the relationship between treatment and outcome in the non-participants.[31]

Every trial needs a 'policeman'[32] — an investigator, co-ordinator or co-ordinating committee who will keep an eye on the study, ensure smooth running and the avoidance of bias, and protect subjects' interests. It may be important to check adherence to randomization plans and 'blind' techniques, and monitor patients' compliance and the completeness and quality of data. In some trials, ongoing monitoring of data is undertaken in order to see whether the study can or should be stopped early, e.g. because of harmful effects or unexpectedly large beneficial effects; this function is best performed by an independent individual or committee, not the investigators.

In the analysis,[21] use should be made of methods that take account of the duration of the subject's participation and the times of end-point events or repeated appraisals. Confounding can be reduced by appropriate analytic techniques, e.g. by subdividing the groups so that similar subjects can be compared (stratification).

Even in the best-run of randomized therapeutic trials, it is unusual for all subjects to have their allocated treatment throughout the study — inevitably, there are withdrawals (generally in the patient's interests), non-compliers and drop-outs. In trials of interventions aimed at changing lifestyles there are always subjects who fail to change their habits, or who change them despite being in a control group. Bias due to withdrawals and drop-outs can be avoided by comparing the outcomes in all the subjects originally allocated to each group (*intention-to-treat analysis*). This stringent approach may underestimate the efficacy of the treatment, and an *on-randomized-treatment analysis* may be performed as well, comparing the experience of subjects while they were still on their allocated treatment.

Clinical trials often yield inconclusive or inconsistent results because of their small size. Results of different trials can, however, be integrated so as to yield firmer conclusions about the effects of the intervention, their consistency, and the factors that influence them (including characteristics of the subjects, variations in the intervention, and the circumstances and methods of the trial). A *meta-analysis*[33] or overview of this sort requires the use of suitable statistical methods. The analysis may bring together studies that test a specific effect of a specific intervention, such as a reduction of mortality by giving aspirin to patients who have had a myocardial

infarction.[34] It may also compare the effects of different interventions—e.g. different ways of reducing blood pressure[35] or preventing dental caries[36]—or the various effects of an intervention,
such as the effects of educational procedures on compliance with
therapy, therapeutic success, and health outcomes.[37]

USING CASE-CONTROL STUDIES TO APPRAISE PROCEDURES

Retrospective case-control studies may be used to evaluate preventive
and therapeutic procedures. For this purpose, a case is defined as a
person who experienced an outcome that the procedure aimed to
prevent, and a control is a person who did not experience this outcome. Cases and controls are then compared, to determine whether
they differed in their prior exposure to the procedure.

For example, in 1979 a report on a case-control study provided
more convincing evidence than was previously available for the value
of Papanicolaou-smear screening in the control of cancer of the
cervix. A history of 'Pap smears' in the previous 5 years was obtained
less than half as often from patients with newly diagnosed invasive
cervical cancer than from carefully matched controls.[38] Similarly,
evidence of the effect of anticoagulants in preventing deaths in
hospital patients with acute myocardial infarction was provided by a
study that compared the prior use of anticoagulants among patients
who died ('cases') and individually matched patients who survived
('controls').[39] Case-control studies have been used to appraise the
effect of prenatal and intrapartum care in the prevention of adverse
outcomes of pregnancy,[40] the effect of screening in the prevention of
deaths from cancer,[41] etc.

The prime problem with this method is that the controls may have
differed from the cases in their prognostic factors or their eligibility
for the procedure in question (resulting in differences in exposure to
the procedure). There may also be bias due to differences in the
recall or reporting of exposure to the procedure. The information
required for properly appraising or controlling these biases is generally difficult to obtain. If it is available, the principles of well designed
clinical trials can be applied in these case-control studies.[42] In the
study of anticoagulants, for example, care was taken to exclude
patients who, on admission to hospital, had strong indications or
contraindications for the use of anticoagulants.[39]

NOTES AND REFERENCES

1. Schwartz D, Flamart R & Lellouch J 1980 (Clinical trials. Academic Press, London) describe in detail how the purpose of a trial (explanatory or pragmatic?) can influence planning, conduct and analysis. In a pragmatic trial the treatment is administered in the manner in which it would be used in practice, to subjects similar to those to whom it would be applied in practice, and appraised in terms of outcomes that are important to patients, rather than biological effects.
2. The proportions of patients who died within 6 weeks of the episode were similar in the two groups (home, 13%; hospital, 11%). The trial included three-quarters of the patients seen by 60 general practitioners in Nottingham. The other quarter were deemed unsuitable for the trial, on predetermined medical and social grounds, and were sent to hospital; their fatality rate was 26%. Hill J D, Hampton J R, Mitchell J R A 1978 A randomised trial of home-versus-hospital management for patients with suspected myocardial infarction. Lancet 1: 837.
3. Symptoms generally attributed to adenoidal hypertrophy (nasal obstruction, snoring, rhinorrhoea, etc.) were very prevalent in both groups before operation, and were seldom found after operation. They were equally common in both groups, both before and after operation. The study was 'blind'; i.e. the examiner did not know what operation the child would have or had had. Hibbert J, Stell P M 1978 Critical evaluation of adenoidectomy. Lancet 1: 837.
4. The proportions who were cured or improved were very similar among patients taking antihistaminic and placebo tablets. This applied to people who started treatment within a day of the onset of symptoms, 1 day after onset, 2 days after, and 3 or more days after onset. Hill A B 1962 Statistical methods in clinical and preventive medicine. Churchill Livingstone, Edinburgh, pp 105–119.
5. Internal mammary ligation was performed on 304 'unselected' patients with angina pectoris and/or a history of myocardial infarction, and symptomatic improvement was reported in 95%; Battezzatti, M, Tagliaferro A, Cattaneo A D 1959 Clinical evaluation of bilateral internal mammary artery ligation as treatment of coronary heart disease. American Journal of Cardiology 4: 180. In a randomized trial in 17 patients with angina pectoris, the results (significant improvement in just over half the cases) were very similar in the patients who had this operation and in those who had a sham operation. One patient, previously unable to work because of his heart disease, was almost immediately rehabilitated and returned to his former occupation, and reported 100% improvement after 6 months; his arteries had not been ligated. The patients were told only that they were participating in a trial of the procedure, and the clinicians who appraised progress did not know which operation had been done. Cobb L A, Thomas G T, Dillard D H, Merendino K A, Bruce R A 1959 An evaluation of internal-mammary-artery ligation by a double-blind technic. New England Journal of Medicine 260: 1115.
6. This experiment was forced on Ambroise Paré one day in 1537, when he ran out of boiling oil. The next morning the soldiers he had treated with boiling oil 'were feverish with much pain and swelling about their wounds', whereas the others had 'but little pain, their wounds neither swollen nor inflamed'; cited by Bull J P 1950 The historical development of clinical therapeutic trials. Journal of Chronic Diseases 10: 218. The trial was not blind, the treatments were not allocated at random, and statistical significance was not tested; but the difference was so convincing that Paré determined 'never again to burn thus so cruelly the poor wounded'; and boiling oil is eschewed to this very day in the treatment of arquebus wounds.

7. 'At the end of ten days their countenances appeared fairer and fatter in flesh than all the children which did eat the portion of the king's meat' (The Book of Daniel 1: 15). Mosteller F, Gilbert J P & McPeek B 1983 [Controversies in design and analysis of clinical trials. In: Shapiro S H, Louis T A (eds) Clinical trials: issues and approaches. Marcel Dekker, New York, pp 13–64] point out methodological flaws in this biblical clinical trial: sample too small, duration too short, no randomization, no control of extraneous factors such as physical activity, ill defined end-point, no information about countenances at start of trial or about changes in countenances.

8. *Study designs for clinical trials*, and their pros and cons, are described by many authors. See, for example, Mosteller F, Gilbert J P, McPeek B (1983; see note 7). For *parallel designs*, see Lavori P W, Louis T A, Bailar J C III, Polansky M 1983 Designs for experiments—parallel comparisons of treatment. New England Journal of Medicine 309: 1291. For *crossover and self-controlled designs*, see Louis T A, Lavori P W, Bailar J C III, Polansky M 1984 Crossover and self-controlled designs in clinical research. New England Journal of Medicine 310: 24. The use of *historical controls* is discussed by Bailar J C III, Louis T A, Lavori P W, Polansky M 1984 Studies without internal controls. New England Journal of Medicine 311: 156 and Dupont W D 1985 Randomized vs historical clinical trials: are the benefits worth the cost? American Journal of Epidemiology 122: 940.

9. The statistics of *factorial experiments* that examine more than two factors and their interaction and Latin squares are discussed by Fleiss J L 1986 The design and analysis of clinical experiments. John Wiley, New York.

10. Hennekens C H, Eberlein K for the Physicians' Health Study Research Group 1985 A randomized trial of aspirin and beta-carotene among US physicians. Preventive Medicine 14: 165. Stampfer M J, Buring J E, Willett W, Rosner B, Eberlein K, Hennekens C H 1985 The 2×2 factorial design: its application to a randomized trial of aspirin and carotene in US physicians. Statistics in Medicine 4: 111.

11. Pocock S J 1977 (Randomised clinical trials. British Medical Journal 1: 1661) found variations of up to 46% in the death rates of control groups (who had the same treatment) used by the same investigators in different cancer chemotherapy trials.

12. Taylor W R 1983 An evaluation of supplementary feeding in Somali refugee camps. International Journal of Epidemiology 12: 433.

13. *Single-patient trials*, like RCTs, are applications of Pickering's counsel to clinicians: 'If we take a patient afflicted with a malady, and we alter his conditions of life, either by dieting him, or by putting him to bed, or by administering to him a drug, or by performing on him an operation, we are performing an experiment. And if we are scientifically minded we should record the results'. Pickering G 1949 Physician and scientist. Proceedings of the Royal Society of Medicine 42: 229.

A typical 'N of 1' trial is based on successive pairs of treatment periods, a treatment being given in one period and another treatment (or a placebo) in the other; the sequence within each pair is decided randomly; where possible, 'blind' methods are used. The greater the number of time periods, the more convincing the results. See Guyatt G, Sackett D, Taylor D W, Chong J, Roberts R, Pugsley S Determining optimal therapy—randomized trials in individual patients. New England Journal of Medicine 314: 889; Polgar S, Thomas S A 1988 Introduction to research in the health sciences. Churchill Livingstone, Melbourne, Chapter 7; Blum M L, Foos P W 1986 Data gathering: experimental methods plus. Harper & Row, New York, p 146.

14. Peto R, Pike M C, Armitage P et al 1975 Design and analysis of randomized clinical trials requiring prolonged observation of each patient. I. Introduction and design. British Journal of Cancer 34: 585; II. Analysis and examples. British Journal of Cancer 1977 35: 1.

15. Wright I S, Marple C D, Beck D F 1954 Myocardial infarction: its clinical manifestations and treatment with anticoagulants. Grune and Stratton, New York, pp 9–11.
16. 'Student' 1931 Biometrika 23: 398.
17. *Using random numbers.* If all the subjects are known in advance, random sampling methods (see p 81) can be used to assign them randomly. If candidates are continuously enrolled during the trial, or if balanced randomization is desired, blocks of subjects can be randomized separately. If the subjects are paired, single-digit random numbers can be used as substitutes for tossing a coin; an even number might mean 'Treat the first member of the pair', and an odd number 'Treat the second'. A similar method can be used for allocating successive cases in a list or series; successive random numbers are used, odd and even numbers being interpreted as 'Group A' and 'Group B' respectively. If the required allocation is 2:1, numbers 1 to 6 might be used for one group, and 7 to 9 for the other (zeros being ignored). If subjects are to be allocated equally to three groups, 1–3 might be taken to mean Group A, 4–6 Group B, and 7–9 Group C (zeros ignored).
18. *Random permutations* are easier to use than random numbers, because each number appears once only. Fleiss J L (1986; see note 9) supplies a table (Table A.7) and instructions (pp 47–51).
19. *Randomization the easy way,* using a microcomputer (see note 3, p 34); *PC-Plan* is a very versatile program that can handle up to 20 blocks (up to 400 subjects per block) and up to 20 treatments; it can permute up to five treatments per subject (for crossover trials). *Epistat* assigns subjects (paired or unpaired) to two groups.

The following simple program performs balanced randomization to two groups; the total sample can be allocated, or each block in turn. A printer must be on-line.

RANDOMZ.BAS

```
10 CLS:RANDOMIZE TIMER:DIM AA(5),BB(5)
20 PRINT "RANDOM ALLOCATION TO GROUPS A AND B."
30 PRINT:PRINT"Enter total number of subjects, or number in block."
40 PRINT:INPUT"How many subjects? (Enter zero to exit).    ",N
50 IF N=O THEN SYSTEM ELSE NN=N/2:ERASE AA,BB:DIM
   AA(NN+1),BB(NN+1):X=0:AT=0:BT=0:PRINT:PRINT"Working..."
60 X=X+1:IF (N−X)*RND<NN−AT THEN AT=AT+1:AA(AT)=X
   ELSE BT=BT+1:BB(BT)=X
70 IF AT+BT<N THEN 60
80 LPRINT"RANDOM ALLOCATION OF"N"SUBJECTS":PRINT
90 LPRINT:LPRINT"Group A:"
100 FOR I=1 TO AT: LPRINT,AA(I):NEXT
110 LPRINT:LPRINT"Group B:"
120 FOR I=1 TO BT: LPRINT,BB(I):NEXT
130 LPRINT:CLS:PRINT"If you wish, use the program again...":PRINT:
    GOTO 20
```

20. Simple instructions for *balanced randomization,* using allocation ratios of 1:1, 1:2 or 1:1:1, are given by Peto et al (1976; see note 14). To obtain a balanced 1:1 allocation to two groups (A and B), for example, list all 30 of the acceptable sequences of six subjects (AAABBB, AABABB, etc.) and then (using random numbers) choose which of these sequences will be applied to each successive set of six subjects.

When allocating patients to three treatments, the groups can be kept equal by ensuring that three of each successive nine patients go into each group. This might be done by denoting treatment A as 1, 2 or 3, treatment B as 4, 5 or 6, and treatment C as 7, 8 or 9. One-digit random numbers are then chosen. Going from left to right in the top line of the table on p 88, the first number is 9. This means that the first case should go into group C. The second number is 6, and the third 2; i.e. the second case should be put in group B, and the third in group A. The fourth number, 2, is ignored, as we have already had a 2. The next number is 7, so the fourth case goes into group C. And so on for the whole series of nine cases; the final sequence is C,B,A,C,B,C,A,A,B. Hill A B 1977 A short textbook of medical statistics. Hodder & Stoughton, London, pp 303–304.

21. For a simple guide to the design and analysis of a randomized controlled trial, see Peto et al (1976 and 1977; see note 14). Practical considerations are discussed by Lavin P T 1983 Practical considerations in the coordination of clinical trials. In: Shapiro & Louis (1983; see note 7), pp 129–154 and Friedman L W, Furberg C D, DeMets D L 1983 Fundamentals of clinical trials. John Wright, Boston. Statistical analysis is considered by (inter many alia) Fleiss (1986; see note 9) and Meier P (Statistical analysis of clinical trials. In: Shapiro & Louis (1983; see note 7), pp 155–190). There is a journal called Controlled Clinical Trials.

22. Bailar J C III Introduction. In:Shapiro & Louis (1983; see note 7), pp 1–12.

23. Zelen M 1969 Play the winner rule and the controlled clinical trial. Journal of the American Statistical Association 64: 131.

24. Pocock S J (1976 The combination of randomized and historical controls in clinical trials. Journal of Chronic Diseases 29: 175) suggests combining the data for the randomized and historical controls in different ways, based on varying degrees of mistrust of the historical data. In a review paper, Louis T A & Shapiro S H (1983 Critical issues in the conduct and interpretation of clinical trials. Annual Reviews of Public Health 4: 25) warn that the inclusion of historical controls 'can compromise a trial's validity, even if the investigators are convinced that it is valid'. See note 11.

25. Armitage P 1975 Sequential medical trials, 2nd edn. Blackwell, Oxford.

26. Zelen M 1979 A new design for randomized clinical trials. New England Journal of Medicine 300: 1242. See debate in 'Variance and dissent' section, New England Journal of Medicine: 1983 36: 609.

27. Weinstein M C 1974 Allocation of subjects in medical experiments. New England Journal of Medicine 291 1278.

28. For a specimen *protocol* outline, see Friedman et al (1983; see note 21), p 6.

29. The organization of *multicentre trials* is described by Friedman et al (1983; see note 21), p 211 and Stanley K, Stjernsward J, Isley M 1981 The conduct of a cooperative clinical trial. Recent Results in Cancer Research no. 77. Springer-Verlag, Berlin. For statistical aspects, see Fleiss (1986; see note 9), p 176.

30. One investigator, scarred by his experiences in collaborative (i.e. multiclinic) clinical trials, cautions that 'consecutive numbering of envelopes alone is inadequate protection against tampering with randomization. The envelopes, if used, should be serially numbered, opaque, and sealed with water-insoluble glue to prevent steaming them open, and all nonopened envelopes should be returned to the coordinating center which should check the integrity of the seal. Still better, the coordinating center should issue an assignment only after the clinic has identified the eligible patient by name'. Ederer F 1975 Practical problems in collaborative clinical trials. American Journal of Epidemiology 102: 111.

31. Olschewski M, Scheurlen H 1985 Comprehensive cohort study: an alternative to randomized consent design in a breast preservation trial. Methods of Information in Medicine 24: 131.

32. Mainland D 1960 The clinical trial—some difficulties and suggestions. Journal of Chronic Diseases 11: 484.

33. The basic text on *meta-analysis* is Glass G V, McGaw B, Smith M L 1981 Meta-analysis in social research. Sage, Beverly Hills. For a detailed consideration of methodological issues, see Yusuf S, Simon R, Ellenberg S (eds) 1987 Proceedings of the workshop on methodological issues in overviews of randomized clinical trials. Statistics in Medicine 6: 217. Simple guidelines are presented by

Gerbarg Z B, Horwitz R I 1988 Resolving conflicting clinical trials; guidelines for meta-analysis. Journal of Clinical Epidemiology 41: 503.

Meta-analysis may embrace non-experimental as well as experimental studies. Jenicek (1989) presents a detailed flowchart, which stresses his view that the quality of the studies should first be appraised ('qualitative meta-analysis'), and taken into account when the statistical analysis ('quantitative meta-analysis') is performed. Jenicek M 1989 Meta-analysis in medicine: where we are and where we want to go. Journal of Clinical Epidemiology 42: 35.

34. Canner P L (1987 Overview of six clinical trials of aspirin in coronary heart disease. Statistics in Medicine 6: 255) performed a meta-analysis of six RCTs of aspirin in coronary heart disease, and concluded that the best estimate of effect was a reduction of total mortality by 8 to 10%.

35. A meta-analysis of 37 trials showed that drug treatment is the most effective way of reducing blood pressure. Weight reduction, yoga and muscle relaxation had smaller effects. Meditation, exercise, biofeedback, salt restriction and placebo treatment had still smaller (and similar) effects. Andrews G, MacMahon S W, Austin A, Byrne D G 1982 Hypertension: comparison of drug and nondrug treatments. British Medical Journal 284: 1523.

36. A meta-analysis showed that fluoride supplementation reduced caries incidence by 53% (milk teeth) or 42% (permanent teeth); acidulated phosphofluoride (AFP) solutions produced a reduction of 38%, and AFP gels reduced incidence by 26%. Clark D C, Hanley J A, Stamm J W, Weinstein P L 1985 An empirically based system to estimate the effectiveness of caries-preventive agents. Caries Research 19: 83.

37. A meta-analysis showed that various educational procedures had a large influence on patient compliance; the effect size (the mean improvement in the outcome measure, expressed as a multiple of the standard deviation in the control group) was 0.67. There was a smaller influence on therapeutic progress (effect size = 0.13) and a very small, although statistically significant, influence on long-term health outcomes (effect size = 0.06). Mazzuca S A 1982 Does patient education in chronic disease have therapeutic value? Journal of Chronic Disease 35: 521. Cited by Louis T A, Fineberg H V, Mosteller F 1985 Findings for public health from meta-analyses. Annual Reviews of Public Health 6: 1.

38. Clarke E A, Anderson T W 1979 Does screening by 'Pap' smears help prevent cervical cancer? A case-control study. Lancet 2: 1.

39. The features of randomized controlled trials that were applied in this retrospective survey, which is described by Horwitz R I & Feinstein A R (1981) in a paper snappily titled 'The application of therapeutic-trial principles to improve the design of epidemiologic research: a case-control study suggesting that anticoagulants reduce mortality in patients with myocardial infarction' (Journal of Chronic Diseases 34: 575), were: (1) The cases (fatalities) and controls (survivors) were treated in the same hospital during the same period. (2) Each case was paired with an individually matched control—the survivor of the same age, sex and race who was nearest in date of hospitalization. (3) Patients who would not have been eligible for random allocation to an anticoagulant or non-anticoagulant group were excluded; i.e. those who died immediately after admission and those who, when admitted, had strong indications for or against the use of anticoagulants (e.g. thrombophlebitis or bleeding). (4) Separate consideration was given to patients for whom anticoagulants were first prescribed *after* the first set of physician order; i.e. where there was a deviation from the original decision. (5) The cases and controls were compared in order to appraise their similarity, and differences were taken into account in the analysis. (6) Cases and controls were stratified according to the severity of the infarct and other prognostic factors, so that 'high-risk' and 'low-risk' groups could be analysed separately.

40. Niswander K, Henson G, Elbourne D et al, 1984 Adverse outcome of pregnancy and the quality of obstetric care. Lancet 2: 827.
41. Collette H J A, Day N E, Rombach J J, De Waard F 1984 Evaluation of screening for breast cancer in a non-randomised study (the DOM project) by means of a case-control study. Lancet 1: 1224.
42. Methodological issues in the use of case-control studies to evaluate procedures are discussed by (inter alia) Feinstein A R 1985 Experimental requirements and scientific principles in case-control studies. Journal of Chronic Diseases 38: 127; 1986 Response. Chronic Diseases 39: 328; Sasco A J, Day N E, Walter S D 1986 Case-control studies for the evaluation of screening. Journal of Chronic Diseases 39: 399 and Horwitz R I 1987 The experimental paradigm and observational studies of cause-effect relationships in clinical medicine. Journal of Chronic Diseases 40: 91.

31. Programme trials

Programme trials are experiments or quasi-experiments that test hypotheses concerning the effects of health programmes. The programme may be directed at a specific problem or population category (e.g. mass screening, anti-smoking, clean air, prevention of AIDS, care of stroke patients or the elderly), or it may be an organizational form—a programme trial may appraise day care hospitals, health centres, the work of a category of health personnel (nurse-practitioners, chiropodists, village health workers), etc.

A programme trial endeavours not only to appraise outcomes, but to determine whether these can be attributed to the intervention, rather than to extraneous factors. In this respect it differs from a simple programme review (see p 20), which aims to appraise the implementation and/or outcome of a specific programme provided for a specific group or community, without necessarily seeking conclusive evidence that the outcome can be ascribed to the programme (if such evidence is required, the techniques used in trials must be employed). Programme trials can provide generalizable knowledge, applicable to settings like the one in which the trial was performed, about the value of a *type* of programme.

OBJECTIVES OF PROGRAMME TRIALS

A programme trial usually focuses on the outcome of care, and its variation in different population groups or different circumstances. There may also be interest in economic efficiency. Appraisals of performance, compliance, satisfaction, facilities and settings (see Ch. 5) usually have the specific purpose of explaining effectiveness or its lack, except in studies that focus on feasibility or acceptability.

Effectiveness can be convincingly demonstrated only if the outcomes used as criteria are clearly desirable ones—i.e. worthwhile 'end-results' in their own right, or stepping-stones to such end-results.

In instances where the benefits to be expected from an activity are certain (e.g. immunization), a measure of its performance may be used as a criterion of effectiveness.

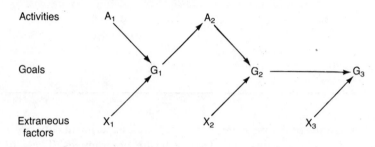

Fig. 31.1   Goal attainment model

The outcomes selected for appraisal are generally those that the programme tries (explicitly or implicitly) to achieve. The goal attainment model[1] is illustrated in Figure 31.1. Every programme goal (G_2) may imply one or more subgoals or intermediate goals (G_1) that must be achieved if the programme goal is to be attained. Activities (A_1 and A_2) are performed in order to achieve the goals. As an example, attaining a reduced prevalence of hypertension (G_2) as a result of antihypertensive treatment (A_2) requires the achievement of an intermediate goal, the identification of hypertensives in the population (G_1), as an outcome of screening activities (A_1).

These activities (A_1 and A_2), which aim at achieving goals G_1 and G_2, constitute the programme. (This is of course an oversimplification; most programmes comprise a number of longer, branched, and interconnecting chains.) It may also be possible to define 'ultimate goals' or end-results (G_3) that may result from the operation of the programme, but without further programme activities—e.g. a reduction in mortality from stroke.

Any outcome that is inherently desirable—in this instance, G_2 or G_3—is a satisfactory criterion of effectiveness in a programme trial. But extraneous factors (X_1, X_2 and X_3) may contribute to each outcome, and their confounding effects must be controlled.

A trial may, of course, aim to appraise undesired as well as desirable outcomes.

Here are three examples of programme trials. The study objectives were:

1. To compare the changes in (a) attitudes to smoking and (b) the prevalence of smoking among boys in the 10th to 12th grades in

two schools, one with an anti-smoking programme and one with-out; controlling for grade, membership of sports teams, parents' smoking habits, and other variables.[2]

2. To compare the changes in the prevalence of specified cardio-vascular risk factors over a 5 year period in two adjacent neighbour-hoods, in one of which a community programme for the control of these factors was conducted by family doctors and nurses; controlling for sex, age, social class, and other variables.[3]

3. To compare the incidence of diarrhoea in children's day-care centres in which a handwashing programme was introduced (handwashing after toilet activities and before handling food or eating) with the incidence in control day-care centres.[4]

STUDY DESIGNS

Programme trials may be individual-based or group-based.

In individual-based trials of programmes, individuals are allocated (preferably randomly) to groups that are exposed (or not exposed) to the programme under study. These trials do not differ in their design from other clinical trials.

In group-based trials the experimental units are not individuals, but groups or communities that are exposed (or not exposed) to the programme. These may be called *community trials*.[5] The basic experimental or quasi-experimental designs are the same as for clinical trials (see p 283): i.e. parallel, externally controlled, and 'self-controlled' (including crossover) studies. Since investigators seldom have the power to decide where or when programmes will be established, most programme trials are quasi-experiments.

A retrospective (case–control) design can also be used. In the Netherlands, for example, the value of a cancer screening pro-gramme was confirmed by a study of women who died of breast cancer and matched living controls, comparing their history of participation in the programme.[6] This use of case-control studies and its intrinsic biases are discussed on p 292.

CLINICAL TRIALS TO EVALUATE PROGRAMMES

It is sometimes feasible to conduct a randomized clinical trial in which some individuals are allocated to a programme and others are used as controls, or individuals are allocated to different programmes.

For example, in a trial of breast cancer screening, members of the Health Insurance Plan of New York were randomly allocated to two groups: some women were offered four annual screening examinations (clinical and mammographic), and others continued to receive their usual medical care. Rates of mortality and other end-points in the two groups were compared. This demonstrated a considerably lower rate of breast cancer mortality in the group assigned to the screening programme, among women aged 50 or more.[7]

As another example, rates of compliance with antihypertensive drug treatment were compared in workers randomly allocated to treatment by industrial physicians during working hours, or by their family doctors. This trial also compared the rates of compliance among men exposed and not exposed to an educational programme (slide-audiotape and booklet) about hypertension. No differences in compliance were found; an unexpected finding was that there was a dramatic increase in absenteeism among workers who were told they had hypertension, especially in the group exposed to the educational programme.[8]

Trials of this kind cannot be 'blind'. Bias caused by the Hawthorne effect (see p 74) may be reduced if an alternative programme is offered to the control subjects. In a trial that showed the effectiveness of physical fitness classes as a way of preventing recurrences of low back pain in hospital workers, for example, a 'back school' (providing instruction on the prevention of back strain) was arranged for the control subjects.[9]

As in other clinical trials, more than one outcome may be studied. In a trial in Seattle, for example, individuals were randomly assigned to a prepaid health maintenance organization or to insurance plans requiring the payment of a fee-for-service, and the outcomes that were compared included changes in blood pressure, functional visual capacity, cholesterol, smoking habits, weight, physical functioning, role functioning, bed-days, serious symptoms, mental health, and other indices of general health.[10]

In trials where there are non-participants, outcomes must of course be measured in the total groups, including their non-participant members. Non-participants are likely to differ from participants,[11] and their exclusion may introduce bias. They may be regarded as a 'hidden study population' (see p 61) requiring special efforts to obtain information. As an example of such bias, if women who did not accept the offer of breast screening made in the Health Insurance Plan study were excluded from the analysis, the results indicated that screening produced a sizeable (but spurious) reduction in mortality from causes other than breast cancer.[7] The crucial comparison in such a study is not between those who participate in the programme and those who do not, but between the randomized groups ('intention-to-treat' analysis; see p 291).

In trials of programmes that require active participation by the subjects, the extent of participation in the trial (as well as in the programme) may have an important bearing on the conclusions. This applies to community as well as clinical trials. In a trial of worksite smoking cessation programmes, where workers at a large installation who consented to participate were randomly allocated to different programmes, the proportions of the randomized groups who quit smoking (measured 12 months later) ranged from 16 to 26% (as compared with a spontaneous quit rate of 5%). But about 64% of the smokers at the plant had not expressed interest in the smoking cessation project, and another 25% had expressed interest but did not agree to participate.[12] Although the results led to a decision to offer the best of the programmes on a regular basis, the overall impact on smoking habits was likely to be small.

When a programme trial is conducted in a single health service, randomization of individuals is generally difficult or impossible. Making a programme available to some patients and not others may be ethically unacceptable, or resented by the patients; this difficulty can sometimes be overcome if the programme is introduced in stages (a shortage of resources may justify this) and will eventually be available to everyone. In a small practice, where patients know and talk to one another, there is likely to be 'contamination' that may interfere with the evaluation of programmes that have an educational component (i.e. that call for changes in behaviour).

COMPARISONS OF GROUPS OR COMMUNITIES

In *parallel community trials* two or more independent groups or communities are studied prospectively and compared (see the three illustrative studies on pp 300–301).

As in clinical trials, randomization (see p 285) is the best way of reducing bias in these trials. It is achieved by the random allocation of groups or communities. Published examples include the random allocation of towns (for fluoridation of water supplies), factories (for programmes for the control of cardiovascular risk factors), villages (for fly control measures), and families (for the provision of primary care by nurse practitioners or physicians). If such studies have few experimental units, randomization may not prevent marked differences. Randomization is of little importance if only two communities are compared—the communities have the same differences, whatever the assignment, and these must be taken into account in the analysis.

Unfortunately, randomization is seldom feasible, since investigators seldom have the power to decide where or when programmes will be established. Most community trials of programmes are quasi-experiments, in which the control groups are purposively selected to be as similar as possible to the intervention groups. The greater this similarity, and the more convincingly it can be demonstrated, the more persuasive are the conclusions. Similarity to the intervention group and the feasibility of obtaining satisfactory data are the main considerations when choosing control groups. There is often a very restricted choice concerning controls.

As in clinical trials, follow-up should be complete; people who do not actively participate in the programme should not be excluded.

'Postmeasure only' studies, where the findings in an intervention group (after exposure to a programme) are compared with those in a control population, are useful only if it can be assumed that the groups were similar before the institution of the programme.[13] A mobile coronary-care service, for example, was evaluated by comparing case fatality rates in two demographically similar communities in Northern Ireland, one of which had such a service. Fatality was higher in the community without a mobile service, although hospital facilities and hospital treatment were similar. The difference could not be attributed to differences in severity or other characteristics of the cases. The results would be more convincing, however, if there was direct evidence that the risk of dying was the same in both communities before the service was instituted or, as the authors point out, if this risk is found to decrease in the control community when such a service is started there.[14]

The minimal requirement is generally a 'premeasure–postmeasure' design, with 'before' and 'after' measurements for both populations. The longer the time series the better, as this permits a fuller comparison of *trends* in both populations. This is especially important if the programme was instituted at different times in different populations. If, for example, cancer screening was started at different times in various regions, its effectiveness may be examined by determining whether and when mortality rates changed in these regions.

A feasible manoeuvre if a service is expanding to a progressively larger population is to compare the 'before' data for each newly admitted chunk with the contemporaneous 'after' data for the population admitted previously (on the assumption that the populations were initially similar), and later with its own 'after' data. In a study in Africa, this technique showed that a reduction in infant mortality could be attributed to a health centre's efforts.[15] In a city in the USA, it demonstrated that a programme for increasing the availability of medical care (by providing services free) apparently led to increased sickness, as measured by self-appraisals of health, the number of symptoms, and limitation of activities because of poor health.[16] A more ambitious multiple-group time-series design (i.e. the use of serial observations in different communities as a basis for both inter-community and within-community comparisons) has been used in community trials of cardiovascular disease prevention programmes.[17]

EXTERNALLY CONTROLLED COMMUNITY TRIALS

In an externally controlled community trial the investigator limits his investigation to groups or communities that are exposed to the programme, and compares the findings with data obtained from other sources. National data may be used, or published reports of surveys or trials in other populations.

The validity of such studies is often in serious doubt. Definitions and study methods may be different, the study population may differ in its characteristics or circumstances from the population from which the control data are derived, and the data may refer to different times.

'SELF-CONTROLLED' ('BEFORE–AFTER') COMMUNITY TRIALS

In 'self-controlled' community trials, observations before and after the institution of the programme are compared. The group or community is its own control. As in clinical trials of this sort, the main biases (see p 284) are those connected with extraneous events or changes that occur between the observations, non-specific effects caused by the trial itself, and changes in methods of measurement. 'Before–after' experiments of this sort, without external controls, are common in public health. 'Infant mortality dropped after the introduction of the programme' is adduced as evidence of effectiveness, although the same change might have occurred without the programme. Salutary testimony to the weakness of this reasoning is provided by McKeown's demonstration that although the introduction of specific immunization procedures and antibiotic treatment was followed by reductions in rates of mortality from tuberculosis, pneumonia, whooping cough, measles and other infective diseases, these changes were continuations of trends that had been observed for many years prior to the introduction of these procedures.[18]

To be reasonably convincing, the 'before–after' trial should be replicated in different populations or at different times—does infant mortality invariably or almost invariably drop when the programme is instituted? It is also helpful to examine data for a number of years *before* the institution of the programme—is there evidence of a *change* in the time trend?

It is also helpful if a 'before–after' study can be extended to an examination of what happens when the programme is withdrawn. It must be very rare, however, for an investigator to have the power or ethical justification for a decision to discontinue a programme that has shown an apparent effect. Such studies are therefore generally opportunistic quasi-experiments. In a rare example of a quasi-experimental crossover community trial, the effects of a programme to encourage the performance of Pap smears were observed in two Indian communities in the USA—one in which such a programme was instituted in 1978, and one in which it was discontinued in the same year.[19]

A WORD OF WARNING

Programme trials are important. Their topics are seldom trivial, and their practical implications may be prodigious. The importance of careful planning and rigorous methods of study and analysis can hence not be underestimated. The fact that most programme trials are quasi-experimental community trials, where the investigator does not have the power to make decisions on the allocation of study groups or (in some instances) on the collection of data, does not mean that the rules can be relaxed. On the contrary, the appraisal of bias and its analytic control become especially important.

Two major principles have been specified for the use of quasi-experimental designs.[20] The first requires that 'all plausible alternative explanations of the relationship between cause and effect or treatment and outcome be specified, and evidence to counter these rival explanations considered or demonstrated'. The second is that of 'assessing the consistency of findings from studies across times and across research settings, methods, and populations'.

The provision of sound scientific evidence about the value of health care cannot ensure that policy for health care will be based on sound scientific evidence, or indeed that there will be *any* policy for health care.[21] But the provision of unsound scientific evidence can hardly improve matters.

NOTES AND REFERENCES

1. The classic paper on the evaluation of programme effectiveness, which presents the *goal attainment model*, is by Deniston O L, Rosenstock L M, Getting V A 1968 Evaluation of program effectiveness. Public Health Reports 83: 323. Also, see note 34, p 27.

2. Using an increased awareness that 'smoking is dangerous to health' as a criterion, the programme was effective. Using changes in smoking habits as a criterion, it was ineffective. Monk M, Tayback M, Gordon J. 1965 Evaluation of an antismoking program among high school students. American Journal of Public Health 55: 994; reprinted in Schulberg H C, Sheldon A, Baker F 1969 (eds) Program evaluation in the health fields. Behavioural Publications, New York, pp 345-359.

3. The prevalence of hypertension, hypercholesterolaemia, smoking and overweight decreased more markedly in the neighbourhood exposed to the programme. Abramson J H, Gofin R, Hopp C, Gofin J, Donchin M Habib J 1981 Evaluation of a community programme for the control of cardiovascular risk factors: the CHAD programme in Jerusalem. Israel Journal of Medical Sciences 17; 201.

4. This study was done in suburban Atlanta, Georgia. During the 35 weeks of the trial the incidence of diarrhoea in the centres where hands were washed was half that in the control centres. Before the handwashing programme was started the incidence was higher in the experimental than in the control centres. Black R E, Dykes A C, Anderson K E 1981 American Journal of Epidemiology 113: 445

5. Community trials may be undertaken to test aetiological hypotheses, not only to evaluate programmes. A classic example is Goldberger's demonstration of the nutritional origin of pellagra, based on experimental dietary changes in orphanages and a mental hospital; Goldberger J, Waring C H, Tanner W F 1923 Public Health Reports 38: 2361. The advantages and limitations of community trials, as compared with clinical trials, are discussed by Farquhar J W 1978 The community–based model of life style intervention trials. American Journal of Epidemiology 108: 103. Also, see Puska P 1985 In: Holland W W, Detels R, Knox G (eds) Intervention and experimental studies. Oxford textbook of public health, vol 3. Oxford University Press, Oxford, Chapter 7.

6. Collette H J A, Day N E, Rombach J J, De Waard F 1984 Evaluation of screening for breast cancer in a non-randomised study (the DOM project) by means of a case-control study. Lancet 1: 1224.

7. Shapiro S, Venet W, Strax P, Venet L, Roeser R 1982 Ten- to fourteen-year effect of screening on breast cancer mortality. Journal of the National Cancer Institute 69: 349.

8. Sackett D L, Haynes R B, Gibson E S et al 1975 Randomised clinical trial of strategies for improving medication compliance in primary hypertension. Lancet 1: 1205; Haynes R B, Sackett D L, Taylor D W, Gibson E S, Johnson A L 1978 Increased absenteism from work after detection and labeling of hypertensive patients. New England Journal of Medicine 299: 741.

9. Donchin M, Woolf O, Kaplan L, Floman Y 1989 Secondary prevention of low back pain. Abstracts: Kyoto, Japan, May 15–19, 1989. International Society for the Study of the Lumber [sic] Spine, Toronto, p 18.

10. This study (part of the Rand Health Insurance Study) found that the outcome of care by an HMO (where costs are lower, mainly because of reduced hospital admissions and hospital days) differed for poor and well-off individuals who had health problems at the outset. Among the well-off, cholesterol levels and general health improved significantly more than in the fee-for-service system; among the poor, those assigned to the HMO had more bed-days and more serious symptoms. Ware J E Jr, Brook R H, Rogers W H et al 1986 Lancet i: 1017.

11. As an example of *differences between participants and non-participants*, in a Swedish trial of a programme aimed at the prevention of coronary heart disease it was found that the men who did not participate tended, at the onset of the trial, to have more chronic illnesses, a higher prevalence of alcoholism, and less favourable social conditions. They subsequently had a higher mortality than participants. Wilhelmsen L, Ljungberg S, Wedel H, Werko L 1976 A comparison between participants and non-participants in a primary preventive trial. Journal of Chronic Diseases 29: 331.

12. Omenn G S, Thompson B, Sexton M et al 1988 A randomized comparison of worksite-sponsored smoking cessation programs. American Journal of Preventive Medicine 4: 261.

13. The lack of baseline information about mortality, morbidity, growth and nutritional status is a serious problem in trials of new patterns of grass-roots primary health care in developing countries. Even discounting ethical considerations, it is difficult to collect such data before community health workers, on whom these care programmes are based, start to function. In the Narangwal project in India, for example (an important controlled study of the comparative effectiveness of nutritional care, medical care, and their combination), no 'before' measurements were available in the villages studied. Information on births and deaths was not collected in a uniform way until the second year of the project. The validity of the conclusions rests on the assurance that the villages were similar in such features as size, education, the distribution of occupational groups, and access to previously available health services. Kielmann A A, Taylor C E, Parker R L 1978 The Narangwal Nutrition Study: a summary review. American Journal of Clinical Nutrition 31: 2040.

14. Mathewson Z M, McClockey B G, Evans A E, Russell C J, Wilson C 1985 Mobile coronary care and community mortality from myocardial infarction Lancet 1: 441.

15. Kark S L, Cassel J, 1952 The Pholela Health Centre: a progress report. South African Medical Journal 26: 101, 132; Kark S L 1981 The practice of community oriented primary health care. Appleton-Century-Crofts, New York, pp 243–245.

16. Diehr P K, Richardson W C, Shortell S M, LoGerfo J P 1979 Increased access to medical care: the impact on health. Medical Care 17: 989.

17. Salonen J T, Kottke T E, Jacobs D R Jr, Hannan P J 1986 Analysis of community-based cardiovascular disease prevention studies—evaluation issues in the North Karelia project and the Minnesota Heart Health program. International Journal of Epidemiology 15: 176.

18. McKeown T 1979 The role of medicine: dream, mirage or nemesis? Blackwell, Oxford.

19. Freeman W L 1987 In: Nutting P A (ed) Community-oriented primary care: from principle to practice. Health Resources and Services. Administration, Public Health, Washington, D C, pp 410–416. In both communities the Pap screening rate was considerably higher when the programme was operative.

20. Patrick D L 1985 Sociological investigations. In: Holland W W, Detels R, Knox G (eds) Oxford textbook of public health, vol. 3. Oxford University Press, Oxford, Chapter 11.

21. 'Do situations exist in which there is health policy without scientific evidence? In fact there are only a few situations in which there is any kind of policy'. Ibrahim M A 1985 Epidemiology and health policy. Maryland, Aspen, Rockville, p 183.

32. Community-oriented primary care

This chapter deals with the collection and use of information by physicians and other health workers who provide health care for individuals or families in the community and also try to 'treat the community as a patient' by appraising its health needs and establishing programmes, in the framework of primary care, to deal with these needs in a systematic way. This kind of integrated practice, which brings personal health care and community medicine together in a primary-care setting, has been termed *community-oriented primary care (COPC)*.[1] COPC programmes deal with selected health problems of the whole community or defined subgroups, and may involve health promotion, primary or secondary prevention, curative, alleviative or rehabilitative care, or any combination of these activities. They may focus on specific disorders or specific risk or preventive factors, may involve individual counselling or clinical care, group or community health education, and other activities, and may require community action or interagency co-operation.

The 'community' in the COPC context may be a true community in the sociological sense, or it may comprise the residents of a defined neighbourhood, the workers at a given place of employment, the students in a given school, or any other defined group of people for whom health care is provided. People registered as potential users of the services of a given general practitioner, group practice, health maintenance organization or neighbourhood health centre may also be regarded as a community for this purpose. Where there is no defined responsibility for a specific population, the practitioner may view the aggregate of people who seek care, or those who seek care repeatedly, as the 'community' for whose welfare he is responsible.

The systematic collection and use of information plays an important role in this form of practice. As shown in Figure 32.1, COPC may be seen as a cyclical process (analogous to the examination–diagnosis–treatment–follow-up–reappraisal cycle in the care of a patient) in

which activities are continuously influenced by epidemiological
and other information. This information provides the basis for the
planning, implementation, monitoring and evaluation of the community health programmes that characterize COPC.

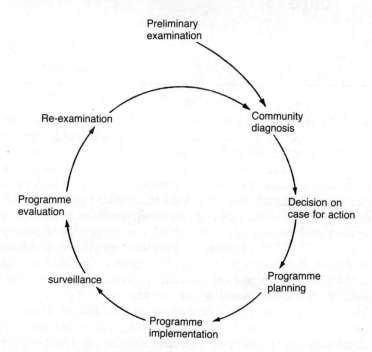

Fig. 32.1 Stages of community-oriented primary care

A distinction is made in Figure 32.1 between a preliminary
examination aimed at 'getting to know' the community and deciding
which of its health problems merit detailed study, and a more detailed
inquiry into selected problems ('community diagnosis'). If it is
decided to set up a programme, the scheme calls for ongoing monitoring of its implementation and ongoing surveillance of changes
in the community's status. Evaluation of the programme and re-
examination of the situation may lead to decisions about the continuation or modification of the programme and about new issues for
study or action.

This chapter will discuss the application in COPC of the principles
and techniques described in previous chapters, with which the reader
is now assumed to be familiar. (If not, return to Square 1.)

STUDY PURPOSES

The prime purpose for which information is collected in COPC is, of course, to help the individuals and community served by the practice. (See the basic questions listed on p 13.)

In the COPC context, survey activities may also be used to promote the community's involvement in its own health care. Meetings with community leaders, designed to learn their views of their health problems and of possible solutions, may also serve to stimulate interest and promote community participation. Whenever a planned survey has obvious implications for the community's health, its purpose can be explained to community members and leaders. Feedback of results can be provided, using meetings, newsletters or other media. A community may sometimes be willing to perform a *community self-diagnosis*—'communities can be helped to look at themselves and to come up with an assessment of their own problems and priorities, and of the causative factors which need tackling'.[2]

Studies in a COPC framework may also provide generalizable new knowledge COPC offers special opportunities for research on the aetiology, natural history and care of disorders handled in the primary-care context, growth and development, the effects of family processes and psychosocial factors on health and health care, and other topics. Probably the most important research challenge facing COPC practitioners today is the need for evaluative studies of COPC itself—how feasible are specific kinds of COPC programmes in different populations and different health-care systems, how effective are they in comparison with ordinary (not community-oriented) care, what is their extra cost, and what hospital or other costs do they save?

STUDY POPULATION

The defined community with whose care the COPC practice is concerned, i.e. the *target population*, is also the study population or denominator population for survey purposes. When COPC is not provided for a total population it is helpful to know what selective factors operate and how the target population differs from the population at large. The criteria for inclusion in the target population require clear formulation.

If the target population is too large to be studied accurately, a part of it may be selected for this purpose. This may be a geographically demarcated *defined area*—'an area of intensive study from which is gathered the data for community diagnosis and in which health action is most easily evaluated'.[3] For health centres serving extensive rural areas or crowded inner-city populations, Kark has suggested that a small 'initial defined area' be selected, preferably demarcated in terms of a census tract or tracts, and that this be widened from year to year.[4]

A health centre with a geographically defined area of responsibility may have to give special consideration to transient residents, such as migrant seasonal labourers and their families, and expectant mothers or ill people who come to live with relatives in order to enjoy the health services available. Measurements of the community's health may be distorted if data concerning temporary residents are included in numerators but not in denominators. If the specific problems and needs of transient residents are to be measured, estimates of numbers and duration of stay are required.

The study population for measurements of the community's health status and the impact of intervention should generally be the target population as a whole, a 'defined area', or (for specific purposes) a defined subgroup, such as infants and their parents, persons with a specific disease, or people to whom a particular programme is offered. If measurements are limited to people who actually use the services that the COPC practice offers, or who use these services in a given period, a biased picture may be obtained. If this limitation is unavoidable, the possible bias should be explored and taken into account (see p 271).

For some purposes, probability samples (see Ch. 8) may be used. The sampling frame for this purpose may be a list of people, families, or dwelling units, or a map showing dwelling units. Sample surveys can yield a satisfactory picture of age and sex composition, habitual practices, the prevalence of common diseases and disabilities, and other characteristics of the community as a whole. The use of a sample is obviously unsatisfactory, however, in surveys that aim (like many surveys in COPC) not only to obtain information at a community level, but also to identify individuals who need care, with a view to offering them this care.

If a controlled programme trial is contemplated, in order to appraise effectiveness experimentally or quasi-experimentally, a control group or population outside the COPC population may be required. This should be as similar as possible to the COPC population, and one that is accessible for study purposes. If the COPC is expanding to serve a progressively larger population, the newly admitted blocs can be used as controls for blocs admitted earlier (see pp 304–305).

STUDY OBJECTIVES

In COPC as elsewhere, sound study design requires decisions as to what knowledge is required, and a clear formulation of the study objectives (see Chs 4 and 5). This applies to the use of data gathered in the clinical situation no less than to special surveys of the COPC population. Primary-care records are generally useful for epidemiological purposes only if special care has been taken in collecting and recording the information this use will require. For evaluative studies in particular, there is usually a need for information that has been systematically collected in order to answer specific questions.

COPC always requires descriptive studies of the community, and often calls for analytic studies as well, i.e. for hypothesis-testing. Hypotheses may be tested to throw light on processes operating in the specific community, or to provide generalizable new knowledge as well, e.g. about the effectiveness of a given type of intervention programme.

The kind of information required, and the appropriate methods for obtaining it, differ in various stages of the COPC cycle. We will therefore give separate consideration to the preliminary examination, community diagnosis, and other specific stages before returning to discuss the selection of variables, and other general aspects of study methods in the COPC context.

PRELIMINARY EXAMINATION

Tasks in the initial phase include defining and 'getting to know' the community and identifying health problems that merit detailed study and possible action. This exploration is generally based on easily accessible data about the characteristics of the population, the extent and impact of various disorders and health hazards, the community's interests and concerns, the availability and use of health and welfare services, and other features that may be relevant to the planning of health care.

A search may be made for published reports and ready-made statistics, including those that deal with a broader population than the specific community served and those that describe epidemiological and other findings in populations that are believed to resemble the target population. Discussions may be held with community members and professionals concerning the community's situation, their perception of its needs, and their interests and concerns (see *qualitative research*, p 134). The use of the nominal group technique (see Ch. 19) has been suggested as a way of exploring laymen's and professionals' perceptions of problems and their possible solutions.

In addition to these steps, easily available clinical and administrative records may be gathered and analysed in order to obtain information about the use of health services, reasons for attendance, infant growth patterns, causes of hospitalization, mortality and its causes, etc. In drawing conclusions from these analyses, it is usually necessary to consider the effects of sample bias, the lack of standardized criteria and methods, incomplete recording, and other shortcomings of the data.

Information about the size and demographic characteristics of the target population is not only essential for the calculation of disease rates and other community health indices, it also carries its own implications for health and health care. Even the simplest of data, concerning only the population's size and age distribution, may be of help in planning the allocation of resources. It may be important to appraise mobility; if there is much flux in the population, this will have obvious implications for the planning of services. Knowledge about educational level, ethnic distribution, religion and other characteristics may add to an understanding of the community's health needs.

Demographic information may be available from the registration system used by the primary-care practice for administrative or fiscal purposes, from other records (e.g. an age–sex register) maintained as a routine in the practice, or (in some circumstances) from official sources (national census, population register, school registers, etc.). If not, a basic demographic survey may be required, a need which is often met by collecting the required data in the course of a household health survey. Sometimes the best that can be done is to use estimates derived from census data for a broad area that includes the COPC population.

A register of the eligible population may be valuable not only as a source of data for epidemiological purposes and as a sampling frame, but as a tool for use in the provision of care, especially if it includes information on age. It might be used, for example, as a checklist for identifying elderly people or infants with whom there has been no contact for some time.

Maps serve useful purposes in COPC; when they are not easy to procure, the practice may itself have to prepare them.

COMMUNITY DIAGNOSIS

The community health diagnosis[5] provides detailed information about selected health problems and their determinants. It can be broad or narrow in its scope; it often deals with only a single topic or a single subgroup of the population.

If the problem under consideration is hypertension, the questions asked might include: What are the frequency distributions of systolic and diastolic pressures in the community? What is the prevalence rate of hypertension? How does it vary in different population subgroups? How common are complications? What contribution do hypertension and hypertension-related diseases make to mortality? How strong is the association with overweight? How prevalent is overweight? What are the community's attitudes to hypertension and overweight? How many of the hypertensives smoke cigarettes, or have other risk factors for coronary heart disease? What proportion of the community has been screened for hypertension? How many of the known hypertensives are under treatment? How many are under adequate control?

The community diagnosis provides a basis for decisions on the need for intervention, the type of intervention needed, and the target groups at whom it should be directed, as well as giving an indication of the resources that intervention will require. It also provides baseline information for the subsequent measurement of change. The study procedures that yield the community picture also serve the needs of patient care more directly, both as a basis for the management of individuals and as an aid in the systematic implementation of a programme. A prevalence survey, for example, not only gives information about prevalence, it also identifies individuals who need care, and can provide a register of cases for use as a framework for the organization and monitoring of a programme.

The community diagnosis may be descriptive, analytic, or both. At a descriptive level, the objectives may be to measure the occurrence or distribution of diseases or disabilities, risk factors, risk markers, or other health-relevant variables, including health and disease behaviour, the use of services, and environmental hazards.

There may be a variety of reasons for examining and measuring associations between variables. The usual purposes are:

1. To identify *groups who require special care*, e.g. social classes or ethnic groups with a high prevalence of a disorder or a harmful practice.

2. To determine the *causal factors* that operate in the COPC population—these may differ in different communities[6]—and to measure their impact. Attention is usually confined to factors known (from studies elsewhere) to be among the determinants of the disease, behaviour, or other characteristic that is under consideration, but a creative mind may find opportunities for original research. When it is believed that an association with a disorder represents a cause-effect relationship, the attributable or preventable fraction (see p 253) in the population may be used to measure the effect.

3. To determine what attributes or combinations of attributes may be of use as *risk markers* for the detection of vulnerable individuals or groups in this population (see p 39).

4. To identify *community syndromes*[7], i.e. sets of associated diseases or other health characteristics. The components of a syndrome may occur together because they possess shared or related causes, or because they are themselves causally inter-related; hence the syndrome points to a nexus of causal processes in the community. Even if these processes are not completely understood, a programme directed at the syndrome as a whole may be more effective and efficient than an endeavour to deal with one or more of the individual components separately.

In COPC, community diagnosis is often a slow and gradual process, based as it generally is on information continuously collected in the clinical situation, supplemented from time to time by surveys performed outside this situation. If the population is small it may be necessary to cumulate several years' experience before satisfactory data, especially on mortality and disease incidence, are available. Moreover, some studies—e.g. of predictors of mortality in the COPC population—are intrinsically long-term. At some point, however, usually sooner than later, it is decided that enough information is available to permit the planning and introduction of an intervention programme. This does not stop the process of community diagnosis, which merges imperceptibly into community health surveillance.

An important function of the community diagnosis in COPC is that it provides a baseline for the subsequent measurement of change, and hence for appraising the effectiveness of intervention. It may be possible to plan intervention without detailed knowledge about the target population, but without such knowledge it is generally not possible to see whether the intervention has achieved its desired effect—a given programme may work well in one community and not in another.

PROGRAMME PLANNING AND IMPLEMENTATION

In deciding whether a case for action exists, consideration should be given not only to epidemiological evidence concerning the nature, extent, causes and impact of the problem, but also to the feasibility of intervention and the likelihood that it will be successful. The competing demands of other health problems must also be taken into account. The decision on the case for action, as well as the detailed planning of the programme, often requires the collection of extra information, e.g. about the community's felt needs and demands, its readiness and capacity to participate in the programme, prevalent attitudes and practices relevant to health care, the nature and extent of the care presently given, and use and availability of time, manpower, and other resources. Published results of evaluative studies of care procedures and programmes tested elsewhere usually play an important part in decisions on the case for intervention and on the nature of the intervention.

Surveillance of health, monitoring of activities and programme evaluation should be planned together with the intervention. As far as possible, the collection of information for these purposes should be built into the planned activities of the programme. Some of this information (Are blood pressure measurements being done as planned? Are hypertensives being investigated for target organ damage?) may be helpful in case management and as a basis for immediate corrections to the intervention plan and the way it is implemented.

SURVEILLANCE

Like the initial community diagnosis, community health surveillance[8] may be broad or narrow in its scope. Its purpose is to detect and measure changes in the community's health status and in its exposure to risk and protective factors. The occurrence of change may be an indication of effectiveness of intervention.

Surveillance brings the community diagnosis up-to-date, and may be seen as a continuation of the same diagnostic process. When study objectives necessitate longitudinal methods—e.g. in studying patterns of child growth and development in the community, or the association between some factor and the subsequent incidence of a disorder—it may be especially difficult to distinguish between community diagnosis and surveillance. Community health surveillance may be based on information collected in the clinical situation or on special procedures, such as repeated surveys of smoking habits.

Updating of the demographic picture requires ongoing surveillance, particularly if a nominal register of the COPC population is maintained. In a neighbourhood practice this surveillance may include the reporting of births, deaths, arrivals and departures. In some circumstances, information may be obtained from official agencies to which births, deaths and movements are reported. In a practice where there are voluntary or other community health workers, notification of these events, and even of pregnancies, often becomes one of their functions. This demographic surveillance obviously serves individual as well as epidemiological needs. The notification can be a signal for action—e.g. for informing newly arrived persons of the services available, for endeavouring to bring a pregnant woman or newly born child into routine preventive care, or for visiting a bereaved family and determining whether crisis intervention or other help is needed.

EVALUATION

In COPC, evaluation is always motivated by concern with the welfare of the specific community served. This kind of evaluation, aimed mainly at determining whether the programme is running well and whether outcomes are satisfactory, is what we have called a *programme review* (see p 20). Evidence may also be sought that the outcomes can be attributed to the intervention (rather than to other factors), using an experimental or quasi-experimental design (see Ch 31). This may require study of a control population as well. If a programme trial is contemplated, it is usually wise to attempt to reduce bias—or accusations of bias—by obtaining the assistance of impartial independent coinvestigators and (for data obtained outside the ordinary clinical context) of independent observers.

The evaluation may embrace the COPC practice as a whole, or it may be limited to a specific programme or programmes, or to specific aspects of programmes. All the basic evaluative questions listed on page 48 may be asked. Questions about the process and outcome of care usually focus on the performance of the activities and the achievement of the goals specified in the plan of the intervention programme. The scope of the inquiry may vary from simple monitoring procedures (Are people with borderline hypertension having regular blood pressure checks? Are hypertensive patients taking their medication?) through a fuller evaluation including the measurement of immediate outcomes and the detection of obvious undesirable effects (What proportion of the known hypertensives have been brought under control? How many of the patients treated with hypotensive drugs complain of impaired sexual functioning?) to a comprehensive appraisal that may include the measurement of long-term outcomes (Have the frequency distributions of systolic and diastolic pressures or the prevalence of hypertension in the community changed? Has the incidence of stroke or other defined complications fallen?).

For practitioners with a crusading interest in the extension of COPC, the importance of evaluative studies cannot be over-emphasized. Pleading for a 'vibrant and compelling data base with which to make a case for COPC', Rogers[9] has pointed out that it may not be enough to demonstrate effects on mortality or morbidity rates. 'Such statistics...lack immediacy and emotional impact...A community or a nation will willingly and instantly spend millions to rescue a trapped coal miner...but it is much harder to get that same community or nation to spend similar sums to reduce infant mortality rates...As with olives or oysters, a taste for vital statistics is an acquired one.' He suggests that new yardsticks, such as measures of the restoration of crippled people to full functioning, may be needed to excite compassion and interest.

SELECTION AND DEFINITION OF VARIABLES

The collection of information that is accurate enough to be useful for epidemiological purposes is far from easy, and a COPC practice ordinarily has limited resources to devote to this task. Attention should therefore be concentrated on data that are of obvious relevance to the practice's needs. There is no point in creating a database that is a cemetery for the interment of useless information, even if some of it will occasionally be exhumed for annual reports or other ritual observances.

A case can be made for the routine collection of standard sets of basic data[10] in all primary care practices of a given kind in a given kind of community, but only as a nucleus or framework for a more useful data set that is custom-made to meet specific needs. In general, the information required will vary from practice to practice. The selection of variables for careful measurement depends on the specific problems that have been chosen for special attention, and on the specific programmes planned or implemented to deal with them.

The definition of variables may need special attention. This applies particularly to standard operational definitions of diseases and disabilities, and especially if diagnoses are made by more than one clinician. It may not be easy to formulate suitable definitions (see Ch. 11), especially in view of the relatively restricted use of diagnostic tests in primary care, and it is certainly not feasible to develop satisfactory definitions for all diagnoses. This should, however, be done for the conditions selected for epidemiological study. For these it may be wise to record the presence or absence of each diagnostic criterion, so as to permit ongoing or spot checks of conformance with the definition. If at any stage it is decided to alter the definition of a disease, an attempt should be made to do this in a way that maintains comparability with earlier data.

If the incidence of disease is to be studied, a 'new case' must be defined (e.g. after what period of freedom from symptoms would a patient be regarded as having a new episode of acute bronchitis?), and so must the date of onset (see p 105).

COLLECTION OF DATA

A characteristic feature of the study methods used in COPC is the use of information to fulfil a double function, to meet the practice's dual responsibilities for individual and community care. When a baby is weighed or a disease is diagnosed—whether in the course of ordinary clinical care or in a special survey—the result may be used both in managing the individual and at a group level.

Often, in fact, one stone may kill more than two birds. An examination, say an ECG or a blood pressure measurement, may be put to a variety of uses other than the immediate management of the individual. Its result may be used in the process of community diagnosis or community health surveillance, e.g. to measure the prevalence or incidence of a disease (or both) or the distribution of ECG findings or blood pressures. If the examination finding indicates disease, the person may be added to a chronic disease register used as a tool in organizing, implementing and monitoring a programme for such patients. The result may also be used in programme evaluation: if there is a programme for primary prevention, say of coronary disease, the incidence data (measured before the programme) may serve as a baseline for the detection of change or (measured later) as an indication of effectiveness; if there is a programme for the care of patients with hypertension, prevalence data may be used as an outcome measure of effectiveness. The mere fact that the test was done may also be used for evaluative purposes, e.g. to measure the extent to which the COPC practice performs the planned activities called for by a programme or to measure compliance with advice to attend for examination.

As a rule, a good deal of the information needed for community diagnosis, surveillance and evaluation is collected in the course of clinical care. It may be a by-product of the ordinary diagnostic investigation and surveillance of patients, or it may be derived from routine tests and questions specially added to clinic procedures for epidemiological purposes. In a practice where periodic health examinations are conducted, these provide an especially useful opportunity for the collection of such information.

This use of clinical data for epidemiological purposes demands methods that are no less rigorous than those in any epidemiological study. The information to be analysed must be as accurate and complete as possible. Standardized procedures should be laid down for the collection of data, especially if questions are asked or examinations done by more than one person. Written instructions are desirable, documenting the procedures and operational definitions, especially if there are frequent changes of personnel. Quality control procedures and tests of validity and reliability should be instituted wherever necessary. Even simple checks on the completeness of recording may yield startling findings.[11]

The clinical context provides special opportunities for the collection of data—e.g. for doing elaborate tests, for asking questions about delicate matters, and for long-term follow-up. But it may also produce various sorts of bias. People differ in their tendency to seek care; the patients seen may give an incomplete picture of morbidity in the community, and may not be representative with respect to other health characteristics. When patients attend, their illness or apprehension may affect their responses or measurements; and they may tend to give the answers they think their health advisors expect of them. Doctors and other health workers, anxious to help the patient rather than to collect standardized data, may diverge from routine examination procedures. When making observations they may be influenced by their prior knowledge of the patient (see 'halo effects', p 147); and they may be biased when appraising the effectiveness of their care. Where possible, these biases should be reduced, e.g. by using standardized objective measures and by making measurements (say of blood pressure or weight) without first referring to the patient's previous values.

Information collected in the course of clinical care may give a biased picture of the prevalence and distribution of chronic disorders or other attributes if there are many non-attenders. In some subgroups, coverage may in the course of time become so high than this bias can be ignored. This may occur with infants and their mothers, pregnant women, the elderly, and hypertensives or other groups of patients for whom periodic health examinations or special care programmes are organized. Often, however, there is a need for supplementary survey procedures. Non-attenders may be identified and invited to attend, or visited at home, or asked to supply information by mail or telephone.

Information collected during the care of people with selected 'tracer' conditions can sometimes be generalized to the total COPC population. In one practice, for example, it was concluded that the results of tests for tuberculosis in diabetic patients (all or most of whom were under care) provided an acceptable estimate of the rate of tuberculosis infection in various age groups of the total population, on the assumption that diabetes does not modify the risk of infection.[12]

Information may also be obtained by special surveys, conducted in the clinic context or outside it. These may range in scope from a small follow-up study of the current status of a group of patients to a comprehensive community health survey. A community survey can provide information that clinical records cannot or do not. It can appraise the health status and needs of people who have not sought care, can measure the use of other health services by the COPC population, and may provide the COPC practice with a considerable amount of new information about its patients.[13] Special surveys performed by or under the auspices of a COPC practice that has a good relationship with the community are generally characterized by high response rates.

To meet the dual obligations of COPC, special surveys are usually designed not only to provide information at a community level but also to identify individuals who need care, and in such instances sampling may not be appropriate. This identification may be based on the presence of disorders, on screening tests that point to a need for further investigation, on the presence of modifiable risk factors, or on the presence of risk markers indicative of vulnerability.

Sackett & Holland[14] have contrasted the roles of 'epidemiological surveys' (studies of population samples aimed at generating new knowledge), 'screening' (of apparently healthy people who have been invited to be examined) and 'case-finding' (examining patients who have sought care, to reveal disorders that may be unrelated to their complaints; sometimes called 'opportunistic' case-finding). In the context of COPC, such distinctions become blurred or vanish. Surveys aim to provide information that will benefit individual participants, as well as providing a basis for decisions about care at a community level, and may be organized in a clinical setting or even based on routine clinical activities. In COPC, people are seldom invited to attend solely for screening purposes. Screening and diagnostic tests may be included as routines for people who attend for treatment, or incorporated in health examinations that provide an opportunity for appraisal of the individual's health status and life situation and for counselling, and that are not concerned solely with discovering disease.

RECORDS AND ANALYSIS

Patients' records should be readily available and easy to use, or recording will tend to be incomplete. Forms and record systems should be designed with an eye to the easy retrieval of data for the purpose of analysis. For some purposes it may be convenient to use special additional records for epidemiological purposes, such as contact sheets (encounter forms) containing diagnostic and other information about each patient seen, and notification forms. Specific intervention programmes may require their own records.[15] If records are computerized, the system should be designed for epidemiological analyses as well as for the more usual purposes of providing feedback about individual patients and information required for administrative and fiscal purposes.

Special efforts are usually needed to ensure that clinical records are complete, and that results of laboratory and other special tests, and reports from consultants and hospitals, get into the patients' files. If disease incidence is to be studied, the record should show whether the diagnosis represents a 'new case', and state the date of onset. Precautions may be needed to ensure that if a diagnosis is changed because of new information, the corrected diagnosis will be used in the analysis. If an analysis is to be done by age, sex, or other characteristics, the requisite information must be recorded for each patient seen—it must be available for numerator data as well as for the denominator.

Ongoing summary records may be maintained to help in the implementation of programmes. These include maps showing places of residence of (say) housebound patients, Pickles charts,[16] which plot new cases of infectious diseases day by day according to their dates of onset, case registers of 'at-risk' individuals or patients with specific disorders, and programme status charts showing what has been done and what still needs to be done in a specific programme.

Coding of diagnoses can be done by any trained personnel, but it may be preferred that doctors do this themselves. The classification should be one appropriate for use in primary care.

Procedures of data processing and analysis do not differ from those in other studies. Data may be analysed in an ongoing way—e.g. by counting visits and diagnoses each day—or accumulated and analysed periodically. The use of a microcomputer has the advantage that it makes data handling relatively easy and inexpensive without dependence on professional computer personnel—'it may be desirable to identify one or more staff members who have a particular interest in becoming somewhat computer literate and obtain extra training for them'.[17]

When interpreting findings, due consideration must be given to possible biases. Caution should be used in generalizing from the findings, both because of the specific features of the given community and because of the specific attributes of the physicians or other health workers in the practice. Practitioners of COPC are, at the present time, a selected group who are not necessarily representative of all practitioners (indeed, their interest in COPC may attest to their sterling quality!).

NOTES AND REFERENCES

1. The concept and practice of *community-oriented primary care* are described by Kark S L 1981 in The practice of community-oriented primary care. Appleton-Century-Crofts, New York. See Abramson J H 1988 Community-oriented primary care—strategy, approaches and practice—a review. Public Health Reviews 16: 35. Also, see Connor E, Mullan F (eds) 1983 Community-oriented primary care: new directions for health services delivery. National Academy Press, Washington, D C; and Nutting P A (ed) 1987 Community-oriented primary care: from principle to practice. Health Resources and Services Administration, Public Health Service, Washington, DC.
2. Bennett F J 1979 Community diagnosis and health action: a manual for tropical and rural areas. MacMillan, London, p 6.
3. Kark S L 1966 An approach to public health. In: King M (ed) Medical care in developing countries. Oxford University Press, Nairobi, Chapter 5; and Kark (1981; see note 1).
4. Kark S L, Abramson J H Community-oriented primary care: meaning and scope. In: Connor & Mullan (1983; see note 1), pp 21–59.
5. See note 10, p 25.
6. In a Jerusalem neighbourhood with a high prevalence of coronary heart disease and a high proportion of deaths (58%) caused by cardiovascular diseases, a multiple logistic analysis of predictors of mortality over a 10-year period revealed that serum cholesterol was not positively associated with mortality, whereas

hypertension was strongly so in both sexes, and smoking was in men. This suggested that intervention to reduce scrum cholesterol in the population as a whole might be unimportant in this community. Kark J D, Donchin M, Gofin R et al 1982 Paper presented at International Symposium on Hypertension Control in the Community, Tel Aviv.

7. *Community health syndromes* described by Kark S L 1974 (Epidemiology and community medicine. Appleton-Century-Crofts, New York, Section 4) who introduced the concept and has emphasized its potential importance for the development of community medicine programmes, include (1) a syndrome of malnutrition, communicable diseases and mental ill-health in a poor rural community undergoing rapid change, and (2) the syndrome of hypertension, coronary heart disease and diabetes frequently found in affluent communities characterized by nutritional imbalance and excesses, limited physical activity and a drive for achievement.

For an example of a study designed to detect community syndromes, see Abramson J H, Gofin J, Peritz E, Hopp C, Epstein L M 1982 Clustering of chronic disorders: a community study of coprevalence in Jerusalem. Journal of Chronic Diseases 35: 221. One syndrome that was detected comprised migraine and other chronic disorders largely based on subjective symptoms. People with one or more of these conditions made particularly heavy use of the primary care service.

8. See Thacker S B, Parrish R G, Trowbridge F L and Surveillance Coordination Group 1988 A method for evaluating systems of epidemiological surveillance. World Health Statistics Quarterly 41: 11.

9. Rogers D E 1982 Community-oriented primary care. Journal of the American Medical Association 248B: 1622.

10. For a limited data set, see National Committee on Vital and Health Statistics 1981 Uniform ambulatory medical care: minimum data set. US Department of Health and Human Services, Hyattsville, Maryland. For an extensive one, see the system used in the University of Rochester's Family Medicine Program, described in a series of papers in Journal of Family Practice 1977 4: 949, 951, 1149; 5: 113, 265, 427, 627, 845, 1007.

11. Checks in three primary care practices in Israel revealed that in two of them less than half the contacts with family doctors were recorded in the patients' files; Weitzman S, Bar-Ziv G, Pilpel D, Sachs E, Naggan L 1981 Validation study on medical recording practices in primary care clinics. Israel Journal of Medical Sciences 17: 213. In England, a study of records from eight general practices showed that 10% of patients' ages were not recorded, for 60% of men there was no record of occupation, and for 99% there was no record of marital status; the proportion of episodes for which diagnoses were reported ranged from 9 to 75%; Dawes K S 1972 Survey of general practice records. British Medical Journal 3: 219. Almost half the patients registered at a health centre in Scotland did not live at their registered addresses; Hannay D R 1972 Accuracy of health-centre records. Lancet 2: 371.

12. The use of clinical data on patients with tracer conditions to obtain estimates for the total population is called 'piggybacking' by Freeman: Freeman W L 1987 'Piggybacking': the selective use of tracer conditions from patient-based data to obtain population-based information useful for COPC. In: Nutting PA (ed) 1987 Community oriented primary care: from principle to practice. Health Resources and Services Administration, Public Health Service, Washington, D C, pp 179–186.

13. A study of the contribution of a population survey to one primary care practice showed that the survey revealed a number of unknown cases of coronary heart disease, diabetes and hypertension. Many people with raised blood pressure values were brought to light, especially adults aged 25–44 years. Half the men and a quarter of the women in this age group had seldom or never attended for

care. The survey yielded the practice's first systematic picture of the prevalence of obesity and smoking. Abramson J H, Epstein L M, Kark S L, Kark E, Fischler B 1973 The contribution of a health survey to a family practice. Scandinavian Journal of Social Medicine 1: 33.

A 'state-of-the-art' summary of the potentials and limitations of local community health surveys is provided by Aday L A, Sellers C, Andersen R M 1981 Potentials of local health surveys: a state-of-the-art summary. American Journal of Public Health 71: 835.

14. Sackett D L, Holland W W 1975 Disease detection. Lancet 2: 357.
15. For examples of records used in COPC, see Kark S L (1974; see note 7), pp 378–381, 389–390, 445–449.
16. Pickles W N 1939 Epidemiology in country practice. John Wright, Bristol. Examples of Pickles charts are given by Kark (1974; see note 7), p 363.
17. Trachtenberg A, Gardner L, Gould J B, Hutchison S In: Nutting (1987; see note 1), pp 109–125.

Appendix: Random numbers

53 74 23 99 67	61 32 28 69 84	94 62 67 86 24	98 33 41 19 95	47 53 53 38 09
63 38 06 86 54	99 00 65 26 94	02 82 90 23 07	79 62 67 80 60	75 91 12 81 19
35 30 58 21 46	06 72 17 10 94	25 21 31 75 96	49 28 24 00 49	55 65 79 78 07
63 43 36 82 69	65 51 18 37 88	61 38 44 12 45	32 92 85 88 65	54 34 81 85 35
98 25 37 55 26	01 91 82 81 46	74 71 12 94 97	24 02 71 37 07	03 92 18 66 75
02 63 21 17 69	71 50 80 89 56	38 15 70 11 48	43 40 45 86 98	00 83 26 91 03
64 55 22 21 82	48 22 28 06 00	61 54 13 43 91	82 78 12 23 29	06 66 24 12 27
85 07 26 13 89	01 10 07 82 04	59 63 69 36 03	69 11 15 83 80	13 29 54 19 28
58 54 16 24 15	51 54 44 82 00	62 61 65 04 69	38 18 65 18 97	85 72 13 49 21
34 85 27 84 87	61 48 64 56 26	90 18 48 13 26	37 70 15 42 57	65 65 80 39 07
03 92 18 27 46	57 99 16 96 56	30 33 72 85 22	84 64 38 56 98	99 01 30 98 64
62 95 30 27 59	37 75 41 66 48	86 97 80 61 45	23 53 04 01 63	45 76 08 64 27
08 45 93 15 22	60 21 75 46 91	98 77 27 85 42	28 88 61 08 84	69 62 03 42 73
07 08 55 18 40	45 44 75 13 90	24 94 96 61 02	57 55 66 83 15	73 42 37 11 61
01 85 89 95 66	51 10 19 34 88	15 84 97 19 75	12 76 39 43 78	64 63 91 08 25
72 84 71 14 35	19 11 58 49 26	50 11 17 17 76	86 31 57 20 18	95 60 78 46 75
88 78 28 16 84	13 52 53 94 53	75 45 69 30 96	73 89 65 70 31	99 17 43 48 76
45 17 75 65 57	28 40 19 72 12	25 12 74 75 67	60 40 60 81 19	24 62 01 61 16
96 76 28 12 54	22 01 11 94 25	71 96 16 16 88	68 64 36 74 45	19 59 50 88 92
43 31 67 72 30	24 02 94 08 63	38 32 36 66 02	69 36 38 25 39	48 03 45 15 22
50 44 66 44 21	66 06 58 05 62	68 15 54 35 02	42 35 48 96 32	14 52 41 52 48
22 66 22 15 86	26 63 75 41 99	58 42 36 72 24	58 37 52 18 51	03 37 18 39 11
96 24 40 14 51	23 22 30 88 57	95 67 47 29 83	94 69 40 06 07	18 16 36 78 86
31 73 91 61 19	60 20 72 93 48	98 57 07 23 69	65 95 39 69 58	56 80 30 19 44
78 60 73 99 84	43 89 94 36 45	56 69 47 07 41	90 22 91 07 12	78 35 34 08 72
84 37 90 61 56	70 10 23 98 05	85 11 34 76 60	76 48 45 34 60	01 64 18 39 96
36 67 10 08 23	98 93 35 08 86	99 29 76 29 81	33 34 91 58 93	63 14 52 32 52
07 28 59 07 48	89 64 58 89 75	83 85 62 27 89	30 14 78 56 27	86 63 59 80 02
10 15 83 87 60	79 24 31 66 56	21 48 24 06 93	91 98 94 05 49	01 47 59 38 00
55 19 68 97 65	03 73 52 16 56	00 53 55 90 27	33 42 29 38 87	22 13 88 83 34
53 81 29 13 39	35 01 20 71 34	62 33 74 82 14	53 73 19 09 03	56 54 29 56 93
51 86 32 68 92	33 98 74 66 99	40 14 71 94 58	45 94 19 38 81	14 44 99 81 07
35 91 70 29 13	80 03 54 07 27	96 94 78 32 66	50 95 52 74 33	13 80 55 62 54
37 71 67 95 13	20 02 44 95 94	64 85 04 05 72	01 32 90 76 14	53 89 74 60 41
93 66 13 83 27	92 79 64 64 72	28 54 96 53 84	48 14 52 98 94	56 07 93 89 30
02 96 08 45 65	13 05 00 41 84	93 07 54 72 59	21 45 57 09 77	19 48 56 27 44
49 83 43 48 35	82 88 33 69 96	72 36 04 19 76	47 45 15 18 60	82 11 08 95 97
84 60 71 62 46	40 80 81 30 37	34 39 23 05 38	25 15 35 71 30	88 12 57 21 77
18 17 30 88 71	44 91 14 88 47	89 23 30 63 15	56 34 20 47 89	99 82 93 24 98
76 69 10 61 78	71 32 76 95 62	87 00 22 58 40	92 54 01 75 25	43 11 71 99 31

Reproduced with permission from Fisher R A, Yates F 1974 Statistical tables for biological, agricultural and medical research. Longman, London.

Index